Manual of
Benirschke and Kaufmann's
Pathology of the
Human Placenta

Rebecca N. Baergen, MD

New York Presbyterian Hospital—Weill Medical College of Cornell University, New York, New York

Manual of Benirschke and Kaufmann's *Pathology of the Human Placenta*

With 447 Illustrations, 120 in Full Color

Foreword by Kurt Benirschke, MD

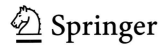 Springer

Rebecca N. Baergen, MD
New York Presbyterian Hospital—Weill
  Medical College of Cornell University
New York, NY 10021
USA

Library of Congress Cataloging-in-Publication Data
Baergen, Rebecca N.
    Manual of Benirschke and Kaufmann's Pathology of the human placenta /
Rebecca N. Baergen.
        p. ; cm.
    Includes bibliographical references and index.
    ISBN 0-387-22089-5 (s/c : alk. paper)
    1. Placenta—Diseases—Handbooks, manuals, etc.   I. Benirschke, Kurt.
Pathology of the human placenta.   II. Title.
    [DNLM: 1. Placenta—pathology—Laboratory Manuals.   2. Specimen
Handling—Laboratory Manuals. WQ 25 B141m 2004]
    RG591.B28 2004
    618.3'4—dc22   2004049198

ISBN 0-387-22089-5   Printed on acid-free paper.

Printed in China.   (BS/EVB)

9 8 7 6 5 4 3 2 1   SPIN 10938584

springeronline.com

To Steve

Foreword

Over the past 50 years the function of the human placenta has gradually become better understood. Simultaneously, pathologic features have been more clearly delineated. Some features are characteristic of certain maternal diseases; others specify fetal conditions. And for still others, although well described with well-characterized consequences, the etiology has remained a mystery. Aspects of placental pathology leading to an understanding of perinatal problems have also been widely used in medicolegal disputes in recent years. When adequately studied, these pathologic findings have often been useful in settling many difficult cases of perinatal mortality and of neonatal diseases, such as the cause of cerebral palsy. All of this has led to a more frequent demand for placental examination—even of "routine" deliveries—of all those leading to premature birth and of neonates who experience perinatal problems.

As the perinatal mortality has decreased substantially over the past decade, largely because of better prenatal care, modern sonographic studies, and the elimination of the common "hyaline membrane syndrome" of premature infants, attention is now focused on understanding preeclampsia and the causes of prematurity, the major obstetric challenges remaining. But as some diseases have now become aspects of the historical past, new challenges are being created, in part through the advent of ART (Assisted Reproductive Technology) and ICSI (Intra-Cytoplasmic Sperm Injection). The multiple gestations created by this technology have produced new challenges in our understanding placentation of multiples, especially the relatively common production of additional multiple offspring from the division of one or more of the transferred blastocysts. All of these features continue to make it mandatory that the detailed study of the placenta after delivery be continued.

The book before us is designed to assist the general pathologist, whose interests have usually been with neoplasms and other diseases, to get a handle on an organ that all too often is described as "mature placenta" when it reaches the pathologist's desk. Dr. Baergen endeavors and succeeds in presenting the essential features of placental pathology to the uninitiated pathologist; she carefully lays out what is a "must-observe" aspect of each of the placental structures and how to assess the findings in the context of normal findings. The book is easily followed, directions and diagnostic features are clearly spelled out, and suggestions for their description in diagnostic terms are provided. The book does not endeavor to be encyclopedic but it is well illustrated—an essential aspect for the morphologist—and the essential references are provided. No doubt this book will be a welcomed addition to the shelves of the practicing pathologist who is looking to find answers to the major questions sought by the neonatologist, to provide answers to obstetricians and parents, and to serve as the basis for possible medicolegal questions of the future.

Kurt Benirschke, MD
San Diego, CA

Preface

The primary objective of this book is to be a concise, practical manual of placental pathology. When I began studying placental pathology, I was intimidated by its complex anatomy and pathology. Although Benirschke and Kaufmann's *Pathology of the Human Placenta* was, and is, a comprehensive text, I often wished for a more basic book that would be appropriate for the neophyte in placental pathology but based on this respected volume. I hope that this book will fulfill this goal. In an effort to be true to this ideal, Kurt Benirschke graciously agreed to review and comment on every chapter—a task for which I am profoundly grateful. Furthermore, each chapter includes references to the fourth edition of *Pathology of the Human Placenta* (PHP4) that direct the reader to the corresponding discussion and references in that book.

The book is designed to be a user-friendly bench manual that can be used in the grossing room as well as at the microscope. To that end, the first section discusses the approach to the placental specimen. These chapters provide suggestions on what to do, as well as when and how to do it. Chapters 3 and 4 include tables of gross and microscopic lesions respectively, which give specific page numbers where the lesions and associated disease processes are discussed and illustrated. Inclusion of page numbers, I believe, make the text quite usable and give quick access to the remainder of the book.

The second section covers detailed development and normal histology of all parts of the placenta for those wanting to learn about specific areas of the placenta. Subsequent sections discuss placental lesions, disease processes related to the placenta, neoplasms and trophoblastic lesions. The subjects discussed in these chapters are all referenced in the tables in Chapters 3 and 4. The last section gives an overview of the legal implications of placental examination and discusses future directions. The last chapter has been kindly written by Kurt Benirschke. Finally, because the study of placental pathology is intimately associated with clinical history and has significant implications for neonatal and maternal health, an appendix is included which provides definitions and explanations of pertinent clinical and pathologic terms.

Specific features have been included throughout the book to enhance readability and usability. Bold type has been used to highlight important lesions, diseases, or concepts; while italic type has been used for features and definitions of bolded items. After discussion of each diagnostic entity, a subheading entitled "Suggestions for Examination and Report" includes key points in gross examination, sectioning, and diagnosis. Suggestions for comments that may be included in the surgical pathology report are included for problematic situations or when the diagnosis or diagnostic implications are unclear. Tables are included in many chapters to summarize pertinent information and to provide easy access to the differential diagnoses of various lesions. Attempts were made to create images of the highest quality, many of them in color. Original art was also created for line drawings to provide a uniform feel to the book.

It is my hope that this book will make examination of the placenta as enjoyable and rewarding for the reader as it has been for me.

Rebecca N. Baergen, MD
New York, NY

Acknowledgments

The implementation of the vision I had for this book would not have been possible without the help of Carol Wang-Mondaca of Springer who supported my ideas and fought to preserve them. I am indebted to our pathology residents for their suggestions and assistance in many aspects of this book and to Dr. Demaretta Rush, Dr. Kay Park, and our pathology assistant, Laura Cervino for their help in the taking of many of the gross photographs. I am immensely grateful to Dr. Kurt Benirschke for many things including providing his invaluable expertise and experience in reviewing each chapter, but most of all for introducing me to the marvel of placental pathology.

Rebecca N. Baergen, MD
New York, NY

Contents

Section I
Approach to the Specimen

The first section of this book is concerned with the approach to gross and microscopic placental examination. The chapters provide a systematic "bench" approach to examination of first, second, and third trimester specimens, which includes initial handling of the specimen, specific steps of the gross examination, sections to submit for microscopic evaluation, special studies, fixation, and storage. A microscopic survey gives the reader a histologic overview and serves as an orientation when more detailed histology is discussed in later chapters. The first chapter covers gross and microscopic evaluation of first trimester abortion specimens. The second chapter covers second trimester specimens and briefly discusses handling of dilatation and evacuation specimens in the setting of fetal anomalies. The third and fourth chapters cover the macroscopic and microscopic examination of the placenta, respectively. Both these chapters feature a series of tables at the end of the chapter, which list pathologic features for each part of the placenta, that is, fetal membranes, umbilical cord, fetal surface, and so on. When the reader is confronted with a particular gross or microscopic finding, the tables provide possible diagnoses, instructions on special handling, and special studies and references to where in the text the lesions are discussed and illustrated. This arrangement enables the reader to diagnose even complex lesions quickly and efficiently.

Chapter 1

Evaluation of the First Trimester Products of Conception

General Considerations

Early abortion specimens are one of the most common specimens submitted to pathology. They are quite varied in their composition; they may consist of blood clot admixed with minimal tissue, fragmented villous tissue and fetal parts, a completely intact gestational sac, or anything in between. Evaluation of these specimens is enhanced by an understanding of the purpose of pathologic examination, and how it may be helpful to both the patient and the clinician. Potential goals of examination include:

- Documentation of **pregnancy**
- Documentation of an **intrauterine** pregnancy
- Documentation of suspected or unsuspected **anomalies**
- Estimation of **gestational age**
- Estimation of the **interval of retention** after embryonic or fetal death
- Exclusion of **gestational trophoblastic disease**

Macroscopic Examination

Macroscopic examination of first trimester products of conception is primarily concerned with the identification of **decidual tissue, villous tissue**, and **embryonic** or **fetal tissue**. Often the components are disrupted and intermixed, but each component should be examined individually. It is convenient to examine the fetal tissues first, and several general questions should be addressed in initial examination:

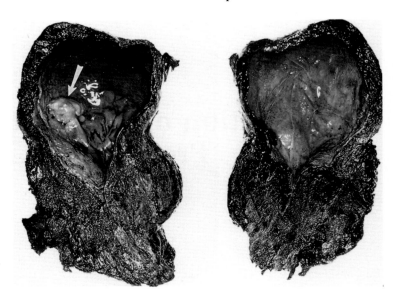

Figure 1.1. Spontaneous abortus with the presence of a fragmented and macerated embryo (arrow).

- Is embryonic or fetal tissue present?
- If present:
  ○ Is the embryo or fetus intact and complete?
  ○ Is the embryo or fetus macerated, and if so, to what extent (Figure 1.1)?
  ○ Is the embryo or fetus the appropriate size for the stated gestational age?
    ■ This is best accomplished by comparison of crown-rump length, foot length, and weight with standard tables (see Table 3.8).
  ○ Does the embryo or fetus have grossly normal features, major growth disorganization, or focal defects such as cleft lip or spina bifida (Figures 1.2, 1.3)?

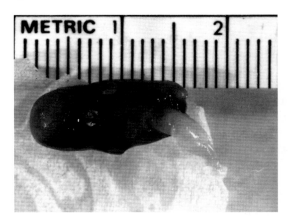

Figure 1.2. Spontaneous abortus at 9 weeks showing major growth disorganization with a cylindrical embryo. It was also small for the gestational age (expected crown-rump length, 2.5 cm).

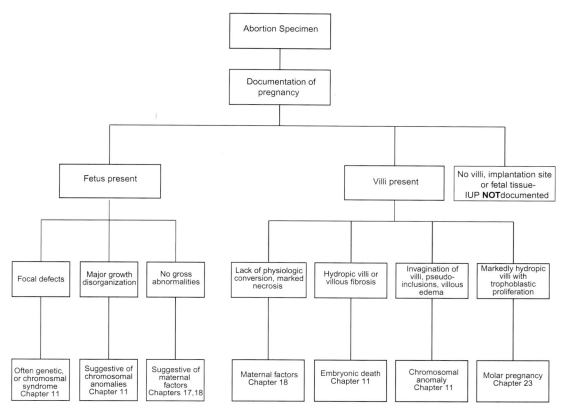

Figure 1.3. Etiologic significance of gross and microscopic findings in abortion specimens. IUP, intrauterine pregnancy.

Each of these points should be addressed in examination and then included in the gross description of the report. Further detailed examination of fetal anomalies is beyond the scope of this text, but the reader is referred to the references for several excellent monographs on the subject.

The nonembryonic tissues are usually more abundant than the embryonic tissue. **Decidual tissue** usually appears as a *small, flattened sheet of tissue that is relatively smooth on one surface and granular or nodular on the opposite surface* (Figure 1.4). Decidual tissue may contain implantation site and so some of this tissue be submitted for histology. **Chorionic villi** are generally *fine, soft, and white, with papillary fronds representative of their villous structure.* Villous tissue is often attached to fragments of *shiny, delicate, and translucent* **fetal membranes** (Figure 1.5). Both should be submitted for microscopic examination along with a fragment of umbilical cord if it can be identified. The blood clot that is often present usually does not contain diagnostic material; however, *if the clot is granular or firm, it may contain fragments of degenerated chorionic villi within.* This may be helpful when villous tissue is not identified grossly. In general, macroscopic examination of nonfetal tissue in

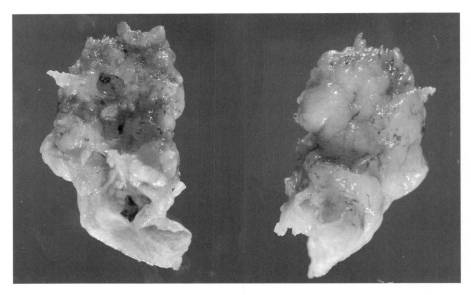

Figure 1.4. Fragment of decidual tissue. Note the membranous character with one smooth (right) and one granular (left) surface.

early products of conception does not provide diagnostic information except in the case of **gestational trophoblastic disease**. Here, the villous tissue shows *enlarged, hydropic vesicles* (see below).

Cytogenetics, Flow Cytometry, and Other Special Studies

In 50% to 60% of spontaneous abortions, chromosomal anomalies are present. Therefore, in spontaneous abortions, it is advantageous to

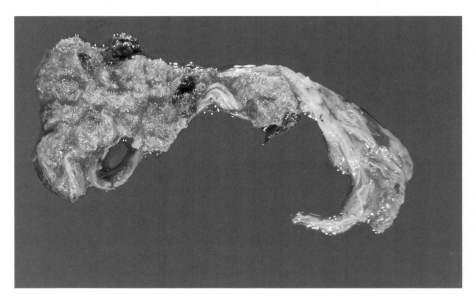

Figure 1.5. Translucent fetal membranes (at right) cover white, papillary villous structures in a typical early abortion specimen (at left).

send material for *cytogenetic analysis*. This may not be possible on every spontaneous abortion for financial or practical reasons. However, in the case of *recurrent or habitual abortion, cytogenetics should always be sent*. Some advocate sending only fetal tissue due to the presence of possible confined placental mosaicism (see Chapter 11) while others point out that fetal tissue may be macerated and then does not grow in culture. For these reasons, it is recommended that *fetal tissue be sent if it appears viable, otherwise villous tissue should be sent*. If resources allow, both tissues may be submitted for optimal results. Then, if the fetal tissue does not grow, the placental tissue may be used for analysis.

Grossly hydropic villi are usually not present except in the case of a partial or complete hydatidiform mole. Hydropic abortuses generally do not show the grossly cystic villi seen in molar pregnancies (see Figure 23.2, page 420). In these cases, it is recommended that the specimen be *sent for flow cytometry* or prepared in such a way that flow cytometry can be done if necessary as differentiation between a molar pregnancy and a hydropic abortus may not be possible on histology alone (see Chapter 23). Flow cytometry can often be done on paraffin-embedded, fixed tissue.

Rarely, requests for molecular testing of fetal tissue are made to rule out a specific disease. In this situation, it is best to communicate directly with the laboratory that will be handling the test **before** receiving the specimen, if possible, because there may be specific handling requirements. Unfortunately, advance notice is not always given. Therefore, if one suspects a special test may be requested, due to either unusual anomalies or clinical information, it is prudent to freeze portions of fetal and placental tissue in liquid nitrogen and store at −70°C. In this way, tissue will be preserved and may be utilized for many types of molecular testing. If tissue is to be frozen, it is recommended that connective tissue and tissue from a fetal organ such as liver be frozen, along with chorionic villi and a portion of chorionic plate.

Submission of Microscopic Sections

In a therapeutic abortion in which no macroscopic abnormalities are noted, one cassette, which includes villous tissue and a small portion of decidua, is acceptable. In a spontaneous abortion, at least two cassettes should be submitted. Additional sections are recommended in a patient with recurrent or habitual abortions. If an ectopic pregnancy is in the differential diagnosis, sufficient tissue should be submitted to ensure the diagnosis of an intrauterine pregnancy. Specifically, if no chorionic villi are grossly identified, or when there is a small amount of tissue, the entire specimen should be submitted. If on initial microscopic examination an intrauterine pregnancy cannot be documented, the remaining tissue should be submitted. Finally, if fetal anomalies are noted, sections should also be taken to optimize diagnosis of those lesions. In cases in which the embryo is small, submission of the entire embryo in a single cassette may be possible.

Microscopic Examination

For the novice in placental pathology, histologic sections of the organ look confusing because they contain not only a broad variety of differently structured villi but, in addition, many nonvillous structures. This section introduces those basic histologic features that leap into the eyes when inspecting a paraffin section of the early placenta. Detailed histology of these features is covered in Chapters 5 through 8.

Overview and Microscopic Survey

Ideally, routine histological examination of the human placenta starts with vertically oriented sections, which cover all placental structures from the chorionic plate, through the intervillous space down to the basal plate (Figure 1.6). Such sections are easily obtained from most second and third trimester placentas, but rarely from first trimester specimens. In tissue from early abortions and curettages, the basal plate together with neighboring tissues such as septa, anchoring villi, and cell columns are often absent or at least difficult to identify as they are often destroyed and/or admixed with the chorionic villi. However, knowledge of the ideal specimen will enhance recognition of structures in the disrupted specimen.

Complete and well-oriented sections of the first trimester placenta (Figure 1.6 A) include the following structures:

- **Chorionic plate** (B),
- **Intervillous space** (A), surrounding the
- **Placental villi** (C to F),
- **Cell islands** (G),
- The **basal plate** (J to M), from which
- **Septae** (H) protrude into the intervillous space, and
- **Anchoring villi** connected via **cell columns** to the septum (H) or to the basal plate (I).

The **intervillous space** (Figure 1.6 A) is the space between the chorionic plate and the basal plate. From the 13th week on it *contains maternal blood*, which flows around the villous trees, chorionic villi, cell islands, septa, and fibrinoid deposits. The **chorionic plate** (Figure 1.6 B) in the first trimester is *usually devoid of amnion* as it is only superficially attached to the chorionic plate. It is commonly removed during preparation. Instead, the fetal surface is covered by an inconspicuous, incomplete layer of mesothelium, *then a thick layer of chorionic mesoderm in which the chorionic vessels (branches of the umbilical vessels) are embedded.* Toward the intervillous space, the surface is covered early on by a layer of syncytiotrophoblast, which, with progressing pregnancy, is replaced by fibrinoid. Fibrinoid is an acellular, eosinophilic material, similar in appearance to fibrin, present in the intervillous space (see Chapter 8).

The **placental villi** arise from the chorionic plate in a *progressive, branching, tree-like arrangement* and protrude into the intervillous space. The outer surfaces of the villi are bathed directly by maternal plasma

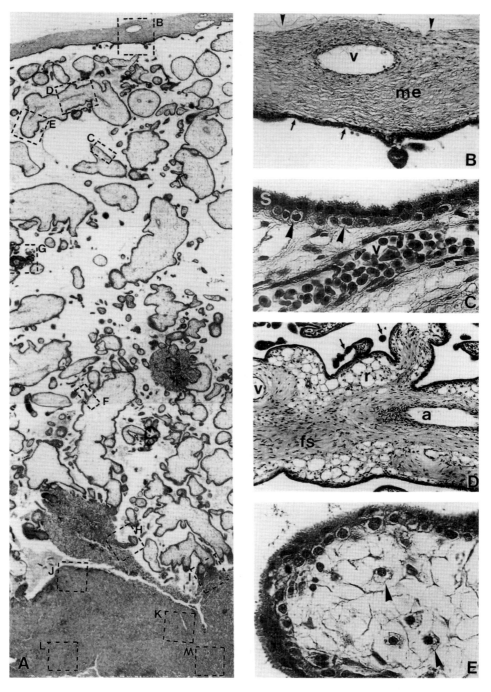

Figure 1.6. Typical features of the first trimester placenta as seen in H&E-stained paraffin sections. All specimens are from the 6th week PM, except when otherwise stated. (A) Vertical survey section of an in situ specimen. The marked frames refer to the following detailed pictures. ×20. (B) Chorionic plate v = vein, me = chorionic mesoderm, arrows = incomplete lager of syncytiotrophoblast, arrowheads = mesothelium. ×100. (C) Surface of an immature intermediate villus with trophoblast and a fetal vessel containing nucleated red blood cells v = fetal vessel, s = syncytiotrophoblast, arrowheads = cytotrophoblast. ×400. (D) Transitional form of an immature intermediate villus to become a stem villus (18th week PM) a = artery, v = vein, r = reticular stroma, fs = fibrous stroma, arrows = sprouts. ×100. (E) Immature intermediate villus showing characteristic reticular stroma with macrophages (arrowheads). ×400.

(Continued)

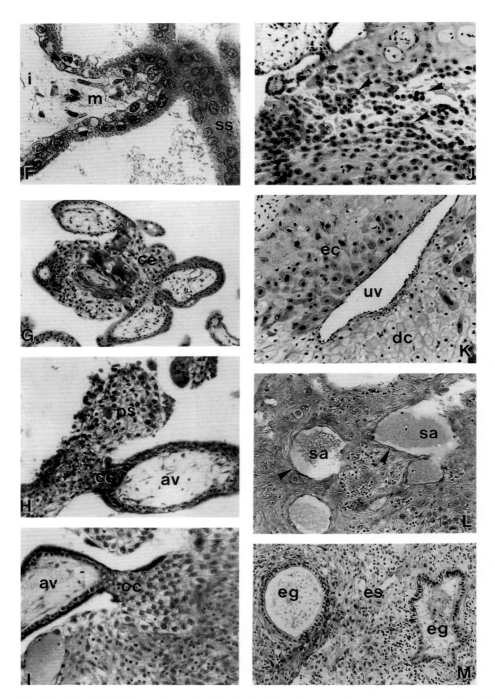

Figure 1.6. *(Continued)* (F) Mesenchymal villus (m) arising from an immature intermediate villus (i) and extending into syncytial sprouts (ss). ×400. (G) Cell island attached to some villi. ×100. (H) Placental septum connected to a villus by a cell column (cc). ×200. (I) Anchoring villus (av) connected to the basal plate by a cell column. ×200. (J) Surface of the basal plate showing extravillous trophoblastic cells (arrowheads) embedded in fibrinoid (10th week PM). ×100. (K) Deep part of the basal plate showing a uteroplacental vein (uv) surrounded by extravillous cytotrophoblast (ec) and decidua (dc) (37th week PM, similar to the first trimester situation). ×140. (L) Multiple cross sections across a spiral artery (sa), the wall of which is replaced by fibrinoid (arrowheads). ×100. (M) Endometrial glands (eg) of the junctional zone embedded in endometrial stroma (es). ×200.

or blood. The trophoblastic surface of the villi is composed of an outer continuous layer of **villous syncytiotrophoblast** beneath which is a discontinuous layer of **villous cytotrophoblast** (Langhans' cells). The villous cytotrophoblast are the proliferating stem cells for the syncytiotrophoblast, which forms the decisive maternofetal transport barrier. The villous **stroma** is *composed of fetal vessels, which are embedded in a mixture of fixed connective tissue cells, macrophages, and connective tissue fibers.* In the first 2 months of pregnancy, nucleated red blood cells are usually found in the villous vessels.

Before the 8th week PM (after the last menstrual period) the villi show a *homogeneous, rather dense cellular stroma* in which arteries and veins are absent. They measure 60 to 200 µm in diameter. These are the **mesenchymal villi**. Peripherally, the mesenchymal villi extend into **syncytiotrophoblastic sprouts**, which often appear as dark cross sections (Figure 1.6 D, arrows), which seemingly do not have contact with the villous surface. After the 8th week PM and through the second trimester, the majority of villi are the **immature intermediate villi** (Figure 1.6 E), which are *large and bulbous with reticular stroma.* Connective tissue cells surround *channel-like spaces within the stroma.* These channels contain stromal macrophages, Hofbauer cells, which are easily identifiable by their rounded shape and their vacuolated or granular cytoplasm. At the periphery of the immature intermediate villi, small branches or sprouts are present, representing the formation of new mesenchymal villi (Figure 1.6 F) from immature intermediate villi. The central stems of the villous trees show fibrotic stroma around larger vessels and form the **stem villi.** See Chapter 7 for discussion of villous development.

Cell islands (Figure 1.6 G) are accumulations of **extravillous trophoblastic cells,** which are adherent to villi and usually embedded in fibrinoid. Parts of the surfaces of these islands may be covered by syncytiotrophoblast. *Cell islands are the proliferating remainders of the primary villi from early pregnancy.* **Placental septa** (Figure 1.6 H) are roughly *pillar-shaped extensions of the basal plate* that protrude into the intervillous space. They are rudimentary and do not completely subdivide the intervillous space. Structurally they have the *same composition as the basal plate, containing mostly extravillous trophoblastic cells admixed with fibrinoid and occasional decidual cells.* Cross sections of tips of septa may look like cell islands, and these two structures are often confused. Very often, **anchoring villi** can be seen attached to the septa. Anchoring villi (Figures 1.6 H,I) are peripheral villi connected to the basal plate or to placental septa (see Figure 1.6 H) via cell columns. *They stabilize the villous trees in the intervillous space.* **Cell columns** are the *trophoblastic feet of the anchoring villi.* Early in pregnancy they consist of several layers of proliferating extravillous trophoblastic cells and serve as a source of proliferation of villous and basal plate cytotrophoblast.

The **basal plate** (Figure 1.6 J) is the bottom of the intervillous space and represents that part of the maternofetal junctional zone that adheres to the placenta after delivery. The deeper portion, the **placental bed,** remains in utero after delivery. The basal plate is composed of an admixture of *extravillous trophoblast, decidual cells, uteroplacental vessels,* and *endometrial glands embedded in abundant fibrinoid.* **Decidual cells** (Figure 1.6 K) are transformed endometrial stromal cells and are *round or ellipsoid with well-defined cell borders and round nuclei with delicate chromatin.* **Uteroplacental veins** consist of endothelium surrounded by few medial and adventitial cells, embedded in decidua and extravillous trophoblast; they are rarely invaded by extravillous trophoblast. **Uteroplacental arteries** (Figure 1.6 L) traverse the basal plate in spiral turns, and connect the maternal uterine arteries to the intervillous space. The *endothelial lining of the arteries, the arterial media, and the adventitia are largely replaced by extravillous trophoblast and fibrinoid.* These cells may form plugs that narrow or even occlude the arterial lumen early in gestation. In the depth of the basal plate, remainders of **endometrial glands** (Figure 1.6 M) may sometimes be found. During the first 2 months, they are surrounded by decidual cells. Subsequently, they disintegrate and only degenerative epithelial remnants remain.

Approach to Microscopic Examination of the Specimen

Therapeutic or Induced Abortion

Therapeutic abortions are performed by dilatation and curettage, dilatation and evacuation, suction curettage, the use of prostaglandins (with or without the use of cervical laminaria), intraamniotic injection of hypertonic saline or urea solutions, and other means. The pathologic findings in the aborted specimen differ to some extent for each procedure but not to a marked degree. For the pathologist, examination generally entails several goals. The most basic is *documentation of the pregnancy.* Confirmation of an intrauterine pregnancy can be accomplished by identification of **chorionic villi, trophoblastic cells,** *or* **portions of implantation site.** The latter consists of *decidual tissue and vessels infiltrated by trophoblast and abundant fibrinoid* (Figure 1.7). The presence of decidualized endometrium alone does **not** confirm **an intrauterine pregnancy** as this change is hormonally dependent and can be seen outside of pregnancy. *Rarely, a few chorionic villi or trophoblastic cells may be transported to the endometrial cavity from an ectopic pregnancy.* Therefore, in these situations, communication with the submitting physician is essential in determining if an ectopic pregnancy is likely. If it is, a comment in the report should indicate that rare trophoblastic elements or chorionic villi do not confirm an intrauterine pregnancy. If an ectopic pregnancy *is* suspected, and microscopic sections do not show villi, implantation site, or trophoblastic cells, the entire specimen should be submitted for microscopic examination. It may be prudent to submit the entire specimen initially as resubmission will result in a delay in diagnosis. Occasionally the remnant of the **yolk sac** may be present in early abortion specimens (Figure 1.8) and cause confusion with other structures. The yolk sac remnant has a lacy, reticular appearance with many glandular-like spaces and the presence of erythropoietic cells.

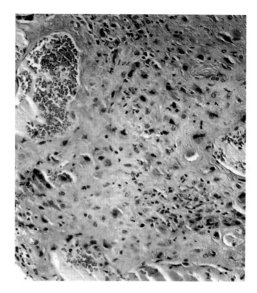

Figure 1.7. Curettings from a placental site of a spontaneous abortion. Note the fibrinoid material admixed with large extravillous trophoblast in the form of placental site giant cells. Despite the absence of chorionic villi and syncytiotrophoblast, this histologic picture suffices for the diagnosis of placental site and thus an intrauterine pregnancy. H&E. ×260.

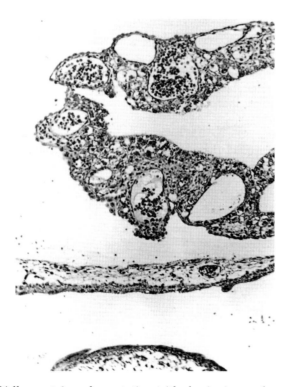

Figure 1.8. Yolk sac at 6 weeks gestation with chorionic membrane, carrying a fetal vessel (below). Note the large sinusoids filled with erythropoietic cells. The tissue is rich in glycogen and occasionally endodermal epithelium may be seen within. H&E. ×240.

Spontaneous Abortions

The spontaneous abortion often arrives with various clinical designations, and these are defined as follows:

- **Threatened**—uterine bleeding without cervical dilatation
- **Inevitable**—uterine bleeding with cervical dilatation or effacement
- **Incomplete**—all tissue (products of conception) has not yet passed
- **Missed**—intrauterine retention after embryonic or fetal death
- **Habitual**—three or more consecutive spontaneous abortions

The goals in examination of these specimens include the goals stated for an induced abortion, except for the increased likelihood of pathologic findings and the fact that special studies are more commonly requested. Unfortunately, however, *the pathologic changes are often more related to the timing of embryonic/fetal death rather than the etiology of the demise*. In previous embryonic death, the **chorionic villi** often show hydropic change and fibrosis, and because many villi are degenerating, there is often much *finely granular mineralization (calcification) along the trophoblastic basement membrane* (see Figure 20.13, page 388).

The early abortion specimen may show abnormalities, which suggest possible etiologies of the pregnancy failure (see Figure 1.3). For instance, trophoblastic pseudoinclusions or invaginations suggest chromosomal anomalies (see Chapter 11). Mild hydropic change in the villi will usually be seen with embryonic death whereas markedly hydropic villi suggest a molar pregnancy (see Chapter 23). A grossly normal fetus is more suggestive of maternal factors rather than fetal factors, whereas anomalies are most suggestive of a genetic or chromosomal disorder. Abnormalities of the implantation site are more consistent with maternal disease. Normally, in the decidua and **implantation site,** there is a mild amount of inflammation; however, *marked inflammation or necrosis is an abnormal finding*. The normal *physiologic conversion of decidual vessels* into uteroplacental vessels should be identified in each specimen (see Figure 1.7). Converted vessels should have *large, irregular lumens and a thin wall composed primarily of fibrinoid and trophoblast*. Small arterioles with persistent muscle and small lumens in an area in which trophoblast is present is diagnostic of **lack of physiologic conversion**. Incomplete conversion may also be identified, and there may be associated thrombosis in decidual vessels. These findings have been associated with spontaneous abortions and are most suggestive of maternal factors such as preeclampsia and other conditions of decreased uteroplacental perfusion (see Chapter 18).

Selected References

PHP4, Chapter 3, pages 16–20; Chapter 21, pages 685–690.

Kalousek DK. Pathology of the abortion. The embryo and the previable fetus. In: Gilbert-Barnass E (ed) Potter's pathology of the fetus and infant. St. Louis: Mosby, 1997:106–127.

Kalousek DK, Lau A. Pathology of spontaneous abortion. In: Dimmick JE, Kalousek DK (eds) Developmental pathology of the embryo and fetus. Philadelphia: Lippincott, 1992:55–82.

Kalousek DK, Pantzar, Tsai M, Paradice B. Early spontaneous abortion: morphologic and karyotypic findings in 3912 cases. Birth Defects 1993;29:53–61.

Kaplan CK. Embryonic pathology of the placenta. In: Lewis SH, Perrin E (eds) Pathology of the placenta. New York: Churchill Livingstone, 1999:89–106.

Szulman AE. Examination of the early conceptus. Arch Pathol Lab Med 1991; 115:696–700.

Chapter 2

Evaluation of the Second Trimester Products of Conception

General Considerations

Specimens involving fetal demise or fetal anomalies in the second trimester require special handling. If the specimen is delivered spontaneously or after labor induction, it may be relatively intact, although some autolysis may be present. Otherwise, various surgical procedures are performed to terminate the pregnancy. In this case, both the placenta and fetus *may be quite disrupted.* This chapter covers the general approach and overview to handling these types of specimens including special studies and suggestions for reporting. However, detailed examination for fetal anomalies is beyond the scope of this text, and the reader is referred to the references for texts on detailed fetal examination in the setting of fetal anomalies.

Gross Examination and Description

The first step in examination is separation of *fetal from the nonfetal tissue.* With practice, the fine papillary villi can be identified and separated from the remaining tissue (see Figure 1.5, page 6). Once the placental tissue is separated, *measurement of the tissue in aggregate, weight, cord length, and cord diameter should be ascertained if possible.* Abnormalities of the cord such as excessive twisting, knots, constrictions, discolorations, or abnormal length should be noted at this time (see Chapter 15). Rarely, cord entanglement may be diagnosable in an intact specimen. The membranes should be evaluated for opacity or discoloration as well as the rare amnionic band (see Chapter 14). The villous tissue should be examined for blood clots, infarcts, or other lesions.

After the fetal tissue has been separated, an attempt to "reconstruct" the fetus should be made, placing the fetal parts in anatomical position (Figure 2.1). This step will provide an opportunity to make an "inventory" of the fetal organs and fetal parts. If any major skeletal structures are missing, it is prudent to contact the clinician, as this may indicate that the tissue is retained in the uterus and may led to bleeding or infection. Disruption and maceration may prohibit identification of all organs, even if they are present. Photographs may be taken at this time. In cases of fetal anomalies and, in particular, fetuses with complex or unusual anomalies, photographs are invaluable for later study or consultation. Radiographs should also be taken at this time, if necessary (see below).

Many specimens show marked disruption, and it is notable that different portions of the fetus are more or less prone to disruption. Usually, the extremities are the most intact portions of the fetus, while the abdomen is usually the most disrupted. The pelvis, chest, and head

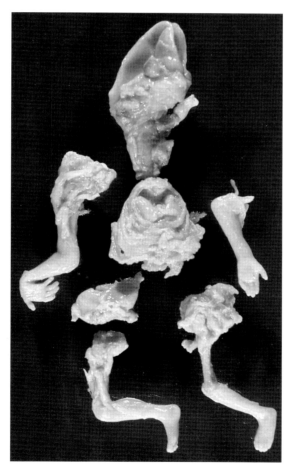

Figure 2.1. Fetus after pregnancy termination procedure with typical disruption. The fetal parts have been arranged such that the normal anatomical position has been approximated. The skull became collapsed during the procedure.

are usually variably disrupted. There is also great variation in the total extent of disruption, and thus examination will also be hindered to a variable degree. Adequate clinical history is extremely helpful in directing examination for anomalies, but this is not always forthcoming. Therefore, *a systematic approach is suggested in which each portion of the fetus is examined* to maximize the information gained.

The external examination is performed first. Measurements should be taken, including crown-rump, crown-heel, and head, abdominal, and chest circumferences. In some cases, because of disruption, the only measurement that is possible is foot length. However, foot length measurements have good correlation with gestational age. After measuring and weighing the specimen, the external appearance of each area of the body is examined, starting with the skull, head, and face. Then, evaluation of the neck, chest, abdomen, pelvis, and external genitalia should be performed, followed by examination of the extremities. For each area, the gross description should indicate whether there is disruption and to what degree. Then, there should be a statement about the presence of anomalies and to what extent evaluation is possible. The limitations of the examination inherent with disrupted specimens should be clearly stated as well. For example:

"The head is markedly disrupted, with collapse of the skull and disruption of the face. Minimal brain tissue is present and therefore examination of the brain for anomalies is not possible. Evaluation of the cranium and upper face is not possible due to disruption. The lower jaw, lower lip, and portions of the upper lip are intact and show no abnormalities. There is no evidence of a cleft lip, but evaluation for a cleft palate is not possible due to disruption."

This format is continued for the remaining areas of the face such as ears, eyes, nose, and so on. Each area of the body is examined and reported in a similar manner. One must be particularly careful in examination of the genitalia because fetuses are often missexed. The large size of the clitoris in female fetuses often gives the impression that they are male. One must not just look at the phallus but *examine the genital folds and identify whether they are fused (scrotum) or separate (labia) and if there is a patent vagina.* It is always helpful to have sections of the gonads to confirm sex as it is often important information both medically and personally for the family.

The same systematic approach is used for the internal organs. *Each visceral organ should be identified, and the organ relationships should be evaluated*, if possible. This is particularly important in the setting of congenital heart defects where relationships with the lungs and great vessels are essential to diagnosis. Finally, anatomical defects in each organ are evaluated. Although each organ and portion of the fetus is examined individually, attempts should be made to integrate the findings and provide as much information about each organ systems as possible. Organ weights should be included for intact organs only.

When specimens are macerated and autolyzed, additional artifacts are introduced. Specifically, the joints may be lax such that abnormalities of positioning of the extremities, such as arthrogryposis, cannot be evaluated. Dehydration also occurs and may make the diagnosis of hydrops or nuchal edema difficult if not impossible. The brain may not be able to be examined due to liquefaction. With fetal death, there is often hemorrhage, discoloration, and softening in many of the fetal tissues. These artifacts may also limit meaningful interpretation.

Special Procedures

In certain situations, special procedures may be required. **Cytogenetic analysis** *is essential in cases of fetuses with multiple malformations.* Sometimes this is done prenatally via amniocentesis or chorionic villus sampling. If one is aware these procedures have been done and has knowledge of these results, cytogenetic testing need not be repeated. In some states, it is required that these results be confirmed by sending a sample from the abortion specimen. Each pathologist should be conversant with the health statutes in their area in order to be compliant. If a specimen is to be submitted for cytogenetic analysis, *it is prudent to send samples of both placenta and fetus.* The rationale for this is the following. The fetal tissue is optimal as it will be most representative of the fetal genetic makeup. In confined placental mosaicism (see Chapter 11), the placental tissue is **not** representative of the fetus. However, if the fetal tissue is macerated, it may not grow in tissue culture. Therefore, it is best if both are submitted so that placental tissue may be used if the fetal cells do not grow. For the fetal sample, a good sample of connective tissue is suggested; chorionic villi and/or chorionic plate tissue is suggested for the placental sample. The specimen should be submitted sterilely in the appropriate medium as required by the specific laboratory.

If the constellation of malformations does not fit into one of the various chromosomal syndromes, for example, trisomies, and the diagnosis is not apparent from prenatal testing or gross examination, it *may be sensible to freeze a portion of fetal tissue.* This procedure requires minimal labor but the rewards are great if tissue for molecular studies is needed to make the diagnosis. If the tissue is found to be unnecessary, it may easily be discarded. Usual recommendations are to snap-freeze organ tissue, such as the liver, and connective tissue in liquid nitrogen and then store at −70°C. Placental tissue may be frozen as well.

If the fetus has obvious limb or bony abnormalities, radiographs should be taken. These images are necessary for the diagnosis of **skeletal dysplasias** as well as many malformation syndromes with bony anomalies. Bony abnormalities include *shortened, missing, or abnormally formed limbs or digits and abnormalities of the spine, ribs, or skull.* On occasion, severe growth restriction of the fetus has been confused with skeletal dysplasias, and radiographs will help differentiate these cases. The fetal parts should be positioned anatomically, and the exposure of the radiograph should be adequate for evaluation of bony structures (Figure 2.2). In cases of suspected skeletal dysplasia, *longitudinal sections of a long bone should also be submitted for routine histology* and a portion of bone should be snap-frozen and stored at −70°C, in addition to organ tissue and connective tissue.

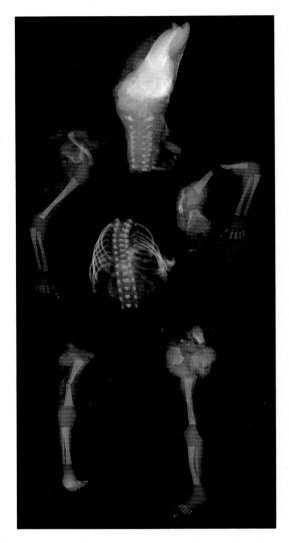

Figure 2.2. Radiograph of the fetus depicted in Figure 2.1. The X-ray has been taken with the fetal parts placed in an approximation of the normal anatomical position. This fetus showed no gross, radiographic, or microscopic abnormalities.

Uncommonly, fetuses may suffer from metabolic disorders. If these are suspected, a small amount of fetal tissue should be fixed for later **electron microscopy.** Finally, in some cases, **bacterial cultures** of the fetus or placenta may be indicated. This is particularly true if the fetal surface of the placenta is opaque, consistent with an ascending infection. In the setting of multiple anomalies, usually bacterial cultures are not helpful. Therefore, unless the clinical history or gross examination suggests an ascending infection or acute chorioamnionitis, bacterial cultures are not recommended.

Microscopic Sections

Sections of each organ identified should be submitted for microscopic examination. At times, marked disruption may make identification of solid organs difficult, particularly the liver, spleen, and adrenals. In this situation, there are often additional fragments of tissue that cannot grossly be identified as a particular organ but are clearly of fetal origin. It is suggested that these fragments also be submitted for microscopic examination. Depending on the type of anomaly identified, special sections of the anomalous part are submitted. For example, in anencephaly sections through the base of the skull are particularly illustrative of the lack of brain tissue and the presence of the cerebrovasculosa. Thus, sectioning must be tailored to the anomalies that are present as well as those that are suspected. Sections of the placenta should also be submitted, including two sections of the membranes, two sections of umbilical cord, and several sections of villous tissue. The latter should include both fetal and maternal surfaces if possible. If grossly identifiable decidual tissue is present, a small fragment should also be submitted for microscopic examination (see Figure 1.4, page 6).

Microscopic Description and Diagnosis

Microscopic sections of each organ should be examined for maturity and appropriateness for stated gestational age as well as the presence of abnormalities. In some cases, this is confirmation of a grossly identified abnormality, while in others it may be primarily a microscopic finding. The gross and microscopic findings should be integrated with the goal of making a specific diagnosis. This diagnosis is important in that different syndromes have markedly different recurrence risks and so have significance to the family in making decisions about future pregnancies.

A statement about whether or not the fetus is the appropriate size for the gestational age is obligatory. Tables of normative values with crown-rump, crown-heel, and foot length can be used for this purpose (see Table 3.8). The sex of the fetus should also be stated if this is known. If the determination of sex is based solely on external genitalia, it is wise to indicate that the fetus is "phenotypically" male or female. Thus, one can state "Phenotypically male fetus, size consistent with 17 weeks gestation." If a diagnosis of a particular syndrome can be made, this should follow in the next statement. If a particular syndrome is suspected clinically, but cannot be confirmed, a statement such as "Clinical history of. . . ." may be used instead. This should be followed by the specific anomalies noted on gross and microscopic examination. Each abnormality indicated in the clinical history should be addressed as either *present, absent, or unable to be evaluated due to disruption and/or maceration.* This is important because lack of specific anomalies may rule out certain syndromes that are in the differential diagnosis. Unfortunately, with disrupted fetuses, limitations in examination often make meaningful diagnosis impossible. In that case, it should be clearly stated that a diagnosis cannot be made and why. A general comment may also be added indicating that pathologic evaluation is limited due to marked disruption.

Selected References

Dimmick JE, Kalousek DK. Developmental pathology of the fetus and infant. Philadelphia: Lippincott, 1992.

Gilbert-Barnass E. Potter's pathology of the fetus and infant. St. Louis: Mosby, 1997.

Kalousek DK, Fitch N, Paradice BA. Pathology of the human embryo and pre-viable fetus. An atlas. New York: Springer-Verlag, 1990.

Keeling JW. Fetal pathology. Edinburgh: Churchill Livingstone, 1994.

Chapter 3

Macroscopic Evaluation of the Second and Third Trimester Placenta

Selection of Placentas for Pathologic Examination

In general, tissue removed or spontaneous passed from the body is required to be sent to surgical pathology. Placentas are the notable exception in that they are the only specimens that are not routinely required to be examined pathologically. The Joint Commission on the Accreditation of Hospitals states that "normal placentas" from "normal deliveries" are not required to be submitted to pathology. However, a definition of what is normal is not forthcoming. Although there are a number of options for placental selection, this task is most often left to the obstetricians or other health care workers involved in the delivery. This is, unfortunately, the least desirable option. Other options are discussed below.

Examination of All Placentas

Most placentas are normal, as are most babies; therefore, examination of all placentas may not be warranted. It may, however, be desirable for the following reasons. First, sporadic examination does not allow the general surgical pathologist or pathology resident *to obtain sufficient background knowledge as to what constitutes a truly normal placenta.* Another reason is today's litigious climate, which makes *the study of placentas highly valuable, particularly in the defense of obstetricians* (see Chapter 26). However, examination of all placentas is often not possible due to time constraints as well as practical, financial, and political considerations, particularly in hospitals with large numbers of deliveries.

Selection Based on Consensus Indications

Triage of placentas based on *relevant indications for submission* of placental specimens is a reasonable compromise. The College of American Pathologists coordinated a multidisciplinary working group on placental pathology that developed indications for submission of placentas for pathologic examination which included **placental, fetal, and maternal indications**. An adapted version is shown in Table 3.1. When delivery personnel are responsible for the selection of placentas, it is recommended that these indications be provided to them.

Initial Selection with Storage of Remaining Placentas

In this approach, *placentas are initially selected for examination* by consensus criteria as above and the remaining placentas are stored in a refrigerator at 4°C. This method is particularly desirable as *a number of neonatal problems are not apparent until several days of life.* One week is usually sufficient time for storage and placentas are almost perfectly preserved for meaningful examination. If this approach is to be implemented, a refrigerator with seven shelves labeled "Monday" through "Sunday" is recommended. The placentas are placed on the shelf corresponding to the day of delivery. Each day, placentas not selected from 1 week prior are discarded. During that week of storage, neonatologists, obstetricians, or other personnel may request placental examination based on development of neonatal or postpartum problems. This method additionally provides a way to "catch" those placentas that *should* have been submitted but for some reason or another, were not. This is the method used in our institution.

Gross Examination of All Placentas with Microscopic Examination on Selected Placentas

In this scheme, *all placentas are initially examined macroscopically.* Based on gross examination and clinical information, a *portion of these is submitted for microscopic examination.* The success of this approach is partially dependent on the skill and experience of the examiner. A variation of this technique is examination of all placentas along with *submission of tissue for processing into blocks only.* Histologic sections are then cut only on cases selected as above. If problems occur in the future, the blocks may then be cut. This approach has not commonly been used and, at some institutions, regulations may prohibit such a system from being implemented. However, in recent years some malpractice insurance companies have shown interest in this approach as a type of "insurance" against future litigation.

Storage

Placentas should ideally be examined *in the fresh state or at least prior to fixation*. Placentas should **never be frozen** before examination, as it makes macroscopic examination difficult and obliterates the most useful histologic characteristics. Specimens that have been previously frozen will show reddish discoloration of the fetal surface, cord, and membranes due to hemolysis. Formalin fixation before examination is not optimal as it obscures many macroscopic features, makes examination more difficult, and causes difficulties in the submission of specimens for tissue culture, cytogenetics, and bacteriologic examination. Although some lesions are better visualized after fixation, examination of unfixed placentas affords the opportunity to view lesions in both fresh and fixed states. If storage is needed, placentas should be stored in tightly sealed containers at 4°C. *During storage, the placenta loses some weight* to a small extent by evaporation but predominantly by leakage of blood and serum. The freshly examined placenta is thus softer, bloodier, and thicker than one that has been stored. Weight loss is most significant in hydropic or edematous placentas. On the other hand, the placenta *gains approximately 5% in weight after formalin fixation*.

Examination

As with examination of any specimen, it is wise to **follow a routine protocol**. This plan not only enhances subsequent interpretation but provides a systematic approach so that nothing is omitted. The following is an example of such a procedure for placental examination. The reader is encouraged to tailor this to his or her personal style and needs. Specific gross lesions are listed by location in tables at the end of the chapter (Tables 3.2 to 3.6), and Figure 3.1 gives an example of a gross reporting form useful for macroscopic evaluation.

Instruments

The instruments needed are basic and consist of a *ruler or tape measure, a long, sharp knife, forceps with teeth, scissors, and a scale*. Mounting the ruler directly over and perpendicular to the cutting board is advantageous as the cord length, placental diameter, and other measurements can be easily made. The knife should be long, relatively thin, and very sharp. Often the best knife for this use is obtained from a butcher supply house or cutlery store rather than conventional sources. The forceps, scissors, and scale are all standard items and easily obtained. In addition, an adjacent sink is optimal as this facilitates rinsing of the placenta for easy, gentle removal of blood and other fluids. This step will assist in accurate identification of lesions and discolorations of the membranes, cord, or surfaces of the placenta and makes for a cleaner work area. The placenta should never be wiped off, as this will damage the surfaces.

REPORT OF PLACENTAL EXAMINATION

Name :_____ Path. #_____ Medical Record #_____

Maternal History:_____
_____

Infant History:_____

GENERAL:

Weight (disk only)_____g   Formalin-fixed _____ Unfixed_____ Size_____ x_____ x_____ cm

CORD:

Insertion: Central_____ Eccentric_____ Marginal_____ Furcate_____ Interpositional_____

Velamentous_____ cm from margin_____

Cord Vessels: 3_____ 2_____ 4_____ Thrombosis: Yes_____ No_____ Knots: Yes_____ No____

Length: _____cm Diameter_____ cm Spiral: left_____ right_____ no or minimal____ marked_____

Discoloration: green_____ yellow_____ opaque_____ brown_____ Other_____

Other lesions_____

MEMBRANES: marginal_____ circumvallate_____ circummarginate_____

Color: green_____ opaque_____ normal_____ other_____

Point of rupture from margin: _____cm   Amnion nodosum_____   Squamous metaplasia_____

Other_____

SURFACE VESSELS:_____

TWINS: Yes_____ No_____   HIGHER MULTIPLES:_____

Fused: Yes_____ No_____   DiDi_____ DiMo_____ MoMo_____

Anastomoses_____

MATERNAL SURFACE:

Intact: Yes_____ No_____ Calcification: Marked _____normal_____

Color: Normal_____ Pale_____ Congested_____

Retroplacental hematoma: Size _____cm, _____% of surface Old_____ Recent_____

CUT SURFACE:

Infarct(s): Yes_____ No_____ Number _____Largest size(cm)_____ % of total

placenta_____ Old_____ Recent_____

Intervillous thrombi_____ Increased Fibrin_____ Other Lesions:_____

Pictures taken? Yes_____ No_____ .

Special Studies _____

OTHER_____

DIAGNOSIS: _____

Pathologist_____

Figure 3.1. Suggested macroscopic worksheet.

Procedure for Examination

After removing the placenta from the container and rinsing briefly in water:

- **Check for odors**—odors often indicate bacterial growth.
- **Ascertain shape**—irregular, discoid, etc. Immersion of the placenta in water will return the placenta to its shape in utero and thus demonstrate the shape of the uterine cavity (see Figure 13.1, page 209).
- **Membranes** (Table 3.2)
  ○ **Check for completeness**—sufficient membranes should be present to enclose the fetus.
  ○ **Measure membrane rupture site**—this is the distance from the placental edge to the nearest rupture site (Figure 3.2). If it is greater than zero in a vaginally delivered specimen, a placenta previa is ruled out.
  ○ **Evaluate color and appearance**—the membranes are normally translucent and shiny, but may be discolored yellow, green, brown, or red-brown.
  ○ **Identify membrane insertion**—the normal insertion is at the margin; insertion other than at the edge indicates circumvallation or circummargination (see Figure 13.4, page 212).
  ○ **Remove fetal membranes**—keep the orientation to rupture site.
  ○ **Make a "jelly roll"**—take a strip approximately 10 cm wide, and with forceps grasp the portion representing the rupture site. Roll the membranes with the rupture site in the center and with the amnion inward (Figure 3.3).

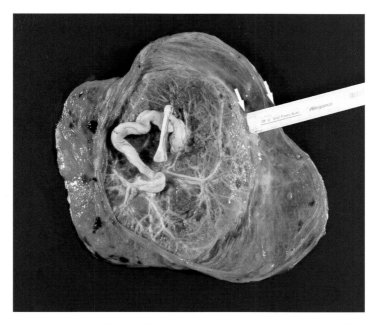

Figure 3.2. Demonstration of the measurement of the rupture site of the membranes. The distance from the closest rupture site to the placental margin is measured. The two arrows along the ruler indicate this measurement.

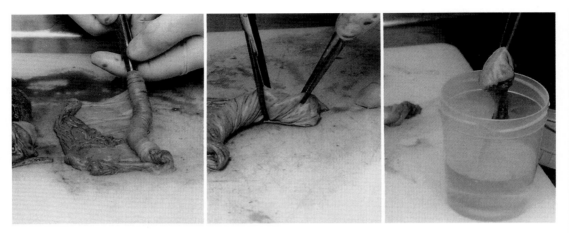

Figure 3.3. Rolling of membranes for fixation and later sectioning. It is best to prepare in a standardized fashion with the amnion inside, starting at the site of rupture and proceeding toward the edge of the placenta as shown at left. A segment is taken from the rolled portion (center) and fixed (right) before sectioning.

- **Fetal Surface** (Table 3.3)
  - **Evaluate color and appearance**—the fetal surface is normally purple-blue and translucent (Figure 3.4).
  - **Examine surface and subchorionic region**—identify nodules, plaques, amnionic bands, hemorrhage, cysts, fibrin, masses and so on.
  - **Inspect the fetal surface vessels**—look for vascular thrombosis, hemorrhage, or disruption; *arteries cross over veins* (Figure 3.5).
- **Umbilical cord** (Table 3.4)
  - **Measure length and diameter.**
  - **Identify spiraling of the umbilical cord**—right or left twist (Figure 3.6); excessive or minimal twisting, focal twisting, or constriction.
  - **Identify insertion of the umbilical cord**—marginal, eccentric, central, paracentral, or velamentous; if velamentous, measure the distance from the insertion to the placental edge, and note hemorrhage, disruption, or thrombosis of vessels (see Figure 15.17).
  - **Knots**—identify true knots; note whether tight or loose and if congestion is present.
  - **Umbilical vessels**—normally three, but two or four vessels may occur.
  - **Other**—discoloration, thrombosis, hemorrhage, cysts, surface nodules, masses, etc.
  - **Remove the cord from the placenta at the insertion site.**
- **Placental Disk** (Tables 3.5, 3.6)
  - **Measure the placenta in three dimensions.**
  - **Weigh the placenta**—without cord or membranes.
  - **Maternal surface**—check for completeness, cotyledonary development, blood clots, calcifications (Figure 3.7).
  - **Retroplacental hematoma (abruptio placentae)**—look for adherent blood clot, compression of villous tissue, underlying infarct.
  - **Serially section the placental tissue at 5-mm intervals**.

Figure 3.4. Normal fetal surface of the placenta showing blue to purple translucent surface and pearly white, eccentrically inserted umbilical cord (top). Normally, subchorionic fibrin/ fibrinoid deposits are present which appear as irregular white patches on the fetal surface (bottom).

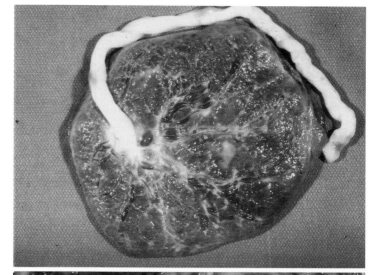

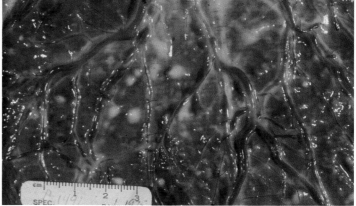

Figure 3.5. Entrance of the vessels on the chorionic plate into the cotyledon. One artery (large arrowhead) brings in the fetal blood and the vein (small arrowhead) returns it to the fetus. Note that the arteries cross over the veins.

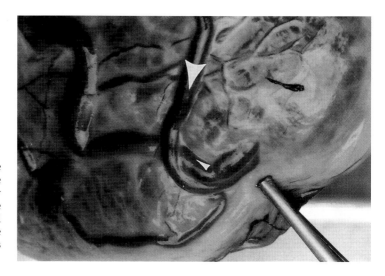

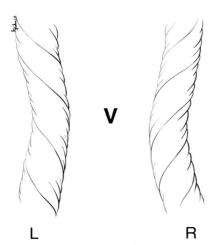

Figure 3.6. Diagram of cord twisting. When cord is placed vertically, the direction of the spiral is compared to the arms of the letter "V." If the spiral is the direction of the left arm, it is a left twist, and if it is in the direction of the right arm, it is a right twist. This method ensures the same results no matter which way the cord is oriented.

- Evaluate the color of villous tissue—pale, congested, or normal.
- Identify and describe villous lesions—measure, note location (fetal versus maternal surface; peripheral versus central), and percentage of placenta involved (Figure 3.8).

Normal Macroscopic Appearance

In 90% of the cases, the placenta is disklike, flat, and round to oval. Abnormalities of shape occur in about 10% of cases and include **bilobed**, **succenturiate lobes**, and **membranacea** (see Chapter 13). At term, the average diameter is 22 cm, thickness is 2.5 cm, and weight is 470 g (Table 3.7). The umbilical cord is normally pearly-white and measures an average of 55 cm in length and 1.0 to 1.5 cm in diameter at term (see Table 3.4). It most commonly inserts **eccentrically** and usually contains three vessels, two arteries, and one vein. It may have

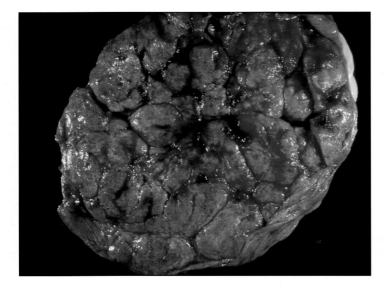

Figure 3.7. Normal maternal surface of the term placenta. Note the divisions into lobules or cotyledons.

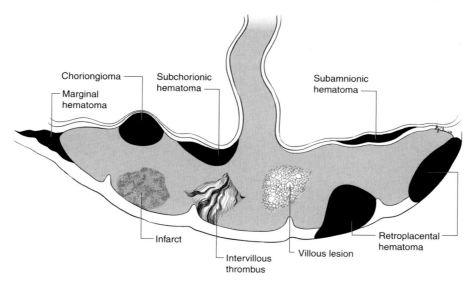

Figure 3.8. Diagram of selected, grossly visible lesions of the placenta. Miscellaneous lesions may include villitis, increased fibrinoid deposition, villous abscesses, metastatic tumors, or choriocarcinoma-in-situ.

a **marginal**, **velamentous**, or **furcate insertion**. Occasionally a single artery or a persistent second vein occurs (see Chapter 15). Care must be taken when evaluating the cord for the presence of a single umbilical artery as the arteries commonly anastomose close to their insertion on the placental surface. The cord is left twisted in about 70% of cases (Figure 3.6).

The **fetal membranes** are generally translucent and shiny but in pathologic conditions may be **opaque or discolored** (see Table 3.2). The **fetal surface**, facing the amniotic cavity, is usually blue to purple with a **glossy** or **shiny** appearance. Pathologic conditions may lead to discoloration or opacity (see Chapter 14). The **chorionic vessels** run underneath the amnion and branch in a starlike pattern, centrifugally from the cord insertion (see Figure 3.4). *Arteries cross over veins* (Figure 3.5, Table 3.3). Around the larger vessels, the **chorionic plate** is more opaque due to increased numbers of collagen fibers. White plaques or nodules are due to **subchorionic fibrinoid** and in moderate amounts are not significant. Occasionally, the remnant of the **yolk sac** can be identified underneath the amnion, consisting of a chalky-white, flattened ovoid of tissue (see Figure 14.7 A, page 228).

After delivery of the placenta, some **decidua basalis** is left in utero and some remains as part of the **basal** plate. The plate is composed of a heterogeneous population of trophoblastic and decidual elements embedded in **extracellular debris**, **fibrinoid**, and **blood clot**. An incomplete system of "grooves" subdivides the basal surface into 10 to 40 lobes or **cotyledons** (Figure 3.7), which correspond to the **septae** seen histologically.

On cut section, the villous tissue is **red** to **red-brown**, and **spongy** on cut section. Its color is almost wholly determined by its content of **fetal blood** (see Tables 3.5, 3.6). If the fetal hemoglobin is high, the villous tissue is dark and congested; if the hemoglobin is low, the villous tissue is pale. In the center of many delivered placentas are "holes," which were filled with blood in utero and thus are of no consequence. At the periphery of many term placentas, the villous tissue may appear "infarcted." These are not true infarcts but rather villous atrophy due to poor circulation at the periphery.

Tissue Sections

Routine sections that should be taken on every placenta are listed below. Additional sections should be taken when abnormalities are present, and the reader is directed to Tables 3.2 to 3.6 for recommendations in the presence of specific lesions. The routine sections should include:

- Two sections of **membrane roll**, one from the rupture site and one from the placental margin
- Two sections of **umbilical cord** from each of two areas
- Two full-thickness sections of **villous tissue** including fetal and maternal surfaces
- Section of the **maternal surface**

Several small sections of the maternal surface in one cassette may enhance one's examination of decidual vessels. The sections of the villous tissue should be *taken away from the margin of the placenta*, as the perfusion is not consistent throughout the placenta and abnormalities exist in peripheral areas of poor perfusion that *may not be reflective of the remainder of the specimen.* Sections of the **fetal surface** or **chorionic vessels** should be included in those sections of villous tissue. This requires taking at least one section near the insertion of the umbilical cord to obtain vessels of sufficient caliber.

Fixation

Pathologists commonly fix tissue for histological study in **10% buffered formalin** solution (a 1:10 dilution of the commercial 40% formaldehyde). However, brief fixation in formalin in usually insufficient for placental tissue, which tends to be quite bloody. Inadequate fixation makes trimming of the tissue and sectioning on the microtome more difficult, giving poor results in final sections. This is particularly true of the sections of the membrane roll. One option is to *fix the initial sections of placental tissue for a longer period*, at least overnight, before trimming and processing. Another option is to *briefly fix the tissue in Bouin's solution* before trimming and processing. Bouin's solution makes tissue considerably harder and allows one to trim the tissue more readily before embedding. Bouin's solution is made by preparing a saturated solution (1.2%) of picric acid in water and adding 40% formaldehyde solution and glacial acetic acid in proportions of 15:5:1. After 1 to 3h fixation, the tissue is ready to be trimmed. Ideally, the Bouin's-fixed sections are immersed in a *saturated lithium carbonate solution* before embedding. This step is not required, but it helps to remove extraneous pigments. Moreover, some intervillous blood is lysed, and pigments derived from blood ("formalin pigment," acid hematin) are more frequently present when lithium carbonate is omitted. This is also important when one wishes to do immunohistochemistry.

Special Procedures

The placenta is a good source of tissue for **chromosome analysis**, particularly when the fetus is macerated and tissue from that source will often not grow in culture. The procedure is to disinfect the amnion with some alcohol and then strip the amnion off a portion of placental surface. With sterile instruments, a piece of chorion is taken, placed in culture medium, and then transferred to the cytogenetics laboratory. Multiple areas of the placenta may need to be sampled if one needs to rule out confined placental mosaicism (see Chapter 11). **For bacterial culture**, tissue swabs or tissue samples from the undersurface of the amnion should be taken as contamination of the amnion is likely.

Photography should be an integral part of any gross examination. The old adage that "a picture is worth a thousand words" is most applicable in this instance and particularly true when the placenta is the subject of future litigation. Any unusual or clinically significant lesion should be photographed, as dissection usually destroys the macroscopic lesion. Photography is particularly important when the macroscopic appearance and not the microscopic appearance demonstrate the lesion best.

Table 3.1. Indications for placental examination

Maternal Indications:	Severe neonatal CNS depression or
History of reproductive failure: 1	neurologic problems such as
or more spontaneous abortions	seizures
(Abs), stillbirths, neonatal	Apgar score of 3 or less at 5 min
deaths, or premature births	Suspected infection
Maternal diseases:	Congenital anomalies
Coagulopathy	Thick meconium
Hypertension (pregnancy	Multiple birth
induced or chronic)	
Diabetes mellitus	*Placental Indications:*
Prematurity (<32 weeks)	Any gross abnormality of the
Postmaturity (>42 weeks)	placental, membranes, or
Oligohydramnios	umbilical cord such as masses,
Fever or infection	thrombi, excessively long, short,
Repetitive bleeding	or twisted umbilical cord
Abruptio placentae	
	Optional Recommendations:
Fetal and Neonatal Indications:	Prematurity between 32 and 36
Stillbirth or perinatal death	weeks
Fetal growth restriction (IUGR)	Low 1-min Apgar score
Hydrops	Fetal distress or nonreassuring
	fetal status

Source: Adapted from the College of American Pathologists (Altshuler G, Deppisch LM. Arch Pathol Lab Med 1991;115:701–703).

Table 3.2. Macroscopic lesions of the fetal membranes

Description	Diagnosis
Discoloration	
Green, green-yellow, or green-brown	Meconium
Opaque, white, yellow, yellow-green	Acute chorioamnionitis
Brown, brown-yellow	Hemosiderin
Red-brown, red-pink	Hemolysis
Focal Lesions	
Hemorrhagic, granular, or necrotic	Retromembranous hematoma
	Decidual necrosis
	Fetus papyraceous
	Vernix caseosa
Strings or bands of membrane tethered to umbilical cord	Amnionic bands

US, usual sections; RS, representative sections; UN, sections unnecessary.
[a] Microscopic picture.

Table 3.3. Macroscopic lesions of the fetal surface and chorionic plate

Description	Category/lesion
Plaques or Nodules	
White, hydrophobic plaques	Squamous metaplasia
Small, translucent, white or yellow nodules	Amnion nodosum
0.5 cm, oval, chalky disk, under amnion	Yolk sac remnant
Firm, white subchorionic nodules or plaques	Subchorionic fibrin/fibrinoid
Bulging, hemorrhage, or fibrous subchorionic nodule	Chorangioma
Cysts	Subchorionic cyst
	Amnionic cyst
Hemorrhage	Subchorionic hematoma
	Subamnionic hematoma
Chorionic Vessels	
Clot or white streak in vessel	Thrombosis of fetal vessels
Dilated and tortuous vessels	Mesenchymal dysplasia

RS, representative section; UN, section unnecessary; AS, additional sections.

Additional gross examination	Additional sections	Figure number	Figure page number	Discussion page number
Note if meconium is only on surface, stains amnion or stains amnion and chorion Examine cord carefully for meconium staining	US	14.14 A	234	233
Note unusual odors or frank pus Look for possible intervillous abscesses	US	16.2	282	280
Note discoloration	US	14.17 A	237	236
Likely due to fetal demise or freezing	US	—	—	385
Note size and location	RS	14.11	231	230
Note presence of associated finding such as hemorrhage or decidual vasculopathy	RS	18.4[a]	336	334
Dissect dividing membranes to establish chorionicity, if possible Measure crown-rump length Identify umbilical cord if possible	RS	10.1 10.2	154 155	153
Describe	UN	14.8	229	228
Note presence and location Examine fetal surface to evaluate absence of amnion Evaluate if there is cord or other entanglement Take photograph	RS	14.24 14.26 14.27 14.28	244 246 246 247	243

Additional gross examination	Additional sections	Figure number	Figure page number	Discussion page number
Differentiate from amnion nodosum	RS	14.20	241	240
Differentiate from squamous metaplasia	RS	14.21	242	240
Note	UN	14.7 A	228	227
Note if excessive	if excessive	3.4	29	361
Note size and extent (% of surface) Note if villous tissue pale	AS of lesion	3.8 22.1 22.2 22.3 22.4	31 406 407 407 408	405
Note size of lesions	RS	14.3 14.4	225 225	223
Note lesion	RS	14.1 A	224	223
Note size and extent (% surface) Note age of hematoma	RS	3.8 14.12 14.13	31 232 233	229
Iatrogenic lesion	UN	3.8 14.10	31 231	229
Describe	AS of fetal surface vessels	21.1 21.2 21.3 21.6	393 393 394 395	392
Look for the presence of cystically dilated villi	AS of vessels and villous tissue	19.18 A	368	368

Table 3.4. Macroscopic lesions of the umbilical cord

Description	Diagnosis
Insertion	
Insertion *at* placental edge	Marginal
Insertion *into* membranes with membranous vessels	Velamentous
Cord divides before insertion	Furcate
Cord inserts and runs in membranes	Interpositional
Length: Normal 55 cm	
<40 cm	Short cord
>70–80 cm	Long cord
Diameter: Normal 1–1.5 cm	
Increased	Thick cord
Decreased	Thin cord
Focal constriction	Stricture
Knot	True knot
	False knot
Twist	
Excessive	Excessive twist
Minimal or no	Minimal twist
Vessels: Normally Three	
Two vessels	Single umbilical artery
Four vessels	Persistent vein
Thinning of vessel wall	Aneurysm
Thrombosis	Thrombosis
Coloration: Normal, White	
Pink, red, or red-brown	Hemolysis
Brown, yellow-brown	Hemosiderin
Green or yellow-green	Meconium
Yellow	Bile
Chalky deposits	Calcification
Masses	
Cysts	Embryonic remnants
White, tan, or yellow surface nodules	Candida infection
Hemorrhage	Hematoma
	Hemangioma
Miscellaneous	
Edema	Edema
Rupture	Rupture

RS, representative section; AS, additional sections; UN, section unnecessary; US, usual sections; FSV, fetal surface (chorionic) vessels.
[a] Microscopic picture.

Additional gross examination	Additional sections	Figure number	Figure page number	Discussion page number
Evaluate for velamentous vessels; if present, see "velamentous insertion"	US	15.17	263	263
Measure distance from insertion to placental margin	AS of velamentous vessels	15.17	263	264
Note hemorrhage in membranes		15.18	264	
Note thrombosis or disruption of vessels		15.21	266	
		15.22	267	
Note thrombosis/disruption of vessels	RS	15.17	263	268
		15.19	265	
Note insertion	RS	15.17	263	268
		15.20	265	
Examine FSV for thrombi	AS of FSV	—	—	255
Examine FSV for thrombi	AS of FSV	15.9	257	255
Note diameter	AS to rule out a cyst	15.10	258	257
Note if focal as it may represent a cyst				
Note diameter	US	15.8	254	257
Note location of stricture	AS of stricture, normal cord and FSV	15.8	254	253
Measure diameter in that region				
Note if loose or tight, or congestion on one side	AS through knot, normal cord and FSV	15.12	260	260
		15.13	260	
Untie cord and note if cord stays coiled		15.16	262	
Differentiate from true knot/thrombus	UN	15.15	261	261
Make note of twisting	AS of FSV	15.6	253	253
		15.7	254	
Make note of twist	US	15.6	253	253
Avoid sections near insertion site due to artery anastomosis	AS of cord	15.23[a]	269	268
Avoid sections with false knots	AS of cord	—	—	270
Serially section to follow dilation and ensure it is not in area of cord clamping	AS (serial) of thinned area	15.27	273	272
		15.28	274	
Measure in three dimensions				
Measure in three dimensions	AS of cord	15.24[a]	271	270
Ensure is not a false knot or area of cord clamping	AS of FSV			
Due to fetal demise or freezing of the placenta	US	—	—	385
Note color	US	14.17 A	237	236
Note whether focal or diffuse	AS of cord	14.14 A	234	233
Note color	US	17.1	321	321
Often due to infection, and necrotizing funisitis	AS of cord	16.21	300	286
Note size and location	RS of cyst	15.2	251	249
Describe lesions	AS of cord (serial)	16.16	296	295
Ensure not due to cord clamping	AS of lesion	15.26	273	272
Measure in three dimensions		15.25*	272	271
Note if localized	AS of cord to rule out cyst	15.10	258	257
Note locations, extent and size	AS (serial) through rupture	15.26	273	274
Note other lesions: meconium, masses, etc.				

Table 3.5. Macroscopic lesions of the maternal surface

Description	Category/lesion
White, chalky, stippled lesions	Calcifications
Focal, shaggy, tan, loosely adherent tissue	Decidual necrosis
Blood clot on surface or at margin	Retroplacental hematoma (abruptio placentae)
	Marginal hemorrhage due to ascending infection
Firm surface with yellow discoloration, corrugated appearance	Maternal floor infarction (massive perivillous fibrinoid)

UN, section unnecessary; AS, additional sections; RS, representative section.
[a] Microscopic picture.

Additional gross examination	Additional sections	Figure number	Figure page number	Discussion page number
Normal finding	UN	3.7	30	30
Note if extensive	AS if extensive	18.4[a]	336	334
Note size and % of maternal surface	AS of clot and underlying placental tissue	3.8 18.13	31 341	340
Note compression of villous tissue		19.5	356	
Note whether clot is recent or old	RS of related infarction	19.6	357	
Note presence of underlying infarct				
Note size and % of surface and compression of villous tissue if present	AS of marginal hemorrhage	16.3	283	283
Note discoloration of fetal surface				
Note size and % involvement of maternal surface and cut surface	AS of normal and abnormal villous tissue	19.13 19.14	364 365	363

Table 3.6. Abnormalities of placental shape and macroscopic lesions of the villous tissue

Description	Category/lesion
Shape Alternations	
Two equal lobes	Bilobed
Two or more unequal lobes	Succenturiate lobe
Extremely large, thin placenta	Membranacea
Membranes do not insert into placental margin	Circumvallate or circummarginate
	Extrachorial or extramembranous pregnancy
Full-thickness defect in placenta	Fenestrata
Ring-shaped placenta	Zonary placenta
Diffuse Lesions	
Increased fibrinoid deposition	Maternal floor infarction/massive perivillous fibrin deposition
Mottling of villous tissue	Chronic villitis
Focal Lesions	
Well-circumscribed, granular surface	Recent infarct
	Old infarct
Well-circumscribed, shiny surface	Intervillous thrombus
Well to poorly demarcated lesion	Tumor
Poorly demarcated white, granular	Intervillous abscess
Cystically dilated villi	Mesenchymal dysplasia
	Hydatidiform moles
Nodular lesion (s)	Chorangioma
	Chorangiomatosis
Color	
Pale	Fetal anemia, hemorrhage, or hydrops
	Twin-to-twin transfusion
Congestion	Villous congestion

RS, representative section; AS, additional sections; UN, section unnecessary.

Gross examination	Additional sections	Figure number	Figure page number	Discussion page number
Note sizes of lobes	RS of any vessels	13.1	209	208
Examine membranous vessels between lobes for abnormalities	between lobes if abnormal	13.2	210	
Note sizes of lobes	RS of vessels	13.1	209	208
Examine membranous vessels between lobes for abnormalities	between lobes if abnormal	13.3	211	
Small lobes may be infarcted	RS of lobe if infarction present			
Describe	AS of placenta	13.1	209	218
		13.12	211	
Note if partial or complete	AS of peripheral	13.4	212	211
Measure distance from insertion to placental margin	placenta not covered by	13.5	212	
	membranes	13.6	213	
Note plication of membrane		13.8	214	
Note size of amniotic sac	AS of peripheral	13.9	215	215
Measure distance from insertion to placental margin	placenta not covered by membranes	13.10	216	
Note size and location	UN	13.1	209	219
		13.13	220	
Note shape	UN	13.1	209	219
		13.14	220	
Note extent, measurement, and % of villous tissue	AS of villous tissue	19.13	364	363
		19.14	365	
Note lesion and extent (%) of villous tissue involved	AS of villous tissue	3.8	31	308
		16.29	310	
Note size	RS	3.8	31	337
If multiple (give % of		18.7	338	
placenta involved)		18.8	330	
Note size, if multiple (give % of placenta involved)	RS	3.8	31	337
		18.9	337	
Note size	RS	3.8	31	351
If multiple, measure each		19.1	352	
		19.2	353	
Note size	RS	3.8	31	405
Note if multiple				
Note size	AS of villous	16.12	291	290
Note if multiple	tissue			
Describe	AS of abnormal	19.19	369	368
Look for dilated, tortuous vessels	placenta and vessels			
Describe	AS	23.2	420	416
		23.3	421	
		23.6	423	
Identify and describe	RS	3.8	31	405
Note if multiple		22.1	406	
		22.2	407	
		22.3	407	
Describe, note if multiple	RS	19.10	362	360
Note color	AS of villous	20.1	373	371
Look for intervillous thrombi	tissue			
Note color	RS	10.12	165	163
Identify vascular anastomoses				
Note color	UN	17.3	325	324
Evaluate if villous tissue is friable (associated with maternal diabetes)				

Table 3.7. Normative values

Pregnancy, week post menstrual	Pregnancy, month	Crown-rump length (mm)	Foot length (mm)	Embryonic/ fetal weight (g)
3	1			
4				
5	2	2.5		
6		5		
7		9		
8		14		1.1
9	3	20		2
10		26		5
11		33		11
12		40		17
13	4	48	12	23
14		56	17	30
15		65	19	40
16		75	22	60
17	5	88	25	90
18		99	28	130
19		112	29	180
20		125	33	250
21	6	137	36	320
22		150	39	400
23		163	42	480
24		176	45	560
25	7	188	47	650
26		200	50	750
27		213	53	870
28		226	55	1000
29	8	236	58	1130
30		250	60	1260
31		263	62	1400
32		276	65	1550
33	9	289	67	1700
34		302	69	1900
35		315	71	2100
36		328	74	2300
37	10	341	76	2500
38		354	78	2750
39		367	80	3000
40		380	81	3400

Portions of this table were modified from Kalousek, DK, Baldwin VJ, Dimmick JE, et al. Embryofetal-perinatal autopsy and placental examination. In: Dimmick JE, Kalousek DK (eds) Development pathology of the embryo and fetus. Philadelphia: Lippincott, 1992:55–82.

Placental weight (g)	Fetal/ placental weight ratio	Placental thickness (cm)	Placental diameter (cm)	Umbilical cord length (cm)
				0.2
				0.4
				0.7
				1.2
6	0.18			2.0
8	0.25			3.3
13	0.38			5.5
19	0.58			9.2
26	0.65			12.6
32	0.72		5.0	15.8
41	0.73	1.0	5.6	18.8
50	0.80	1.1	6.2	21.5
60	1.00	1.2	6.9	24.0
70	1.29	1.2	7.5	26.4
80	1.63	1.3	8.1	28.7
101	1.78	1.4	8.7	30.9
112	2.23	1.5	9.4	33.0
126	2.54	1.5	10.0	35.0
144	2.78	1.6	10.6	36.9
162	2.96	1.7	11.2	38.7
180	3.11	1.8	11.9	40.4
198	3.28	1.8	12.5	42.0
216	3.47	1.9	13.1	43.5
234	3.72	1.9	13.7	45.0
252	3.97	2.0	14.4	46.4
270	4.19	2.0	15.0	47.7
288	4.38	2.1	15.6	49.0
306	4.58	2.1	16.2	50.2
324	4.78	2.2	16.9	52.0
342	4.97	2.2	17.5	53.0
360	5.28	2.3	18.1	54.0
378	5.56	2.3	18.7	54.9
396	5.81	2.4	19.4	55.7
414	6.04	2.4	20.0	56.5
432	6.37	2.4	20.6	57.2
451	6.65	2.5	21.3	57.9
470	7.23	2.5	22.0	58.5

Selected References

PHP4, Chapter 1, pages 1–12; Chapter 2, pages 13–15.

Altshuler G, Hyde S. Clinicopathologic implications of placental pathology. Clin Obstet Gynecol 1996;39:549–570.

Baergen RN. Macroscopic examination of the placenta immediately following birth. J Nurse Midwifery 1997;42:393–402.

Benirschke K. Examination of the placenta. Obstet Gynecol 1991;18:309–333.

Booth VJ, Nelson KB, Dambrosia JM, et al. What factors influence whether placentas are submitted for pathologic examination? Am J Obstet Gynecol 1997; 176:567–571.

Gruenwald P. Examination of the placenta by the pathologist. Arch Pathol 1964; 77:41–46.

Langston C, Kaplan C, MacPherson T, et al. Practice guidelines for examination of the placenta. Developed by the placental pathology practice guideline development task force of the College of American Pathologists. Arch Pathol Lab Med 1997;121:449–476.

Naeye RL. Functionally important disorders of the placenta, umbilical cord, and fetal membranes. Hum Pathol 1987;18:680–691.

Chapter 4

Microscopic Evaluation of the Second and Third Trimester Placenta

Overview and Microscopic Survey

Sections of the placenta have a complex configuration. Therefore, a low-power survey is essential for orientation and identification of the specific structures comprising the mature placenta. The following is a list of those structures (letters in parentheses refer to Figure 4.1):

- **Chorionic plate** (C), including
  - **Amnion** (B),
  - **Chorion** (C),
  - **Fibrinoid** (Langhans' fibrinoid stria) (C)
- **Chorionic villi** of various types (D to G),
- **Intervillous space** (A),
- **Fibrinoid deposits** in various locations (C, F, H to L),
- **Cell islands** (J),
- **Septa** (K), and
- **Basal plate** including
  - **Anchoring villi** and
  - **Cell columns** (I).

The **amnion** (Figure 4.1 B) covers the chorionic plate toward the amniotic cavity. It consists of a *single layer of cuboidal to columnar cells*. Beneath the amnionic epithelium is a thin layer of amnionic mesoderm, which is only loosely applied to the next layer, the chorionic mesoderm, via a reticular zone with large clefts (Figure 4.1 C). Due to this unstable connection, the amnion may "detach" from the chorion or even become lost during preparation.

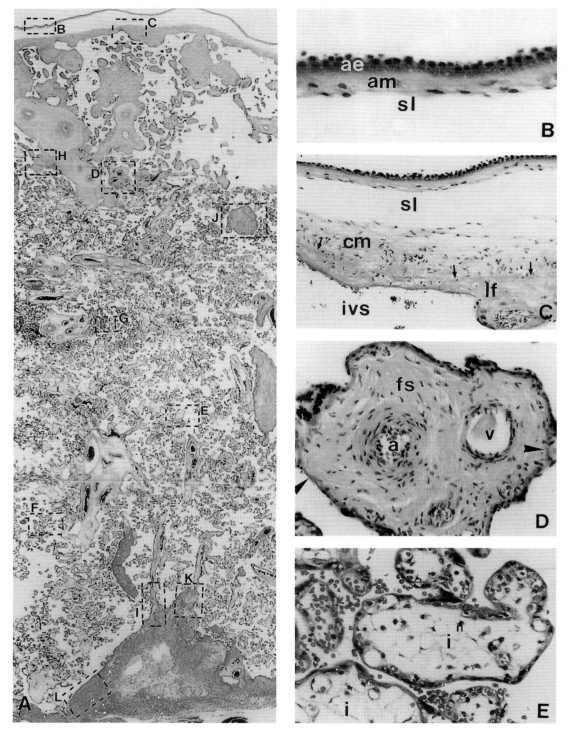

Figure 4.1. Typical features of the third trimester placenta in paraffin sections following H&E staining. All specimens are from the 40th week PM (after last menstrual period). (A) Vertical survey section. The marked frames refer to the following detailed pictures. ×10. (B) Amnion. ×120. (C) Chorionic plate, covered by the amnion. ×60. (D) Peripheral stem villus. ×180. fs = fibrous stroma; a = artery, v = vein, ae = amnionic epitheilium, am = amnion, sl = spongy layer, ivs = intervillous space, lf = Langhan's fibrinoid, cm = chorionic mesoderm, arrowheads = syncytiotrophoblast. (E) Two immature intermediate villi (i) surrounded by some mature intermediate and terminal villi (t). ×180.

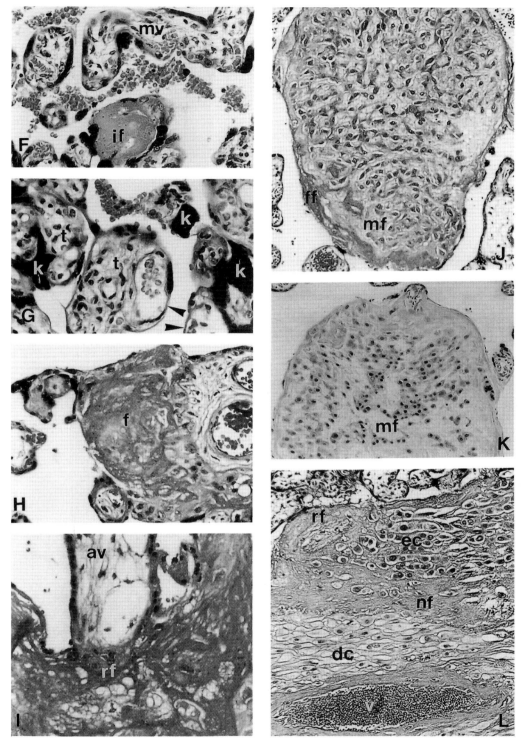

Figure 4.1. (F) A longitudinally sectioned mature intermediate villus (mv) together with some terminal villi and villous fibrinoid (if). ×180. (G) A group of terminal villi(t) showing considerable syncytial knotting (k). ×360. (arrowheads = syncytiotrophoblast). (H) A small stem villus (sv), the trophoblastic cover of which is partly replaced by perivillous fibrinoid (f). ×180. (I) An anchoring villus (av), connected to the basal plate by fibrinoid (rf) as the originally connecting cell column has vanished. ×180. (J) Cell island, mf = fibrinoid. ×90. (K) Tip of a placental septum. ×90. (L) Basal plate with obvious layering. rf = Rohr's fiorinoid, nf = Nitabuch's fibrinoid, dc = decidual cells. ×90.

The **chorionic plate** (Figure 4.1 C) is the cover of the intervillous space, which is directly below. The chorion consists of the *spongy layer with clefts, then a compact layer of chorionic mesoderm, a rudimentary basement membrane, and finally fibrinoid.* On the lower side of this basement membrane, highly variable amounts of extravillous trophoblast can be found. In early pregnancy, they form a complete and usually multilayered stratum. In later pregnancy, this layer becomes rarified. Attached to or extending from the fibrinoid one finds numerous stem villi, *representing the first branches of villous trunks branching off from the chorionic plate* (see upper third of Figure 4.1 A).

Different from the first trimester situation, the width of the **intervillous space** (Figure 4.1 A) is highly variable with large "subchorionic lakes" of maternal blood below and narrow intervillous clefts between the terminal villi. In the term placenta, the width of the clefts is somewhat dependent on the mode of delivery and how much maternal blood is expelled during the process. The **villous trees** (Figure 4.1 D) measure 1 to 4 cm in diameter. Their central branches consist of **stem villi**, which are the largest caliber villi. They are found in highest concentration near the chorionic plate, particularly near the insertion of the umbilical cord. Histologically, they are characterized by one or several *arteries and veins, or arterioles and venules, with clearly visible muscular walls surrounded by a fibrous stroma containing only a few paravascular capillaries.* Near term, the trophoblastic cover is focally or largely replaced by fibrinoid (arrowheads) (see Chapter 8). This process is more pronounced in larger stem villi. The immature forerunners of the stem villi are the **immature intermediate villi** (Figure 4.1 E). They are easily identifiable by their large-caliber; pale-staining, minimal collagen and *loose reticular network with connective tissue cells surrounding stromal channels* containing *Hofbauer cells* (see Chapter 6). **Mature intermediate villi** (Figure 4.1 F) are the forerunners of the terminal villi. They are slender, multiply curved branches of stem villi with diameters ranging from 60 to about 100 μm. They differ from stem villi by the absence of both stromal fibrosis and stem vessels with an identifiable media. *Their stroma is composed of slender capillaries embedded into a loose connective tissue that is rich in cells but poor in fibers.* **Terminal villi** (Figure 4.1 G) are the grapelike terminal side branches of the mature intermediate villi, which range 40 to about 80 μm in diameter. The dominating structures within the *loose stroma* are *sinusoidally dilated and highly coiled fetal capillaries.* A typical feature of terminal villi is the syncytial knotting, which are clusters of syncytial nuclei at the villous surfaces and are mostly due to tangential sectioning. They are more common toward term (see Chapter 7 for discussion of villous types).

Fibrinoid (Figure 4.1 H) is an *acellular, eosinophilic material* present in the intervillous space (Figures 4.1 C,D,F,H). When it replaces the trophoblastic cover of villi, it is called perivillous fibrinoid. When it replaces the stroma beneath the trophoblastic surface, it is called intravillous fibrinoid (Figure 4.1 F). Areas of prominent fibrinoid deposition are below the chorionic plate (Langhans' fibrinoid, lf, Figure 4.1 C), at the surface of the basal plate (Rohr's fibrinoid, rf, Figures 4.1 I,L), Nitabuch's fibrinoid in the depth of the basal plate (Figure 4.1 L), and in the extracellular matrix of cell islands (Figure 4.1 J) and septa (Figure 4.1 K). Despite the fact that fibrinoid appears to be homogeneous histologically, it has two different compositions (see Chapter 8), which may be deposited close together or separately:

1. **Fibrin**: consisting of blood clotting products free of extravillous trophoblast cells; and
2. **Fibrinoid**: which embeds extravillous trophoblast cells and is primarily a secretory product of these cells.

Cell islands (Figure 4.1 J) are *composed of extravillous trophoblastic cells and fibrinoid* (see Chapter 8). They increase in size throughout pregnancy due to continuous trophoblastic proliferation and an increase in the fibrinoid embedding these cells. Large cell islands may contain central cavities or "cysts," which result from degeneration of trophoblast cells and subsequent liquefaction. Occasionally, cell islands may contain decidual cells and thus may represent cross sections of placental septa. **Placental septa** (Figure 4.1 K) are the result of folding of the basal plate, probably supported by tension of anchoring villi (see Chapter 8). They are *rudimentary pillar-shaped structures* and are not true septa. They are attached only to the basal plate (Figure 4.1 A) and are composed of *extravillous trophoblast and decidual cells embedded in fibrinoid*. Sometimes large cysts, similar to those of the cell islands, can be found. The septal tips are often difficult to distinguish from cell islands in histologic sections.

Only in a few exceptional places is the **basal plate** (Figure 4.1 L) of the term placenta as clearly layered as depicted here. The figure shows the layers of the basal plate starting with a *superficial layer of Rohr's fibrinoid, followed by extravillous cytotrophoblast, a layer of Nitabuch's fibrinoid, and a compact decidual layer* (see Chapter 8). In most cases, there is no clearly defined fetomaternal border, and extravillous trophoblast, decidual cells, uteroplacental vessels, and endometrial glandular residues are intermingled with fibrinoid in a somewhat haphazard manner. In the last trimester, anchoring villi (Figure 4.1 I) become less prominent but *are still connected to the basal plate or to septa* by cell columns. As the proliferative activity of the cell columns slows down, the cells are rarified to one layer that is sometimes incomplete or even replaced by fibrinoid. Some *cell columns maintain their proliferative activity and thus act as growth zones for the anchoring villi and basal plate*, even near term.

Microscopic Survey of the Fetal Membranes

The term "membranes" is usually taken to be synonymous with the amnion and the chorion laeve or the extraplacental membranes. They are the "bag of waters" that contain the amniotic fluid and enclose the fetus. The structure and function of the membranes include *turnover of the water* and *enzymatic activity during the initiation of labor*. The membranes have three *distinct* layers (Figure 4.2), the **amnion, chorion**, and **decidua capsularis**. The inner layer (toward the fetus) is the amnion composed of amnionic epithelium and amnionic mesoderm, which

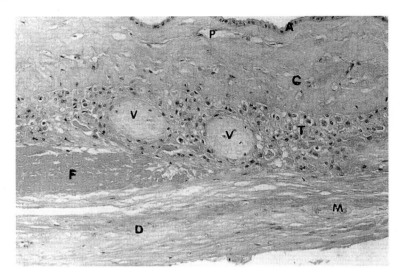

Figure 4.2. Microscopic appearance of normal "membranes." Amnionic epithelium (A) sits on a thin layer of connective tissue that is separable from chorionic connective tissue (C) in an ill-defined plane (P) representing the intermediate spongy layer. The following layer of extravillous trophoblastic cells (T) is irregularly studded with atrophic or "ghost" villi (V). At the periphery is the decidua capsularis (D) with maternal vessels (M) and frequent fibrinoid (F) deposits. H&E. ×16.

includes a basal lamina. The **amnionic epithelium** is a *single layer of flat, cuboidal, or columnar epithelial cells*, derived from the fetal ectoderm and contiguous with the amnion over the umbilical cord and with the fetal skin. The amnion is *passively* attached to the next layer, the chorion, by the internal pressure of the amniotic fluid and can usually be easily separated from it. As it does not contain its own blood vessels, *the amnion obtains its nutrition and oxygen form the surrounding chorionic fluid, the amniotic fluid, and from the fetal surface vessels*. The **chorion** is a tough fibrous tissue layer that *carries the fetal blood vessels*. It is composed of an intermediate (spongy) layer, blood vessels, and chorionic mesoderm. The **intermediate spongy layer** is in between the two layers and is composed of *a few fibroblasts, an occasional macrophage, and loosely arranged bundles of collagen fibers separated by a communicating system of clefts*. The collagen composition of both amnion and chorion contribute to the mechanical stability and tensile properties of the membranes. Because the villi of the chorion frondosum originate from the chorion, one often finds *atrophied villous remains in the free surface of the membranes* even in term pregnancy specimens. These former villi appear as round "balls" of degenerated connective tissue, usually lacking trophoblastic cover, and possessing no vessels (Figure 4.2).

A highly variable layer of **extravillous trophoblastic cells** persists until term. These consist of *small, undifferentiated; proliferating trophoblastic cells admixed with larger, more differentiated, nonproliferating cells*. Fibrinoid may also be present. The extravillous trophoblast are intimately intermingled with the outermost layer, the **decidua capsu-**

laris, which is the only maternal component of the membranes. The decidua capsularis contains very few maternal vessels but normally contains *some macrophages, lymphocytes, and other inflammatory cells in addition to decidualized endometrial stromal cells*. At the edge of the placenta, the decidua capsularis is contiguous with the decidua basalis and delimits the "marginal sinus" (see Chapter 8). One often finds inflammation, degenerative changes, and hemorrhage at this location.

Microscopic Survey of the Umbilical Cord

The umbilical cord (Figure 4.3) consists of the **amnionic epithelium**, **Wharton's jelly**, and **umbilical vessels**. The cord is completely covered by amnionic epithelium. Near the umbilicus, it is largely *unkeratinized, stratified squamous epithelium*, then becomes *stratified columnar epithelium* and finally simple columnar epithelium that is contiguous with the epithelium of the fetal surface. In contrast to the amnion of the membranes, the amnion of the cord *grows firmly into the central connective tissue core* and cannot be dislodged.

The connective tissue of the cord, or **Wharton's jelly**, is a jelly-like material composed of a *ground substance of open-chain polysaccharides distributed in a fine network of microfibrils*. Extracellular matrix molecules are present, often accumulated around stromal clefts. These clefts should not be misinterpreted as lymphatic vessels, which do not exist in the cord or in the placenta, nor should they be confused with pathologic changes such as edema or cyst formation (see Chapter 15). Wharton's jelly is sparsely cellular, containing a few macrophages, mast cells, and myofibroblasts.

There are normally two arteries and one vein in the human umbilical cord (see Figure 4.3). The second umbilical vein normally atrophies during the second month of pregnancy. The mean intravital diameter of the arteries is around 3mm, while the venous diameter is around twice this. *The muscular coat of the arteries consists of crossing spiraled fibers. The venous muscular coats are thinner than those of the arteries and are composed of separate layers of longitudinal or circular fibers.* Each vessel

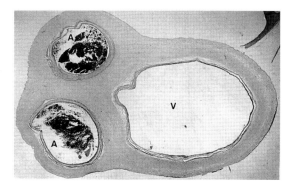

Figure 4.3. Cross-section of mature umbilical cord, near its placental insertion. Wharton's jelly is compressed by the expanded umbilical vein (V) and two arteries (A).

is surrounded by crossing bundles of spiraled collagen fibers that form a kind of adventitia.

Approach to the Specimen

An easy approach to examination of the slides is to review each part of the placenta sequentially, that is, the fetal membranes, umbilical cord, and placental disk. To this end, each component of the placenta is listed below followed by the specific features that should be evaluated and possible abnormalities which may be present. Reference to the tables at the end of the chapter is also given in each section. The tables (Tables 4.1–4.6) list lesions with a brief microscopic description, possible diagnosis, additional studies that may be needed, and references to the location in the text where figures and additional information can be found. Table 4.7 lists placental lesions that may be found in certain important clinical conditions such as fetal demise and growth restriction.

Fetal membranes (Table 4.1):
- **General**
  - Accumulation of macrophages containing pigment such as meconium or hemosiderin
  - Acute or chronic inflammatory infiltrate, associated bacteria
  - Hematoma or other masses.
- **Amnionic epithelium** (Figure 4.4):
  - Metaplastic change to keratizined squamous epithelium
  - Nodules of keratinous debris
  - Degenerative changes, piling up of cells, sloughing, or
  - Cytoplasmic vacuolization.
- **Decidua capsularis:**
  - Necrosis, inflammation
  - Abnormalities of vessels such as thickening of vessel walls, fibrinoid necrosis, inflammation, foamy macrophages in the endothelium, or thrombosis

Epithelial Abnormalities

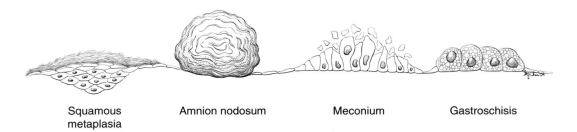

Squamous   Amnion nodosum   Meconium   Gastroschisis
metaplasia

Figure 4.4. Various epithelial abnormalities of the amnionic epithelium are depicted. These lesions are referenced and described in Table 4.1.

Umbilical Cord (Table 4.2):
- **General**
  - Abnormal thickness, abnormal length, edema, or focal constriction
  - Surface lesions, ulceration
  - Inflammation, calcification
  - Masses including hematoma, tumors, cysts, or epithelial remnants
- **Umbilical vessels:**
  - Single umbilical artery or second umbilical vein
  - Disruption, thinning of the wall, degeneration of smooth muscle, or
  - Thrombosis

Placental Disk
- **Chorionic Plate** (Table 4.3):
  - Masses, cysts, hematomas, or
  - Excessive fibrinoid
- **Chorionic and Stem Vessels** (Table 4.3):
  - Inflammation or thrombosis
- **Intervillous Space** (Table 4.4):
  - Thrombosis
  - Excessive fibrinoid
  - Cellular infiltrate such as inflammatory cells, or atypical cells
- **Chorionic Villi** (Table 4.5):
  - Size and morphology, appropriateness for gestational age: enlarged (delayed maturation) or small (hypermature), increased or decreased syncytial knots
  - Simplified outlines, invaginations or irregularities of the surface, hydropic change
  - Ischemic change or infarction
- **Villous stroma** (Table 4.5):
  - Inflammatory cell infiltrate
  - Microcalcification
  - Edema, hyalinization, or hemorrhage
- **Villous capillaries** (Table 4.5):
  - Increased or decreased
  - Thrombosis, disruption or extravasation of red blood cells into the stroma
- **Basal plate including decidua basalis** (Table 4.6):
  - Excessive fibrinoid
  - Necrosis, marked chronic inflammation with plasma cells, or
  - Hematoma
- **Decidual vessels** (Table 4.6):
  - Thrombosis, fibrinoid necrosis, or atherosis

Routine and Special Stains

For histologic examination, the standard hematoxylin and eosin (H&E) stain is usually adequate. On many occasions, however, it is useful to employ special stains for microorganisms. These include tissue Gram stains, silver stains such as Warthin–Starry, Steiner, or Gomori methenamine silver stains, periodic acid–Schiff (PAS), Geimsa, and acid-fast stains. In general, bacterial organisms causing acute chorioamnionitis are difficult to identify in tissue sections even if special stains are performed. Specific immunohistochemical stains that disclose the presence of viruses, for example, cytomegalovirus and herpes antigens, are sometimes used.

Immunohistochemical Markers

Immunohistochemistry may be used to differentiate trophoblast from other cells. The following immunohistochemical reactions may be useful for histologic examination of placental paraffin sections.

Anticytokeratin stains epithelial cells such as the *amnionic epithelium* and all *trophoblast*. It is a useful marker in distinguishing extravillous trophoblast from decidual cells or intraarterial trophoblast from maternal endothelium. Syncytiotrophoblast stains strongly for human chorionic gonadotropin **(hCG)** while extravillous trophoblastic cells are either negative or weakly positive. Extravillous trophoblast stains for human placental lactogen **(hPL)**, **α-inhibin**, **Mel-CAM**, and placental protein 19 **(PP19)**. Some markers may be able to differentiate different

Table 4.1. Lesions of the fetal membranes

Description of feature	Lesion
Pigmented Macrophages	
Yellow-brown	Meconium
Brown, particulate, refringent	Hemosiderin
Inflammation	Acute chorioamnionitis
	Chronic chorioamnionitis
	Subacute chorioamnionitis
Hemorrhage	Retromembranous hematoma
Cysts	
Epithelial	Amnionic cyst
Squamous	Epidermoid cyst
Extravillous trophoblast	Subchorionic cyst
Masses	
Cartilage, bone, skin	Teratoma
	Embryonic remnants
	Fetus papyraceous
Anucleate squames and debris	Vernix caseosa

types of extravillous trophoblast (see Chapter 25). **Antivimentin** stains all mesenchyme-derived cells such as *connective tissue cells, macrophages, decidual cells, smooth muscle cells, and endothelial cells.* Generally, cells in the placenta will be positive for either cytokeratin or vimentin. As with cytokeratin, it is a useful tool to identify decidual cells as opposed to extravillous trophoblastic cells or to discriminate maternal endothelium from intraarterial trophoblast, and these two stains may be used together.

The antibodies **Ki-67**, MIB-1, and anti-PCNA (clones PC10, 19A2, 19F4) bind to nuclear proteins and are expressed in proliferating cells. Ki-67 is only applicable on cryostat sections. MIB-1 is its analogue for carefully fixed paraffin sections and can also be applied on cryostat sections. Anti-PCNA can be used only for paraffin material. These antibodies are useful markers *to distinguish proliferating stem cell populations from differentiated ones and identifying growth zones.*

Other immunohistochemical stains may be helpful when abnormal or atypical cells are present in the intervillous space. These may represent choriocarcinoma or tumors metastatic from the fetus or mother (see Chapter 22). In this case, characterization of these cells with immunohistochemistry is often necessary. Finally, immunohistochemistry may be helpful in identification of specific organisms causing chronic villitis and congenital infections (see Chapter 16).

Comment	Additional studies	Figure number	Figure page number	Discussion page number
Meconium-filled macrophages in fetal membranes or meconium histiocytosis	May use iron stain to rule out hemosiderin	14.14 B	234	233
Hemosiderin-laden macrophages in fetal membranes May be secondary to decidual bleeding	May use iron stain to confirm	14.17 B	237	236
Involvement of extraplacental membranes, chorionic plate, chorionic plate vessels should be mentioned Bacteria should be mentioned if present	Gram stain rarely	16.4 16.5	284 285	280
May be associated with chronic villitis		16.32	312	312
Acute chorioamnionitis of longer duration	Gram stain rarely	16.10	289	288
Nonspecific finding		14.11[a]	231	230
No clinical significance		14.1 B	224	223
No clinical significance		14.2	224	223
No clinical significance		14.5	226	223
May represent acardiac twin		—	—	156
No clinical significance		14.6	227	227
Identify membrane relationships		10.3	155	153
No clinical significance Occurs with membrane rupture		14.9	230	228

Table 4.1. *Continued*

Description of feature	Lesion
Masses	
Necrotic tissue	Decidual necrosis
Epithelial Changes: See Figure 4.4	
Squamous change	Squamous metaplasia
Loss of epithelium with nodules on surface	Amnion nodosum
Degenerative change of epithelium	Meconium
Vacuolization	Gastroschisis
Decidua	
Inflammation	Acute deciduitis
	Chronic deciduitis
Abnormal vessels	Decidual vasculopathy

[a] Gross picture.

Table 4.2. Umbilical cord

Description of feature	Lesion
Tumors/Masses	
Skin, cartilage, bone	Teratoma
Vessels	Hemangioma
	Vitelline vessels
Epithelial elements	Embryonic remnants
Edema	Edema
	Embryonic cyst
Calcification	Necrotizing funisitis
Cellular Infiltrate	
Acute inflammation	Acute funisitis
	Candida infection
	Necrotizing funisitis

Comment	Additional studies	Figure number	Figure page number	Discussion page number
May be associated with decidual vasculopathy or hemorrhage		18.4	336	334
Normal finding		4.4	52	240
		14.19	240	
Usually secondary to chronic, significant oligohydramnios and often associated with renal anomalies in infant		4.4	52	240
		14.22	242	
		14.23	243	
Degenerative change may indicate that meconium discharge is more remote	Iron stain to rule out hemosiderin if necessary	4.4	52	233
		14.15	235	
Specific finding in gastroschisis not seen in other anomalies		4.4	52	239
		14.18	239	
May be associated with acute chorioamnionitis, otherwise is nonspecific		16.6	285	289
May be associated with chronic villitis Diagnosis usually made only with intense infiltrate and/or presence of plasma cells		16.20	299	298
May be associated with other changes of placental malperfusion (see Chapter 18)		18.1	334	333
		18.2	335	
		18.3	335	
		18.4	336	
		18.5	337	

Comment	Additional studies	Figure number	Figure page number	Discussion page number
May represent an acardiac twin		—	—	156
Similar to hemangiomas elsewhere May be associated with hematoma or rupture		15.25	272	221
Embryonic remnant		15.5	252	249
Allantoic duct remnant		15.1	250	250
Omphalomesenteric duct remnant		15.3	251	250
Vitelline vessel remnants		15.4	252	250
If localized, may represent cyst		15.10	258	257
Usually develop from embryonic remnants		15.2	251	250
Classically seen in syphilis but may be seen with other infections	Warthin–Starry or Steiner to rule out syphilis	16.8	287	297
		16.22	300	
May involve all vessels and extend into Wharton's jelly Fetal inflammatory response	Gram stain rarely	16.7	286	284
Usually not associated with acute chorioamnionitis	GMS or PAS demonstrates organism	16.17	297	295
May be associated with calcification Often seen in infection with syphilis	Silver stains and other stains for organisms	16.8	287	286
		16.22	300	

Table 4.2. *Continued*

Description of feature	Lesion
Cellular Infiltrate	
Pigmented macrophages	Meconium
Vascular abnormalities	
Single umbilical artery	Single umbilical artery
Four umbilical vessels	Supernumerary vessel
Thrombosis	Thrombosis
Hemorrhage	Hematoma
Thinned vessels	Varix or aneurysm
	Segmental thinning
Vascular necrosis	Meconium-induced vascular necrosis

[a] Gross picture.

Table 4.3. Chorionic plate

Description of feature	Lesion
Miscellaneous	
Lacy structure	Yolk sac remnant
Fetal skeleton	Fetus papyraceus
Fibrinoid	Subchorionic fibrinoid
Cyst	Subchorionic cyst
Hematoma	Subchorionic hematoma
	Subamnionic hematoma
Vascular mass	Chorangioma
Chorionic Vessels	
Thrombosis	Thrombosis
Inflammation	Acute chorioamnionitis
	Chronic chorioamnionitis
	Subacute chorioamnionitis
Degeneration of muscle	Meconium-induced damage

[a] Macroscopic picture.

Comment	Additional studies	Figure number	Figure page number	Discussion page number
Meconium-filled macrophages rarely identified in cord despite gross staining	May use iron stain to rule out hemosiderin	—	—	233
Associated with other fetal anomalies		15.23	269	268
Rare, may be associated with fetal anomalies		—	—	
Often associated with thrombosis in chorionic or stem vessels		15.24	271	270
May be associated with other cord lesions		15.26[a]	273	274
May compress umbilical vessels (particularly the umbilical vein) leading to vascular embarrassment				
May lead to umbilical cord rupture		15.27[i]	273	274
May be associated with congenital anomalies		15.29	275	274
Usually due to prolonged meconium exposure in utero		14.16	236	236

Comment	Additional studies	Figure number	Figure page number	Discussion page number
No clinical significance		1.8 14.7 B	11 228	227
Note membrane relationship if possible		10.3	155	157
If excessive, may be associated with placental malperfusion or maternal floor infarction		3.4[a]	29	232
No clinical significance		14.5	226	223
If large, may be associated with stillbirth		14.12[a]	232	232
Artifact secondary to excessive traction on cord during delivery		14.10[a]	231	239
Benign neoplasm		22.5 22.6 22.7	408 409 409	405
Other findings may include villous congestion		21.4 21.7 21.8 21.10 21.11	394 396 397 398 399	392
Ascending infection	Gram stain rarely	16.4	284	283
Note involvement of chorionic vessels and possible associated thrombosis		16.5	285	
Often associated with chronic villitis		16.32	312	312
Due to long standing ascending infection	Gram stain rarely	16.10	289	288
Usually due to long-standing meconium		14.16	236	235

Table 4.4. Intervillous space

Description of feature	Lesion
Blood clot	Intervillous thrombus
Fibrin/fibrinoid	Increased perivillous fibrin
	Maternal floor infarction
Inflammation	Intervillous abscess
	Chronic intervillositis
Abnormal or atypical cells	Metastatic malignancy
	Choriocarcinoma-in-situ
Collapse of intervillous space	Early villous ischemic change
Expansion of intervillous space	Hypoplasia or terminal villus deficiency

Table 4.5. Chorionic villi

Description of feature	Lesion
Villous Morphology	
Increased syncytial knots	Increased syncytial knots
Delayed maturation	Delayed maturity
Straight, unbranched villi	Terminal villus deficiency
Invagination, irregular contour	Possible chromosomal defect
Degeneration, smudging of nuclei	Ischemia/infarction
Ghost villi	Infarction
Vacuolization of trophoblast or other cells	Storage disorder

Comment	Additional studies	Figure number	Figure page number	Discussion page number
May be associated with fetomaternal hemorrhage	If extensive or large, Kleihauer-Betke stain on maternal blood	3.8 19.3	31 353	351
Moderate amounts normal If excessive may represent maternal floor infarction		19.12	364	361
Marked deposition Often involves full thickness of placenta and not just maternal floor		19.15 19.16 19.17	365 366 367	363
Generally due to *Listeria* infection	May use Gram stain	3.8 16.13	31 292	290
Infiltrate consists of histiocytes and lymphocytes		16.33	313	313
Cells may present as clusters in intervillous space or invade villi	Immunohistochemistry to determine origin of atypical cells	3.8 22.8 22.9 22.10	31 413 414 415	412
Markedly atypical syncytiotrophoblast and cytotrophoblast	Immunohistochemistry may be needed to determine differentiation	24.10 24.11 24.12	443 444 445	443
Often associated with infarction		18.10	338	338
Often associated with other changes of placental malperfusion		18.16	344	344

Comment	Additional studies	Figure number	Figure page number	Discussion starting page number
Associated with placental malperfusion		18.15 18.17	343 345	342
Associated with maternal diabetes		17.4	326	324
Indicative of profound decrease in perfusion Usually associated with abnormal Doppler (absent or reversed end-diastolic flow)		18.15 18.16	343 344	344
Suggestive of chromosomal defect Also seen in moles		11.7	181	181
Evidence of early infarction Associated with placental malperfusion		18.11	340	337
Old infarction		18.12	341	337
Various cells may show vacuolization See Table 20.1	EM, various other tests	20.9	383	382

Table 4.5. *Continued*

Description of feature	Lesion
Villous Morphology	
Trophoblastic proliferation	Hydatidiform mole
Villous Stroma	
Inflammation	Acute villitis
	Chronic villitis
Fine stippled calcification of stroma of basement membrane	Microcalcification
Hyalinization of stroma	Avascular villi
Hemorrhage	Intravillous hemorrhage
Red blood cells in stroma	Hemorrhagic endovasculitis (HEV)
Edema or hydropic change	Mesenchymal dysplasia
	Molar pregnancy
	Hydropic abortus
	Hydrops
	Immature intermediate villi
	Beckwith-Wiedemann syndrome
Villous Capillaries	
Increased vessels	Chorangiosis
	Chorangiomatosis
	Chorangioma

Comment	Additional studies	Figure number	Figure page number	Discussion starting page number
Associated with hydropic villous change	Ploidy analysis	23.4	421	416
		23.5	422	
		23.9	426	
		23.10	427	
		23.12	430	
Most commonly due to *Listeria* infection	May do Gram stain	16.13	292	290
Differential diagnosis is chronic villitis of unknown etiology versus infectious etiology	Stains for organisms, immunohistoch emistry	16.18	298	297
		16.19	299	
		16.23	301	
		16.30	310	
		16.31	311	
Seen in fetal death, twin–twin transfusion, and hydrops		20.13	388	385
Associated with thrombosis in fetal circulation		21.9	397	396
May be secondary to acute injury		19.4	354	354
Generally associated with other findings of HEV such as disruption of vessels		21.12	399	398
		21.13	400	
Developmental abnormality of villous tissue		19.19	369	368
Trophoblastic hyperplasia is also necessary for the diagnosis	Flow cytometry, ploidy analysis	23.4	421	416
		23.5	422	
May be partial or complete mole		23.9	426	
Rule out twin with mole		23.10	427	
		23.12	430	
Seen in early pregnancy and may be confused with a hydatidiform mole	Flow cytometry, ploidy analysis	11.5	179	175
		23.11	429	
Placental and/or fetal hydrops	Kleihauer-Betke if hemorrhage suspected	20.2	373	371
May be secondary to fetomaternal hemorrhage		20.3	374	
		20.4	374	
		20.5	375	
Residual immature villi in term placenta may be confused with villous edema		7.4	101	99
Also associated with mesenchymal dysplasia, placentomegaly, chorangiosis, and long umbilical cords		20.6	377	377
Associated with chronic hypoxia and poor perinatal outcome		19.8	359	358
Focal, segmental, or multinodular diffuse		19.11	363	360
Is a localized area of increased capillaries representing a benign neoplasm		22.5	408	405
		22.6	409	
		22.7	409	

Table 4.5. *Continued*

Description of feature	Lesion
Villous Capillaries	Congestion
Disruption of vessels or thrombosis	Hemorrhagic endovasculitis (HEV)
Nucleated red blood cells	Nucleated red blood cells

Table 4.6. Basal place

Description of feature	Lesion
Increased fibrinoid	Increased fibrinoid
	Maternal floor infarction
Necrosis	Decidual necrosis
Inflammation	Acute deciduitis
	Chronic deciduitis
Hemorrhage	Retroplacental hematoma
Abnormal vessels	Decidual vasculopathy
Adherent myometrium	Placenta accreta

Comment	Additional studies	Figure number	Figure page number	Discussion starting page number
Not true increase in vessels but may be confused with chorangiosis		19.9	360	358
Associated with decreased venous return and maternal diabetes				
Associated with disruption of vessels and extravasated red blood cells		21.12 21.13	399 400	398
Associated with intrauterine hypoxia		20.7	379	381

Comment	Additional studies	Figure number	Figure page number	Discussion page number
Normal, if not excessive		19.12	364	361
If excessive		19.15	365	363
May be present throughout villous tissue		19.16	366	
May be associated with proliferation of extravillous trophoblast		19.17	367	
Look for associated lesions such as hemorrhage or decidual vasculopathy		18.4	336	334
May be associated with acute chorioamnionitis		16.6	285	284
May be associated with chronic villitis		16.20	299	298
Underlying tissue may be ischemic or infracted		3.8 18.14	31 342	355
May be associated with other changes of placental malperfusion		19.7	357	
Usually associated with other changes of placental malperfusion		18.1 18.2 18.3 18.4 18.5	334 335 335 336 336	333
Diagnosis based on lack of deciduas between chorionic villi and myometrium	Cytokeratin to differentiate trophoblast from decidual cells	12.5	200	197

Table 4.7. Placental lesions in specific clinical situations

Clinical situation	Placental conditions	Maternal conditions	Fetal conditions
Preterm delivery	Placental malperfusion Infarction Decreased weight Retroplacental hematoma Circumvallate membrane insertion Maternal floor infarction Acute chorioamnionitis	Poor nutrition Uterine anomalies	Fetal anomalies

Intrauterine growth restriction	Maternal floor infarction
	Villitis of unknown
	    etiology
	Fetal thrombotic
	    vasculopathy
	Shape abnormalities
	Umbilical cord
	    Excessively long cord
	    Velamentous insertion
		Drug use
		    Tobacco
		    Alcohol
		Poor nutrition
		Uterine anomalies
		Systemic disease
		    Diabetes mellitus with
		        vascular disease
		    Preeclampsia
		    Gestational hypertension
		    Renovascular disease
		    Autoimmune disease
		    Thrombophilias
			Genetic conditions
			Confined placental
			    mosaicism
			Chromosomal
			    disorders
			Genetic disorders

Intrauterine fetal demise	Maternal floor infarction
	Villitis of unknown etiology
	Fetal thrombotic vasulopathy
	Abruptio placentae
	Umbilical cord
	    Entanglement
	    True knots
	    Torsion
	    Constriction
	    Rupture
	    Excessive length or twisting
	    Velamentous insertion and
	        rupture
			Infection
			TORCH
			    Ascending infection
			Fetomaternal
			    hemorrhage

Selected References

PHP4, Chapter 3, pages 20–29.

Bourne GL. The microscopic anatomy of the human amnion and chorion. Am J Obstet Gynecol 1960;79:1070–1073.

Bourne GL, Lacy D. Ultrastructure of human amnion and its possible relation to the circulation of amniotic fluid. Nature (Lond) 1960;168;952–954.

Gill P, Jarjoura D. Wharton's jelly in the umbilical cord: a study of its quantitative variations and clinical correlates. J Reprod Med 1993;38:611–614.

Hertig AT. On the development of the amnion and exocoelomic membrane in the previllous human ovum. Yale J Biol Med 1945;18:107–115.

Khong TY, Lane EB, Robertson WB. An immunocytochemical study of fetal cells at the maternal-placental interface using monoclonal antibodies to keratins, vimentin and desmin. Cell Tissue Res 1986;246:189–195.

Nanaev AK, Kohnen G, Milovanov AP, Domogatsky SP, Kaufmann P. Stromal differentiation and architecture of the human umbilical cord. Placenta 1997;18:53–64.

Takechi K, Kuwabara Y, Mizuno M. Ultrastructural and immunohistochemical studies of Wharton's jelly umbilical cord cells. Placenta 1993;14:235–245.

Section II

Normal Development and Histology

This section presents the development and histology of the normal placenta. It starts in Chapter 5 with a discussion of the early development of the placenta, umbilical cord, and fetal membranes. Detailed normal histology of the chorionic villi, the cells comprising the villi, the fetal membranes, and the umbilical cord follows in Chapter 6. In Chapter 7, the development of the different types of chorionic villi is presented; these include the mesenchymal villi, immature intermediate villi, mature intermediate villi, stem villi, and terminal villi. The placentone (placental lobule) and the intervillous space are also briefly discussed. Finally, due to the complexity of the nonvillous parts of the placenta, an entire chapter is devoted to their discussion. This chapter, Chapter 8, covers detailed histology of placental structures introduced in Chapter 5 such as the chorionic plate, basal plate, marginal zone, cell columns, cell islands, septae, fibrinoid, decidua, and extravillous trophoblast.

Chapter 5

Early Placental Development

General Considerations

For many years, it was thought that the understanding of placental pathology required only a limited knowledge of implantation and early placental development, as disturbances of these early steps of placentation seemed to cause abortion, rather than affecting placental structure and function. Increasing experience with assisted reproductive technology (ART), however, has taught us that improper conditions during implantation can handicap early development and result in inappropriate functioning of the fetoplacental unit and impaired outcome. For this reason, basic understanding of early placental development has become increasingly important.

Prelacunar Stage: Day 1 to 8 Post Conception

The **prelacunar stage** is defined as the period from conception to day 8 PC (post conception). After fertilization, the zygote develops into a **blastocyst**, a flattened vesicle composed of between 107 and 256 cells. The cells of the outer wall are the **trophoblast**, which surround the **blastocystic cavity** (Figure 5.1 A). The **inner cell mass** is a small group of larger cells on the inner surface. The trophoblast is the forerunner of the placenta while the inner cell mass forms the **embryoblast**. The

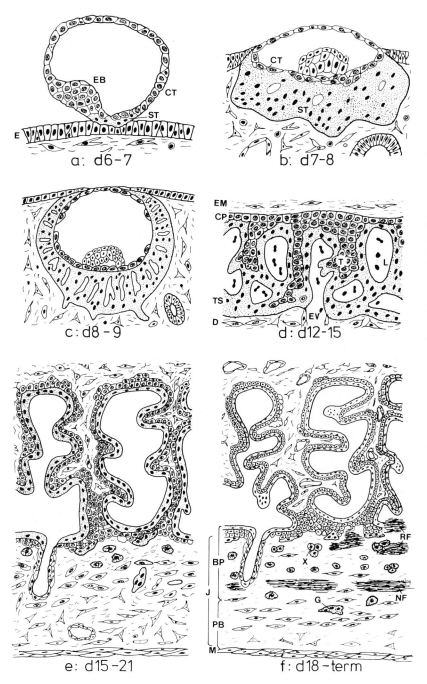

Figure 5.1. Simplified drawings of the stages of early placental development. (A, B) Prelacunar stages. (C) Lacunar stage. (D) Transition from lacunar to primary villous stage. (E) Secondary villous stage. (F) Tertiary villous stage. Note that the basal segments of the anchoring villi (E, F) consist only of trophoblast and form cell columns. E = endometrial epithelium; EB = embryoblast; CT = cytotrophoblast; ST = syncytiotrophoblast; EM = extraembryonic mesoderm; CP = primary chorionic plate; T = trabeculae and primary villi; L = maternal blood lacunae; TS = trophoblastic shell; EV = endometrial vessel; D = decidua; RF = Rohr's fibrinoid; NF = Nitabuch's or uteroplacental fibrinoid; G = trophoblastic giant cell; x = X-cells or extravillous cytotrophoblast; BP = basal plate; PB = placental bed; J = junctional zone; M = myometrium. (From Kaufmann P., Scheffen I. I. Placental development. In: Neonatal and Fetal Medicine: Physiology and Pathophysiology. Vol. I. R.A. Polin and W.W. Fox, eds. Orlando, FL: Saunders; 1992;7–55, with permission.)

embryo, umbilical cord, and amnion are derived from the latter. Both embryoblast-derived mesenchyme and embryoblast-derived blood vessels contribute to the formation of the connective tissue and blood vessels of the chorionic villi.

The first step in implantation of the **blastocyst** is called apposition and takes place around day 6 to 7 PC.

In most cases, the blastocyst is oriented so that the **embryonic pole** attaches to the endometrium, thus forming the **implantation pole**. If, during implantation, the blastocyst rotates so that the embryonic pole and the implantation pole are not identical, abnormal cord insertions will occur (see Chapter 15). The "**implantation window**" is a short, specific phase during which attachment of the blastocyst occurs. To find or to generate this window is the most important prerequisite for successful implantation in in vitro fertilization and other forms of ART.

In the following days, the trophoblastic cells proliferate to form a double layer as they progressively invade the endometrial epithelium. *The inner layer, which does not initially contact the maternal tissues, is composed of* **cytotrophoblast**. *The outer layer, facing the maternal tissue, is transformed to* **syncytiotrophoblast** by fusion of neighboring cytotrophoblastic cells (Figure 5.1 B). The syncytiotrophoblast is a continuous system, not interrupted by intercellular spaces and is composed neither of individual cells nor of individual syncytial units (see Chapter 6). At the implantation pole, the syncytial mass forms branching, finger-like extensions that deeply invade, and interdigitate with, the endometrium. This is the **trophoblastic shell**.

Lacunar Stage: Day 8 to 13 Post Conception

On day 8 PC, *small vacuoles appear in the syncytiotrophoblastic mass*. The vacuoles grow and become confluent, forming a system of **lacunae** (Figures 5.1 B,C). The lacunae are separated from each other by bands of syncytiotrophoblast, called **trabeculae**. The syncytiotrophoblastic mass and the lacunar system expand circumferentially over the entire blastocystic surface. By day 12 PC, the blastocyst is deeply implanted and the uterine epithelium closes over the implantation site. The cytotrophoblastic cells extend into the trabeculae and, by day 13 PC, reach the trophoblastic shell, eventually coming into contact with the endometrium (Figures 5.1 D,E,F).

Trophoblastic proliferation and syncytial fusion start at the implantation pole, making the trophoblast thicker here. This area of preferential growth is *later transformed into the placental disk*. The opposing thinner trophoblastic circumference only initially attempts to establish the same structure. Eventually, it *atrophies and becomes the smooth chorion*, or the **chorion laeve**. At this point, the trophoblastic covering of the blastocyst is divided into three layers (Figures 5.1 C,D):

- The **primary chorionic plate**, facing the blastocystic cavity,
- The **lacunar system** including the trabeculae, and
- The **trophoblastic shell**, facing the endometrium.

The Primary Chorionic Plate

The **primary chorionic plate** is composed of cytotrophoblast covered by syncytiotrophoblast on the "maternal" side (Figure 5.1 D). On day 14 PC, **embryonic mesenchyme** spreads around the inner surface of the blastocyst cavity and cytotrophoblast layer. This forms a *triple-layered chorionic plate composed of mesenchyme, cytotrophoblast, and syncytiotrophoblast*. At the same time, the first villous outgrowths form from the trabeculae (Figures 5.1 D,E). The trabeculae are henceforth called the **villous stems**, which later become the **stem villi**. The lacunar system is transformed into the **intervillous space**. The chorionic plate creates a "lid" over the intervillous space and serves as the base from which the villous trees are suspended.

The Lacunar System

Below the primary chorionic plate is the **lacunar system** (Figure 5.1 C). Around day 12 PC the trabeculae are invaded by cytotrophoblastic cells (Figure 5.1 D) from the primary chorionic plate. At the maternal surface, *the trabeculae join together to form the* **trophoblastic shell**. The syncytiotrophoblast is present at the "luminal" surface of the lacunae; below that is a zone of cytotrophoblast. Below the latter, and facing the endometrial connective tissue, is an additional discontinuous layer of syncytiotrophoblastic elements.

During the early stages of implantation, erosion of the maternal tissues occurs under the lytic influence of the syncytial trophoblast. Subsequently, there is proliferation and migration of trophoblast, resulting in deep invasion of the endometrium and superficial myometrium. This is accomplished by *multinucleated and mononucleated tropohoblastic elements far removed from the trophoblastic shell*—the **extravillous trophoblast**. The extravillous trophoblast are intimately involved in development of the implantation site including invasion and remodeling of the decidual vessels (see Chapter 8). Meanwhile, the endometrial stromal cells transform into the **decidual cells**. On day 12 PC, invading trophoblast cause disintegration of the endometrial vessel walls and the expanding extravillous trophoblast replaces the capillary walls in a stepwise fashion, from beginning to end.

The Trophoblastic Shell

Around day 12 PC, as the cytotrophoblast expands into the trabeculae, *the distal ends of the trabeculae join together and form the outermost layer of the trophoblast*, the **trophoblastic shell**. Initially, this is a syncytiotrophoblastic structure, but when the cytotrophoblast reaches the shell at about day 15 PC, the shell becomes more heterogeneous (Figure 5.1 E). The syncytiotrophoblast face the lacunae, followed by cytotrophoblast and then a discontinuous layer of syncytiotrophoblastic elements facing the endometrial connective tissue. From day 22 PC onward, the term "**trophoblastic shell**" is usually replaced by "**basal plate**," a term that includes the base of the intervillous space together with all placental and maternal tissues that adhere to it after parturition.

Early Villous Stage: Day 13 to 28 Post Conception

In the early villous stage, cytotrophoblast invades the trabeculae, and "**trophoblastic sprouts**" grow into the lacunae to form the **primary villi** (Figures 5.1 D,E). *Primary villi are composed only of an outer layer of syncytiotrophoblast and a core of cytotrophoblast.* Their presence marks the beginning of the villous stages of placentation. Further proliferation and subsequent branching initiate the development of primitive **villous trees**, the stems of which are derived from the former trabeculae (Figure 5.1 E). The villi that keep their contact to the trophoblastic shell are called **anchoring villi**. Subsequently, cells derived from the mesenchymal layer of the primary chorionic plate invade the villi, transforming them into **secondary villi** (Figure 5.1 E). *Secondary villi consist of an outer layer of syncytiotrophoblast, an inner layer of cytotrophoblast, and a core of connective tissue.* Within a few days, the mesenchyme expands peripherally to the villous tips. The expanding villous mesenchyme does not completely reach the trophoblastic shell. Clusters of cytotrophoblast surrounded by an incomplete layer of syncytiotrophoblast persist as **cell columns** (Figures 5.1 E,F). They are places of *longitudinal growth of the anchoring villi as well as sources of extravillous trophoblast.* Focally, the villous tips of free-floating villi may not be invaded by villous mesenchyme, and these become the **trophoblastic cell islands** (see Chapter 8).

The first **fetal capillaries** appear in the villi on day 18 to day 20 PC. They are derived from hemangioblastic progenitor cells, which locally differentiate from the mesenchyme. *The appearance of capillaries in the villous stroma marks the development of the first **tertiary villi**.* When enough capillary segments are fused with each other to form a capillary bed, a complete fetoplacental circulation is established. This occurs at the beginning of the fifth week.

The early villous trees expand in the following way: At the surfaces of the larger villi, cytotrophoblastic cells proliferate and subsequent syncytial fusion produces **syncytial (trophoblastic) sprouts**. These *sprouts are comparable to the early primary villi* as they consist of only cytotrophoblast and syncytiotrophoblast. Most degenerate, but a few are invaded by villous mesenchyme and transformed into **villous sprouts**, *which are comparable to the secondary villi*. Fetal vessels then form within the stroma, *similar to the development of tertiary villi*. Fetal and maternal blood comes into close contact with each other as soon as a fetoplacental circulation is established. The two bloodstreams are always separated by the **placental barrier** (see Figure 6.1, page 81), which is composed of **syncytiotrophoblast, cytotrophoblast, basal lamina, connective tissue**, and **fetal endothelium**. In the last trimester, the cytotrophoblast is discontinuous and the fetal endothelium is surrounded by endothelial basal lamina.

The Second Month and Beyond

Starting with the second month PC (Figure 5.2), the connective tissue layer of the chorionic plate becomes more densely fibrotic and fibrous tissue extends into the villous stems. Subsequently, the tertiary villi undergo a complex process of differentiation that results in various villous types which differ from each other in structure and function (see Chapter 7). With maturation, the *syncytiotrophoblast is reduced in thickness and the cytotrophoblast becomes rarified*. The *mean villous diameter decreases, and the fetal capillaries are more numerous and closer to the villous surfaces*. This change results in considerable reduction of the thickness of the placental barrier and thus a reduction in the mean maternofetal diffusion distance.

Development of the Fetal Membranes

With the appearance of the first villi, the trophoblast at the implantation pole becomes the **chorion frondosum**, the forerunner of the placenta. The **capsular chorion frondosum**, which is opposite the implantation pole, initially undergoes a corresponding, although delayed, development. However, beginning at the end of the third week PC, regression of newly formed villi and obliteration of the surrounding intervillous space begins and then spreads laterally over the blastocyst surface. Ultimately, *the chorion, the obliterated intervillous space, the villous remnants, and the trophoblastic shell fuse, forming the* **smooth chorion** or **chorion laeve**. This process gradually spreads over about 70% of the surface of the chorionic sac, continuing until approximately the fourth month.

Depending on its spatial relation to the implanting chorionic sac, the decidua is subdivided into several segments (Figure 5.3). The decidua at the implantation site, below the blastocyst and later the placenta, is the **basal decidua** or **decidua basalis**. When the embryo becomes completely embedded in the endometrial wall, the decidua closes over the blastocyst. Growth of the embryo and placenta causes the decidua to *protrude* into the uterine cavity. This protruding portion of the decidua is the **capsular decidua** or **decidua capsularis**. The remaining decidua, that which is without contact with the blastocyst (i.e., on the opposite uterine wall), is the **parietal decidua** or **decidua vera**. With growth of the chorionic sac, the capsular decidua focally degenerates, and eventually touches the parietal decidua (Figure 5.3 C). Between the 15th and 20th weeks PC, *the smooth chorion, together with its attached residual capsular decidua, locally fuses with the parietal decidua, thereby largely obliterating the uterine cavity* (Figure 5.3 C). From this date onward, the smooth chorion has contact with the decidual surface of the uterine wall over nearly its entire surface. However, there is no true fusion between the decidua capsularis and the decidua vera.

Small cells lining the inner surface of the trophoblast, the *amniogenic cells*, are the forerunners of the **amnionic epithelium**. A cleft separates these cells from the embryoblast, which ultimately becomes the

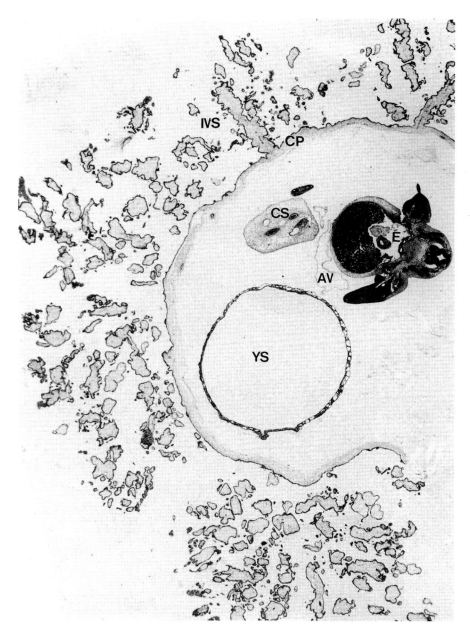

Figure 5.2. Semithin section across embryo and placenta of the fourth week after conception. Underneath the embryo (E) one can identify the connective stalk (CS) as precursor of the cord, the yolk sac (YS), and a small amnionic vesicle (AV). The chorionic cavity is surrounded by the chorionic plate (CP); from the latter, numerous placental villi protrude into the surrounding intervillous space (IVS). The basal plate is missing in this specimen. ×9.5. (From Kaufmann P. Placentation and Placenta. In: Humanembryologie. K.V. Hinrichsen, ed. Heidelberg: Springer-Verlag; 1990, with permission.)

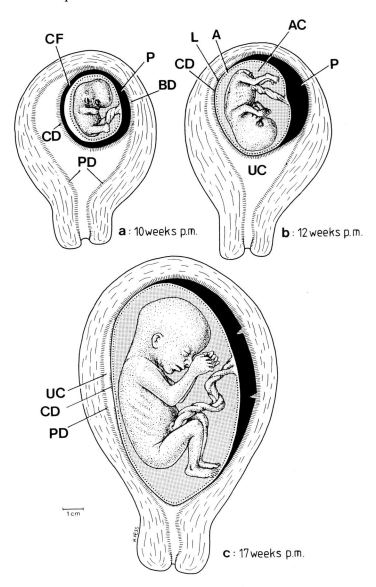

Figure 5.3. Development of the fetal membranes. (A) Up to 10 weeks PM (after last menstrual period), the embryo is surrounded by the chorion frondosum (CF); its later specialization into chorion laeve and the placenta (P) is indicated by only a slight increase in thickness at this stage. The capsular part of the chorion frondosum is covered by the capsular decidua (CD), which is continuous with basal decidua (BD) at the placental site, and with the parietal decidua (PD), which lines the uterine cavity. The amnion (dotted line) is not fused in most places with the chorion frondosum. (B) Two weeks later (12th week PM), the original chorion frondosum has differentiated into the placenta (P) and the fetal membranes that surround the inner amniotic cavity (AC). At this stage, the membranes are composed of the amnion (A), chorion laeve (L), and capsular decidua (CD). Because of the embryo's small size, the uterine cavity (UC) still is quite large. (C) From 17 weeks on, the membranes come into close contact with the uterine wall. The remainder of the capsular decidua (CD) fuses with the parietal decidua (PD) and obliterate the uterine cavity (UC). From then on, the chorion laeve contacts the parietal decidua. (Modified from Kaufmann, P. Entwicklung der Plazenta. In: Die Plazenta des Menschen. V Becker. ThH Schiebler, F Kubli, eds. Stuttgart: Thieme; 1981, with permission.)

amniotic cavity (Figure 5.4, day 13). Before the 12th week PC, the amniotic cavity is separated from the chorion by chorionic fluid, the **magma reticulare**. Extraembryonic mesenchyme expands to cover the surface of the amnionic epithelium and becomes the **amnionic mesoderm**. During the 6th to 7th week PC, the amnionic mesoderm fuses with the chorionic mesoderm, starting at the cord insertion site at the chorionic plate (Figure 5.4, day 28 and day 40). This process is completed in the 12th week PC. However, *fusion of the amnion and chorion is never complete,* and thus the two membranes can always easily slide against each other. This is different from the situation in the umbilical cord where the *expanding amnion becomes closely attached to the surface of the cord and firmly fuses with it.*

Development of the Umbilical Cord

The development of the umbilical cord is closely related to that of the amnion. At the end of the second week PC, the embryoblast within the blastocystic cavity is surrounded by a loose meshwork of mesodermal cells (Figure 5.4, day 13). The double-layered embryonic disk is between the **amnionic vesicle** and the **primary yolk sac**. Basal to the amnionic vesicle, the mesodermal cells condense and form the **connecting stalk** (Figure 5.4, day 18), which is the *early forerunner of the umbilical cord*. During the same period, a ductlike extension of the yolk sac, originating from the future caudal region of the embryo, grows into the connecting stalk. This structure is the transitory **allantois**, the *primitive extraembryonic urinary bladder*. Remnants of allantoic elements may be found in sections of the umbilical cord at term (see Chapter 15).

The subsequent weeks are characterized by three developmental processes. First, the **embryo rotates** so that the yolk sac is turned toward the implantation pole rather than away from it. Second, the **amniotic cavity enlarges** and extends around the embryo. Last, the originally **flat embryonic disk is bent in both anteroposterior and lateral directions** and thus "herniates" into the amniotic cavity. As the embryo bends, it subdivides the yolk sac into an intraembryonic duct (the gut) and an extraembryonic part (the omphalomesenteric duct), which is dilated peripherally to form the extraembryonic yolk sac vesicle.

Both the allantois and the extraembryonic yolk sac extend into the mesenchyme of the connecting stalk (Figure 5.4, day 22). Between days 28 and 40 PC, the expanding amniotic cavity surrounds the embryo and *the connecting stalk, allantois, and yolk sac become compressed to a slender cord covered by amnionic epithelium* (Figures 5.2, and 5.4, day 28, day 40), the **umbilical cord**. The cord lengthens as the embryo "prolapses" backward into the amniotic sac. During the same process of expansion, the amnionic mesenchyme locally touches and finally fuses with the chorionic mesoderm, thus obliterating the exocoelomic cavity. This phase is completed at 12 weeks.

During the third week PC, the **extraembryonic yolk sac**, or the **omphalomesenteric duct**, which connects with the embryonic gut, and

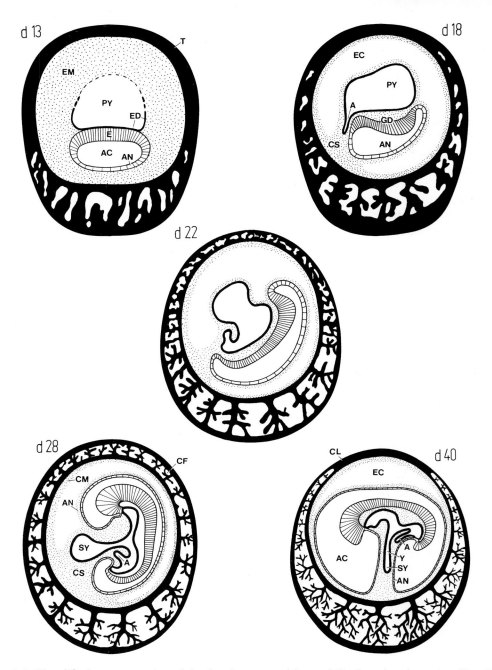

Figure 5.4. Simplified representation of the development of the umbilical cord and amnion. Day 13 PC. The embryonic disk consists of two epithelial layers: the ectoderm (E), which is contiguous with the amnionic epithelium (AN), and the endoderm (ED), which partially surrounds the primary yolk sac cavity (PY). Both vesicles are surrounded by the extraembryonic mesoderm (EM), T = trophoblast. Day 18 PC. At this stage, the endoderm has become closely applied to the periphery of the yolk sac; and at the presumptive caudal end of the germinal disk (GD), the allantoic invagination (A) has occurred. In the extraembryonic mesoderm, the exocoelom (EC) has cavitated. A mesenchymal bridge, the "connecting stalk" (CS), has developed that will ultimately form the umbilical cord. Day 28 PC. The embryo has begun to rotate and fold. The primary yolk sac is being subdivided into the intraembryonic intestinal tract and the secondary (extraembryonic) yolk sac (SY). Secondary yolk sac and allantois extrude from the future embryonic intestinal tract into the connecting stalk. The amnionic sac largely surrounds the embryo because of its folding and rotation. Villous formation has occurred at the entire periphery of the chorionic vesicle, forming the chorion frondosum (CF). Day 40 PC. The embryo has now fully rotated and folded. It is completely surrounded by the amniotic cavity (AC) and is attached to the umbilical cord. The latter has developed from the connecting stalk as it has become covered by amnionic membrane. The exocoelom has become largely compressed by the expansion of the amniotic cavity. At the anembryonic pole of the chorionic vesicle, the recently formed placental villi gradually atrophy, thus forming the chorion laeve (CL). Only that portion that retains villous tissue, that which has the insertion of the umbilical cord, develops into the placental disk.

the **allantois** become supplied with fetal vessels. Two allantoic arteries originate from the internal iliac arteries, and one allantoic vein enters the hepatic vein. These allantoic vessels invade the placenta and become connected to the villous vessels. The allantoic participation in placental vascularization is the reason that the human placenta is a "chorioallantoic" placenta.

Selected References

PHP4, Chapter 5, pages 42–49.

Boyd JD, Hamilton WJ. The human placenta. Cambridge: Heffer & Sons, 1970.

Castellucci M, Scheper M, Scheffen I, et al. The development of the human placental villous tree. Anat Embryol (Berl) 1990;181:117–128.

Enders AC, King BF. Formation and differentiation of extraembryonic mesoderm in the rhesus monkey. Am J Anat 1988;181:327–340.

Hertig AT, Rock J. Two human ova of the previllous stage having an ovulation age of about eleven and twelve days respectively. Contrib Embryol Carnegie Inst 1941;29:127–156.

Heuser CH, Streeter GL. Development of the macaque embryo. Contrib Embryol Carnegie Inst 1941;29:15–55.

Leiser R, Beier HM. Morphological studies of lacunar formation in the early rabbit placenta. Trophoblast Res 1988;3:97–110.

Luckett WP. Origin and differentiation of the yolk sac and extraembryonic mesoderm in presomite human and rhesus monkey embryos. Am J Anat 1978;152:59–97.

Pijnenborg R, Robertson WB, Brosens I, Dixon G. Trophoblast invasion and the establishment of haemochorial placentation in man and laboratory animals. Placenta 1981;2:71–92.

Chapter 6

Histology of the Chorionic Villi, Fetal Membranes, and Umbilical Cord

Histology of the Chorionic Villi

The **chorionic villi** are the site where virtually all *maternofetal and feto-maternal exchange* takes place. In fact, *most metabolic and endocrine activities* of the placenta are localized there as well. The villi are the only components of the placenta that have a dual blood supply from both the fetal and maternal circulations. Despite the diversification of villous types, *all chorionic villi exhibit the same basic structure* (Figure 6.1). They are covered by **syncytiotrophoblast**, an epithelial surface layer (Figure 6.1 A) that is in direct contact with the maternal blood and *functions as an endothelium*. Between syncytiotrophoblast and the basement membrane are the **villous cytotrophoblast**, or **Langhans' cells**. These are the *stem cells of the syncytium*, supporting its growth and regeneration. The **trophoblastic basement membrane** separates the trophoblast from the villous stroma. The stroma is composed of *connective tissue cells, connective tissue fibers, ground substance, and fetal vessels*. In the larger stem villi, the vessels are mainly arteries and veins, while in the peripheral branches most fetal vessels are capillaries or "sinusoids." The human placenta is **hemochorial** in that the maternal blood has

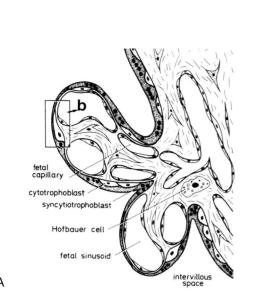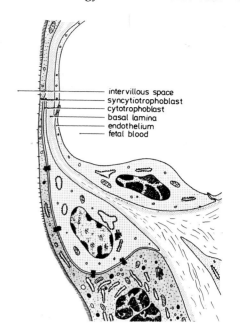

Figure 6.1. Morphology of human placental villi. (A) Simplified light microscopic section of two terminal villi, branching off a mature intermediate villus (right). (B) Schematic electron-microscopic section of the placental barrier, demonstrating typical layers. (Modified from Kaufmann P. Vergleichend-anatomische und funktionelle Aspekte des Placenta-Baues. Funkt Biol Med 1983;2:71–79, with permission.)

direct contact with trophoblast. The layers separating maternal from fetal blood are these (Figure 6.1 B):

- **Syncytiotrophoblast,**
- An incomplete layer of **cytotrophoblast**,
- The **trophoblastic basement membrane**,
- **Connective tissue,**
- The **endothelial basement membrane**, and
- The fetal **capillary endothelium**.

Syncytiotrophoblast

The **syncytiotrophoblast** is a continuous, normally uninterrupted layer that extends over the surfaces of all villous trees and villi as well as over parts of the inner surfaces of chorionic and basal plates. It thus lines the *entire intervillous space and is a **single** continuous structure for every placenta.* Therefore, terms such as "syncytial cells" and "syncytiotrophoblasts," which are often used, are inappropriate and should be avoided. Their use indicates a misunderstanding of the true nature of the syncytiotrophoblast. The syncytium is involved in *complex, active maternofetal transfer mechanisms,* including catabolism and resynthesis of proteins and lipids, synthesis of hormones such as human chorionic gonadotropin, human chorionic somatotropin, human placental lactogen, and human growth hormones, diffusional transfer of gases and water, the facilitated transfer of glucose, and active transfer of amino acids and electrolytes.

The syncytium is composed of **two plasmalemmas** with an intermediate layer of **syncytial cytoplasm**. It varies in thickness from 2 to about 10 μm (Figure 6.2). The syncytiotrophoblast at the villous surface is nearly completely covered by **microvilli** forming an enormous maternofetal contact zone that multiplies the total villous surface area by a factor of 7.67 at term. Remnants of syncytial fusion such as fragments of cell membranes and desmosomes are sometimes present in the cytoplasm. On routine tissue sections of first trimester placentas (Figure 6.3), the syncytiotrophoblast appears as a single layer surrounding the cytotrophoblast with no cell border. The *nuclei are small, with moderately dense chromatin. The cytoplasm is homogeneous to finely*

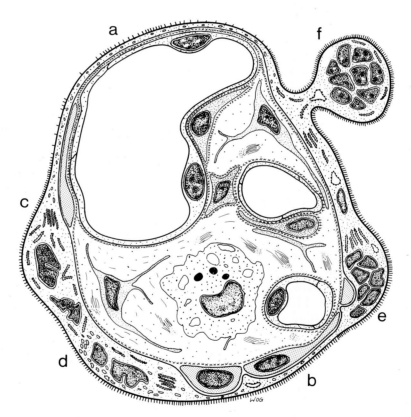

Figure 6.2. Simplified drawing of a cross section of a terminal villus demonstrating the structural variability of the syncytiotrophoblast. (a) Vasculosyncytial membrane. (b) Thin syncytial lamella covering villous cytotrophoblast. (c) Syncytiotrophoblast with well-developed rough endoplasmic reticulum. (e) Syncytiotrophoblast with well-developed smooth endoplasmic reticulum. (e) Syncytial knot. (f) Syncytial sprout. (From Kaufmann P, Schiebler ThH, Biobotaru C, Stark J. Enzymhistochemische Untersuchungen an reifen menschlichen Placentazotten. II. Zur Gliederung des Syncytiotrophoblasten. Histochem 1974;40_191–207, with permission.)

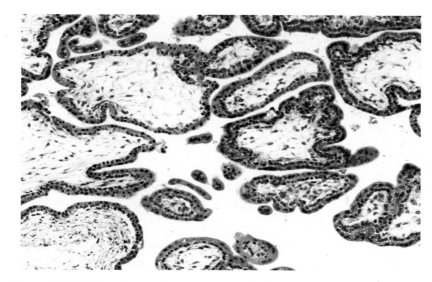

Figure 6.3. Light microscopic appearance of a first trimester chorionic villus with relatively thick syncytiotrophoblast and well-defined cytotrophoblastic layer. H&E. ×100.

granular, somewhat basophilic, and is often vacuolated. Later in pregnancy, the syncytiotrophoblast (Figure 6.4) has a variable thickness as it surrounds the villous structures. Focally, it is thinned to almost invisibility, forming the **vasculosyncytial membrane** (see Figure 6.2 a), in other areas it appears as a single layer of cells, while in still other areas, the nuclei are piled up forming **syncytial knots** (Figure 6.2 e). The nuclei

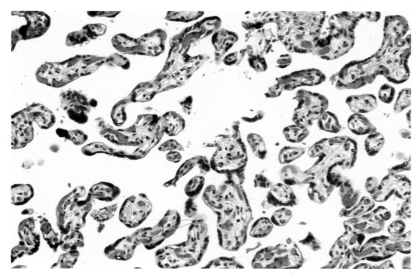

Figure 6.4. Light microscopic appearance of third trimester chorionic villi with irregularly thinned syncytiotrophoblast and focally incomplete cytotrophoblastic layer. H&E. ×100.

may focally show degenerative change. Mitotic figures are not identified in syncytiotrophoblast.

Syncytial Knots, Sprouts, and Bridges

Syncytial knots, sprouts, and **bridges** are names for a heterogeneous group of syncytiotrophoblastic specializations *characterized by a group of aggregated nuclei at the trophoblastic surface*. The general term **syncytial knots** is often used to refer to this entire group as they are often indistinguishable on light microscopy. Most commonly, accumulations of syncytial nuclei in sections of placental villi are the result of *tangential sectioning across syncytiotrophoblastic surfaces*. For these accumulations, "**syncytial knots**" is the most appropriate term (Figure 6.4).

Throughout the first half of pregnancy, a limited number of true **syncytial sprouts or trophoblastic sprouts** (Figure 6.5) can be found. These are characterized by a vermiform extension from the villous surface with *loosely arranged, large ovoid syncytial nuclei at the tip*. Toward the villous stroma, portions of villous cytotrophoblast and connective tissue may also be present. These are true proliferative outgrowths of the chorionic villi. A minority of "syncytial knots" show apoptotic changes and are the sites of *shedding of apoptotic nuclei* into the maternal circulation. For these, the term "**apoptotic knots**" is recommended. Apoptotic knots are characterized by *densely packed nuclei with condensed chromatin and occasional degenerative change, separated from each other by slender strands of cytoplasm*. The surrounding cytoplasm also usually exhibits degenerative changes. These apoptotic knots are eventually pinched off together with some surrounding cytoplasm. **Syncytial bridges** are uncommonly seen. They are true bridges and develop

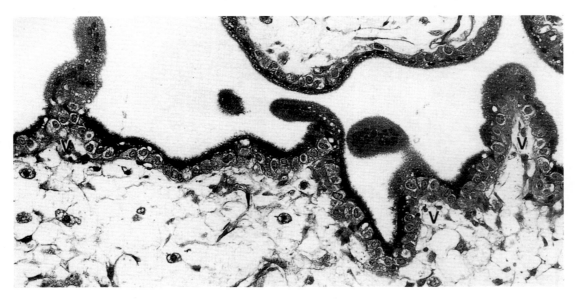

Figure 6.5. Placental villi from sixth week PM (after last menstrual period). Below is a large mesenchymal villus with several true syncytial sprouts protruding into the intervillous space. At the tips, they consist only of syncytiotrophoblast, but at the base there is cytotrophoblast and even loose connective tissue. ×390.

from fusion of adjacent villi. Fetal vessels may be identified within these bridges, connecting the circulations of the two villi.

Generally, in the **young placenta**, most syncytial knots are attached to immature intermediate and mesenchymal villi and are signs of *villous sprouting and thus villous growth*; less often are they sites of extrusion of apoptotic nuclei. Only a minority of these are due to tangential sectioning. In contrast, in the **mature placenta**, the vast majority of knots are caused by tangential sectioning (see Chapter 18). Far fewer are accumulations of apoptotic nuclei, and only a very small minority represents true villous sprouting.

Villous Cytotrophoblast (Langhans' Cells)

The **Langhans' cells** or **villous cytotrophoblastic cells** form a second trophoblastic layer beneath the syncytiotrophoblast. During early pregnancy, this layer is nearly complete (Figure 6.3), and later it becomes *discontinuous* (Figure 6.4). As the villous surface expands, the cytotrophoblastic cells become widely separated, and so are less numerous in sectioned material. During all stages of pregnancy, Langhans' cells have the characteristic features of undifferentiated, proliferating stem cells. On light microscopy (Figures 6.3, 6.4), they generally are *cuboidal, polyhedral, or ovoid cells* with *well-demarcated cell borders, and large, lightly staining nuclei containing finely dispersed chromatin*. The cytoplasm is usually clear to slightly granular and somewhat basophilic. In contrast to syncytiotrophoblast, mitotic figures are occasionally found.

Villous Stroma

The **trophoblastic basement membrane** separates the trophoblastic epithelium from the **villous stroma**. Under normal conditions the average thickness of the trophoblast basement membrane ranges from 20 to 50 nm and consists of collagen IV, laminin, heparan sulfate, and fibronectin. The amount of collagen varies with villous type. The **fixed connective tissue cells** form a network that enmeshes the *connective tissue fibers, free connective tissue cells (Hofbauer cells), and fetal vessels*. The stroma forms a supportive matrix for the cytotrophoblast and, where the latter is lacking, for the syncytiotrophoblast. Another important function is a *filtration barrier* between maternal and fetal circulations.

Mesenchymal cells, or undifferentiated stromal cells, are the prevailing cell type until the end of the second month. In later pregnancy, they are generally found only in stem villi and in the few remaining villous precursors, that is, mesenchymal villi and immature intermediate villi (see Chapter 7). They are *small spindled cells with little cytoplasm, measuring 10 to 20 μm long and 3 to 4 μm wide* (Figure 6.6). Throughout pregnancy they continue to proliferate and may be found beneath the trophoblastic surface of large-caliber villi.

At the end of the second month, dramatic changes in stromal architecture and composition take place. Starting in the centers of the villi and spreading toward the surface, the mesenchymal cells differentiate into **fibroblasts**. The newly formed fibroblasts have *elongated, bizarre-shaped cell bodies that measure about 20 to 30 μm in length*. From the cell

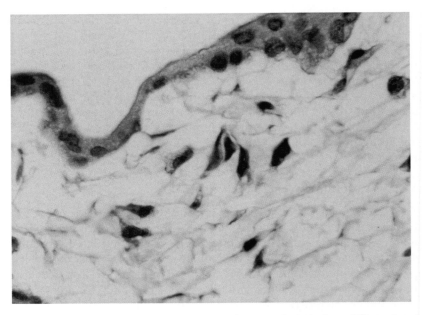

Figure 6.6. Immature chorionic villus with several typical undifferentiated mesenchymal cells present underneath the trophoblastic cover. H&E. ×400.

bodies, several long, thin, branching cytoplasmic processes extend forming flat sails of cytoplasm. These form the **stromal channels** of the immature intermediate villi (see Figures 7.1, 7.4, pages 97, 101). *Fetal vessels and connective tissue fibers are present in the spaces between the channels.* Later in pregnancy the mesenchymal cells differentiate into **myofibroblasts**. The myofibroblasts have abundant cytoplasm and are 30 to 100 µm long by 5 to 8 µm wide. In contrast to the fibroblasts, they have *only few short, filiform, or thick processes.* The myofibroblasts are arranged parallel to the longitudinal axis of the villi, and in large stem villi they form a clearly defined **perivascular contractile sheath**. Contraction of these cells may be important for villous turgor, thus influencing the width of the intervillous space and regulation of maternal intervillous blood pressure.

Most free connective tissue cells of placental villi are *tissue macrophages*, the **Hofbauer cells**. However, there are a few **mast cells** and **plasma cells**. **Hofbauer cells** are numerous in both the villous stroma and the chorionic plate throughout pregnancy. Initially, they are derived from *chorionic mesenchymal cells*, but once fetal circulation is established, they likely derive, as other macrophages do, from fetal bone marrow-derived monocytes. They share with other macrophages the expression of surface immunoglobulin receptor and the expression of major histocompatibility complex, class II antigens. On microscopic examination (Figure 6.7), Hofbauer cells are large, isolated cells that vary from 10 µm to 30 µm in diameter. They are *round, ovoid, reniform, or stellate in shape* and have an eccentric nucleus. Early in pregnancy, *the cytoplasm is coarsely vacuolated; later it is more granular.* At term, Hofbauer cells are difficult to identify and to differentiate from other cells, in part because they become compressed by the condensing villous stroma. Villous edema actually "unmasks" the Hofbauer cells, making them easier to appreciate. The placenta lacks a lymphatic system to return proteins from the interstitial space to the vascular system, and therefore the Hofbauer cells are involved in *water balance*. They also have a role in *maintaining host defenses*.

Fetal Villous Vessels

Extraembryonic mesenchyme invades the villi and forms the villous stroma. **Hemangioblastic cells** differentiate locally from these cells. Initially, they form cords of cells connected by primitive tight junctions. Then capillary sprouts, without blood cells, develop at around 21 to 22 days PC (post conception). Intercellular clefts appear and form the early capillary lumen. Then, around day 28 PC, *the first hematopoietic stem cells develop by delamination from the primitive vessel wall into the early lumen.* At the same time, some of the cells attached to the endothelial cells on the abluminal side acquire the characteristics of pericytes. A complete endothelial basement membrane between the endothelial cells and pericytes is not observed until the third trimester. In stem vessels and vessels of the chorionic plate, *elastic lamina are largely absent, the muscular coats are thinner,* and the muscle cells are more dispersed than in corresponding vessels of other organs.

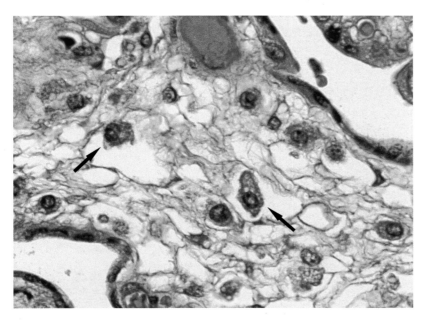

Figure 6.7. H&E stained section of an immature chorionic villus with prominent Hofbauer cells (arrows). ×400.

Structure and Histology of the Fetal Membranes

The term "membranes" is usually taken to be synonymous with the **amnion** and the **chorion laeve** of the extraplacental membranes. They are distinct from the chorion frondosum, which refers to a specialized, thickened part of the membranes, otherwise known as the placental disk. The membranes are the "bag of waters" in which the fetus is enclosed. Their structure and function include *turnover of water and enzymatic activity during the initiation of labor*. The structure of the membranes remains constant from the fourth month until term. The mean thickness after separation from the uterine wall is about 200 to 300 μm, but because of local edema of the amnionic mesoderm, considerably thicker membranes are sometimes observed. After birth, the following layers can be seen histologically (Figure 6.8):

- **Amnion**
  - **Amnionic epithelium** (20 to 30 μm)
  - **Amnionic mesoderm** (15 to 30 μm)
    - Basal lamina or basement membrane
    - **Compact stromal layer**
    - **Fibroblast layer**
- **Intermediate spongy layer** (highly variable in thickness)

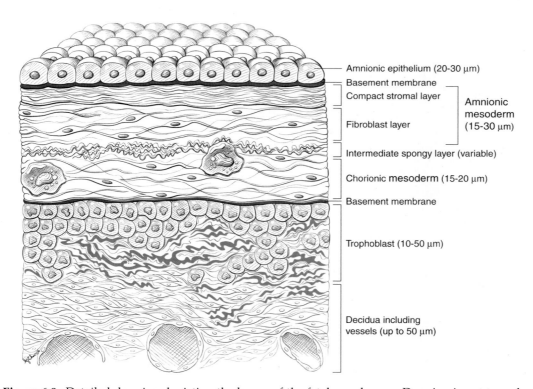

Figure 6.8. Detailed drawing depicting the layers of the fetal membranes. Drawing is not to scale.

- **Chorion laeve**
  - ○ **Chorionic mesoderm** (15 to 20 μm)
    - ▪ **Blood vessels**
    - ▪ **Basal lamina or basement membrane**
- **Trophoblast** (10 to 50 μm) and
- **Decidua capsularis** (up to 50 μm)

The Amnion

Macroscopically, the amnion is a translucent structure, easily separated from the underlying chorion. It never truly fuses with the chorion, cellularly speaking, as it is only passively attached by the internal pressure of the amniotic fluid. It is important to recognize that the amnion *does not possess its own blood vessels and obtains its nutrition and oxygen from the surrounding chorionic fluid, amniotic fluid, fetal surface vessels*, and, during early gestation, from the magma reticulare. The **amnionic epithelium** is derived from the fetal ectoderm and is thus contiguous over the umbilical cord and fetal skin. The epithelium is composed of a *single layer of flat, cuboidal to columnar cells*. Taller, columnar cells are usually present near the insertion of the membranes at the placental margin, whereas flatter cells are generally present in the periphery. Defects in the epithelial layer may be due to expulsion of dying cells into the amniotic fluid. The amnionic epithelium rests on a **basement membrane**, which is connected to a **thin connective tissue layer** by filamentous strands (see Figure 6.8). The latter consists of a compact stromal layer and a fibroblast layer. The compact stromal layer contains bundles of collagen and scattered elastic fibers. The fibroblast layer consists of a network of fibroblasts and a few macrophages (Figure 6.8). Although the amnionic mesoderm is divided into a compact stromal layer and fibroblast layer, these are difficult to appreciate on histologic section.

The amnion has multiple functional roles in the placenta. It is essential for the *structural integrity and junctional permeability* of the membranes, serving as a *permeability barrier to anionic macromolecules*. It is thought to have a *role in the onset of labor* including the initiation and maintenance of uterine contractions. The amnion is also involved in the *turnover of the amniotic fluid* including *resorption and secretory activity*. It also appears to be responsible for *regulating the pH of the amniotic fluid* and thus is involved in *fetal pH regulation* because the fetus delivers considerable amounts of proteins and bicarbonate via its kidneys into the amniotic fluid.

Amniotic Fluid

The amniotic fluid is derived from multiple sources: *filtration from fetal blood* via the chorionic plate, the umbilical cord, and the fetal urine, *secretory processes* of the amnionic epithelium, *filtration from maternal blood* via the parietal decidua and the chorion laeve, and *filtration from intracorporeal fetal vessels* via the fetal skin in early pregnancy. The amniotic fluid is *resorbed by the fetal digestive tract, the amnion, pressure-dependent fetomaternal filtration across the membranes, and inhalation*. The volume of the fluid varies with the stages of pregnancy with the

Table 6.1. Constituents of amniotic fluid

Component[a]	Concentration	Specific components
Glucose	5–20 mg/100 mL	
Proteins		α_1-Albumin, α_2-albumin, β-globulin, τ-globulins (IgA, IgG, IgM), α_1-fetoprotein, lipoproteins
Lipids		Cholesterol, triglycerides, diglycerides, free fatty acids, phospholipids
Urea	20–40 mg/100 mL	
Hormones		Progesterone, estradiol, estriol, testosterone, aldosterone, cortisol, thyroid hormones, parathyroid hormone, oxytocin, glucagons, insulin, hypothalamic-releasing hormones, and neurophysin
Gonadotropins		Luteinizing hormone, follicle-stimulating hormone, human chorionic gonadotropin, human placental lactogen, prolactin, adrenocorticotropic hormone, growth hormone, somatomedin, and thyrotropin
Enzymes		Activators and inhibitors of proteases such as tissue-type plasminogen activator, urokinase-type plasminogen activator, and their respective inhibitors PAI-1 and PAI-2
Cells	Increase throughout pregnancy	Anucleate squamous cells, nucleated squamous cells (probably from fetal mucous membranes or the amnion), fetal urothelial cells (both mononuclear and multinuclear)
Miscellaneous		Amino acids, creatinine, bilirubin

[a] Also present are amino acids, uric acid, creatinine, and bilirubin.

maximum volume of 984 ml at about 33 to 34 weeks. At term, the mean is 836 ml while at 42 weeks the mean is 544 ml. The pH is around 7.10 and the osmotic pressure is about 255 mosmol. The constituents of the amniotic fluid are listed in Table 6.1.

Chorion Laeve

The **chorionic membrane** is a tough *fibrous layer carrying the fetal blood vessels*. The amnion and chorion are easily separated and will readily slide along one another. This is due to the existence of the **spongy layer**, which is the result of incomplete fusion of the amnionic and chorionic mesoderm and is thus between the two layers. It is composed of *loosely arranged bundles of collagen fibers with a few scattered fibroblasts, separated by a communicating system of clefts* (Figure 6.8). Fibroblasts, macrophages, or remainders of amnionic and chorionic mesothelium occasionally line the clefts. The collagen composition of both amnion and chorion contributes to the mechanical stability and tensile properties of the membranes.

The spongy layer continues without sharp demarcation into the next layer, the **chorionic mesoderm**. Its composition is similar to the fibroblast layer of the amnion, as it consists of a *coarse network of collagen bundles intermingled with finer argyrophilic fibrils. Fibroblasts, myofibroblasts, and macrophages* are also regular findings (Figure 6.8). Chorionic vessels are present in the mesoderm of the chorionic plate. Occasional remnants of atrophied chorionic villi may also be found. These former villi appear as round "balls" of loose connective tissue, without a trophoblastic cover (Figure 6.9). Finally, there is a **basal lamina** that is highly variable in thickness and structure.

Trophoblast Layer

A highly variable layer of **trophoblastic cells** persists until term. These cells are the residues of the former villi of the chorion frondosum, inter-mingled with the trophoblastic residues of the primary chorionic plate and the trophoblastic shell. They constitute a population of *extravillous trophoblastic cells that are not involved in implantation*, commonly referred to as **migratory trophoblast** (see Chapter 8, Extravillous Trophoblast, Invasive Phenotype). *Proliferating, small, undifferentiated trophoblast* may be present as well as *nonproliferating, large, differentiated trophoblast*. With advancing gestation, some of these cells may show degenerative change and foci of fibrinoid (see Chapter 8) are often observed between the cells. *Toward the uterine wall, the trophoblast inter-digitates intensely with the decidua.*

Decidua

The decidual layer is the only maternal component of the membranes. The decidual tissue attached to the membranes after birth is largely

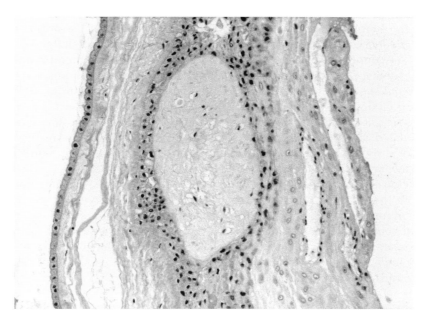

Figure 6.9. Macroscopic appearance of normal "membranes." The amnionic epithelium (at the left)sits on a thin layer of connective tissue that is not easily discernible from the chorionic connective tissue. The following layer of extrav-illous trophoblastic cells contains an atrophic or "ghost" villus. At the right of the figure is the decidua capsularis with maternal vessels visible. H&E. ×200.

derived from the **parietal and capsular decidua** (see Figure 5.3, page 76). Whether the individual cells are derived from one or the other layer cannot be distinguished. The deeper layers of the parietal decidua, which remain in utero, are richly supplied with maternal blood vessels. *In the superficial parts of the decidua, maternal vessels are the exception.* Generally, only a few capillaries, smaller arterioles, and venules can be identified (Figure 6.9). Macrophages, lymphocytes, and other inflammatory cells may also be present. At the edge of the placenta, the decidua capsularis is contiguous with the decidua basalis and delimits the "marginal sinus" (see Chapter 8).

Structure and Histology of the Umbilical Cord

The umbilical cord contains two arteries and a vein suspended in Wharton's jelly. The surface of the cord consists of a layer of **amnionic epithelium**, which is contiguous with the surface of the placenta and the fetal skin. The amnionic epithelium, near the umbilicus, is largely *unkeratinized, stratified squamous epithelium.* This layer provides a transition to the keratinized stratified squamous epithelium of the abdominal wall. Farther away from the umbilicus, the epithelium becomes *stratified columnar epithelium* (two to eight cell layers) and finally *simple columnar epithelium* as it continues onto the fetal surface. The basal cells of the stratified portions resemble the epithelium of the membranes, whereas the superficial cells sometimes are squamous and are occasionally pyknotic. The amnion of the cord is structurally similar to that described in the membranes, the one difference being that the amnion of the membranes is easily detached whereas *the amnion of the cord grows firmly into the central connective tissue core* and cannot be dislodged.

The connective tissue of the cord is derived from the **extraembryonic mesoblast**. The jelly-like material of **Wharton's jelly** is composed of a *ground substance* (collagen, laminin, heparan sulfate, hyaluronic acid, carbohydrates with glycosyl and mannosyl groups) *distributed in a fine network of microfibrils.* Extracellular matrix molecules are often accumulated around "stromal clefts." The clefts should not be misinterpreted as lymphatic vessels, which do not exist in the cord or in the placenta, nor should they be confused with pathologic changes such as edema or cyst formation (see Chapter 15). The stromal spaces together with the surrounding meshwork of contractile cells serve as a mechanism for turgor regulation of the cord, avoiding compression of umbilical veins and counteracting bending or kinking of the cord. The cord is sparsely cellular (Figure 6.10). There are a **few macrophages** and somewhat greater numbers of **mast cells**. **Myofibroblasts** are present around vessels and underneath the cord surface.

Umbilical Vessels

There are normally **two arteries** and **one vein** in the human umbilical cord (Figure 6.10). Originally, two veins are present, but the second normally atrophies during the second month of pregnancy. A **single**

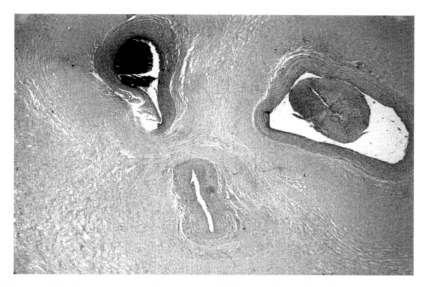

Figure 6.10. Cross section of mature umbilical cord, near its placental insertion showing a sparsely cellular Wharton's jelly, an umbilical vein and two arteries. H&E. ×20.

umbilical artery, which may be associated with multiple fetal malformations, is present in approximately 1% of cases (see Chapter 15). Rarer anomalies include local fusion of the two arteries and persistence of the second (right) umbilical vein, the latter also being associated with malformed fetuses. The mean intravital diameter of the arteries is around 3 mm, and the venous diameter is around twice this size.

Human umbilical vessels differ from the major vessels of similar caliber in the body in the following ways. Transudation of fluid occurs in these vessels and this contributes to the formation of amniotic fluid. *The muscular coat of the arteries consists of crossing spiraled fibers. The venous muscular coats are thinner than those of the arteries and are composed of separate layers of longitudinal or circular fibers.* Each umbilical vessel is surrounded by crossing bundles of spiraled collagen fibers that form a kind of adventitia. The *endothelial cells are unusually rich in organelles* and thus structurally different from the endothelium of the villous vessels. Endothelial extensions interdigitate with adjacent muscle cells to form an endotheliomuscular system. *The arteries possess no internal elastic membrane* and have much less elastica than in other similar caliber arteries. The vein, on the other hand, has an elastic subintimal layer (Figure 6.11). The umbilical vessels also *lack vasa vasorum*, except for the intraabdominal portions in fetuses beyond 20 weeks of gestation. In general, *no nerves traverse the umbilical cord from fetus to placenta and the placenta has no neural supply.*

After delivery, umbilical cords show irregular constrictions of the arteries, but the mechanism is not clear. It is known that increased transmural pressures exerted on the umbilical arteries led to vasoconstriction. In addition, many substances induce vasodilatation

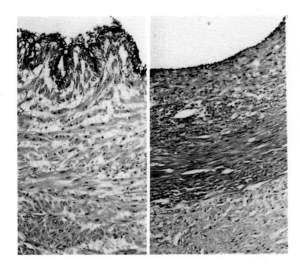

Figure 6.11. Umbilical cord sections of one umbilical artery (right) and a vein (left). In these sections, one may observe the presence of a delicate subendothelial elastica only in the vein at left. von Gieson ×160.

or vasoconstriction of the umbilical vessels. Vasodilators include serotonin, angiotensin, oxytocin, prostaglandins, nitrous oxide, and atrial natriuretic peptide. Vasoconstrictors include angiotensin II, 5-hydroxytryptamine (5-HT), thromboxane, neuropeptide Y, and endothelin-1. The functions of these vasoconstrictors are still under discussion, and they may function as mediators of closure of the placental circulation at birth.

Selected References

PHP4, Chapter 6, pages 50–115.

Bourne G. The microscopic anatomy of the human amnion and chorion. Am J Obstet Gynecol 1960;79:1070–1073.

Bourne G. The human amnion and chorion. London: Lloyd-Luke, 1962.

Bourne GL, Lacy D. Ultrastructure of human amnion and its possible relation to the circulation of amniotic fluid. Nature (Lond) 1960;168:952–954.

Boyd JD, Hamilton WJ. Electron microscopic observations on the cytotrophoblast contribution to the syncytium in the human placenta. J Anat 1966;100:535–548.

Cantle SJ, Kaufmann P, Luckhardt M, et al. Interpretation of syncytial sprouts and bridges in the human placenta. Placenta 1987;8:221–234.

Castellucci M, Zaccheo D. The Hofbauer cells of the human placenta: morphological and immunological aspects. Prog Clin Biol Res 1989;269:443–451.

Demir R, Kaufmann P, Castellucci M, et al. Fetal vasculogenesis and angiogenesis in human placental villi. Acta Anat 1989;136:190–203.

Enders AC, King BF. The cytology of Hofbauer cells. Anat Rec 1970;167:231–252.

Fox H, Khong TY. Lack of innervation of human umbilical cord. An immunohistochemical and histochemical study Placenta 1990;11:59–62.

Graf R, Schoenfelder G, Muehlberger M, et al. The perivascular contractile sheath of human placental stem villi: Its isolation and characterization. Placenta 1995;16:57–66.

Nanaev AK, Kohnen G, Milovanov AP, et al. Stromal differentiation and architecture of the human umbilical cord. Placenta 1997;18:53–64.

Takechi K, Kuwabara Y, Mizuno M. Ultrastructural and immunohistochemical studies of Wharton's jelly umbilical cord cells. Placenta 1993;14:235–245.

Chapter 7

Villous Development

General Considerations

The ramifications of the villous trees can be subdivided into five villous types based on caliber, stroma, vasculature, position within the villous tree, and development (Figures 7.1 A–E). The five types are these:

- **Mesenchymal villi,**
- **Immature intermediate villi,**
- **Mature intermediate villi,**
- **Stem villi,** and
- **Terminal villi.**

The **mesenchymal villi** are the first generation of the tertiary villi and *are the precursors from which all other villous types arise.* **Immature intermediate villi** develop from maturation of mesenchymal villi during the first two trimesters and are later transformed into **stem villi** (Figure 7.2 A). The **mature intermediate villi** derive from mesenchymal villi during the third trimester and are later transformed into **terminal villi** (Figure 7.2 B). Thus, both types of "intermediate" villi are transitions from mesenchymal to mature villi. These intermediate villi topographically lie between the centrally located stem villi and the most peripheral terminal villi.

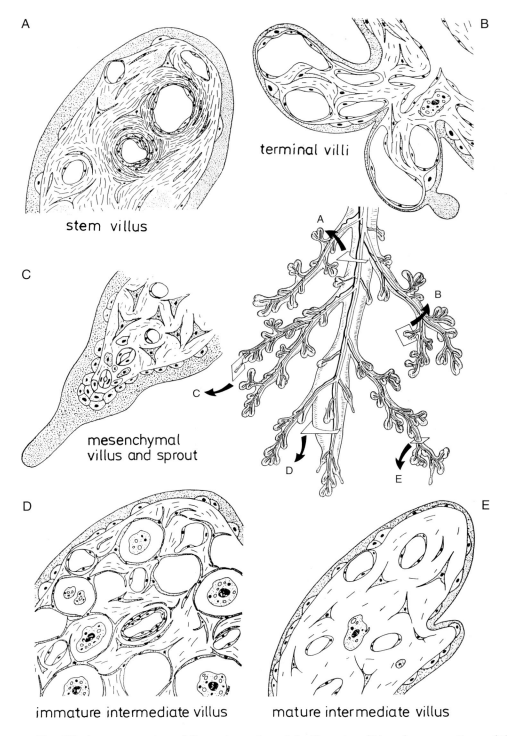

A

B

terminal villi

stem villus

C

mesenchymal
villus and sprout

D

E

immature intermediate villus   mature intermediate villus

Figure 7.1. Simplified representation of the mature placental villous tree (A) and cross sections of the various villous types (B–E). For further details see text. (From Kaufman P, Scheffen I. I. Placental development. In: Neonatal and Fetal Medicine: Physiology and Pathophysiology. Vol. I. R.A. Polin and W.W. Fox, eds., Orlando, FL: Saunders, 1992; 7–55, with permission.)

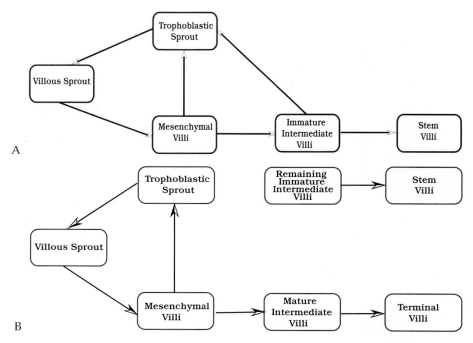

Figure 7.2. Routes of villous development during the first and second trimester (A) and third trimester (B). (A) Trophoblastic sprouts are produced along the surfaces of mesenchymal and immature intermediate villi. Via villous sprouts, they are transformed into mesenchymal villi. The latter differentiate into immature intermediate villi, which produce new sprouts before they are transformed into stem villi. (B) Throughout the third trimester, the mesenchymal villi differentiate into mature intermediate villi, which then may produce terminal villi. Mesenchymal villi no longer produce immature intermediate villi, but those still remaining continue to differentiate into stem villi. Thus, their number decreases with increasing gestational age. The source of new sprouts is also then reduced, and therefore the growth capacity of the villous trees gradually slows.

Mesenchymal Villi

Mesenchymal villi are the forerunners of all other villous types. They develop beginning in the fifth week PM (from last menstrual period) at the onset of villous vascularization. From the fifth to the sixth week PM they develop from the tertiary villi via primary and secondary villi. After the sixth week PM, the primary and secondary villi are exhausted and new mesenchymal villi develop by a different method. First, the villous surface of the mesenchymal villi develops syncytial outgrowths called **syncytial sprouts**. Ingrowth of cytotrophoblast forms **trophoblastic sprouts** and then ingrowth of connective tissue forms **villous sprouts**. Finally, fetal capillaries form in the connective tissue core. From early gestation through the second trimester, mesenchymal villi differentiate into **immature intermediate villi**, which ultimately form **stem villi**. In the third trimester, mesenchymal villi primarily differentiate into **mature intermediate villi**, which are the forerunners of the **terminal villi** (Figures 7.1, 7.2, Table 7.1).

Table 7.1. Villous characteristics

Villous type	When present	When maximum	% volume at term	Size	Characteristic features
Mesenchymal villi	Throughout gestation	0 to 8 weeks	<1	120–250 µm (0–8 weeks) 60–100 (8 weeks to term)	Primitive stroma, thick trophoblastic cover, few vessels
Immature intermediate villi	8 weeks to term	14 to 20 weeks	5 to 10	Usually 100–200 µm; may be up to 400 µm	Reticular stroma with fluid-filled stromal channels
Stem villi	12 weeks to term	Term	20 to 25	150–300 µm	Dense fibrotic stroma and myofibroblastic perivascular sheath, large vessels
Mature intermediate villi	Third trimester	Third trimester	25	80–150 µm	Dense, cellular stroma with >50% capillaries
Terminal villi	Third trimester	Term	40 to 50	60 µm	>50% capillaries

Mesenchymal villi have a *thick trophoblastic cover* with prominent Langhans' cells. They have the most Langhans' cells and the highest mitotic index of all villous types. There is a *primitive stromal core with loosely arranged collagen, fibroblasts and a few Hofbauer cells* (Figures 7.1 C, 7.3). *Fetal capillaries are poorly developed* and do not show sinusoidal dilatation. Occasionally, the capillaries are occluded at the villous tips. During the first weeks of pregnancy, mesenchymal villi are not only the source of *villous proliferation* but also the site of *maternofetal exchange* and *endocrine activity*. With advancing pregnancy and the development of more advanced villous types, their functional importance is reduced to villous growth. At term, they are generally only found in small numbers on the surfaces of immature intermediate villi in the center of the villous trees and comprise less than 1% of the placental volume.

Immature Intermediate Villi

The **immature intermediate villi** appear around the 8th week PM and comprise the majority of villi from the 14th to the 20th week. At term, only rare clusters are present in the center of the villous trees where they comprise less than 5% of the placental volume. They mature into stem villi, a transformation that is a gradual process resulting in many intermediate forms. Morphologically, immature intermediate villi are *bulbous* in shape with a *thick tropohoblastic cover* and a distinctive *reticular stroma containing fluid-filled stromal channels* (Figures 7.1 D, 7.4). The stroma contains *Hofbauer cells*, and there are prominent *Langhans' cells*

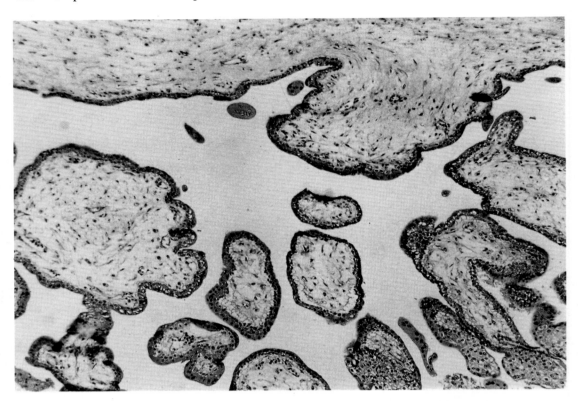

Figure 7.3. Mesenchymal villi. Eighth week PM. As can be seen from the diffuse stromal structure, the villi still belong to the mesenchymal type. ×125. (From Kaufmann P. Entwicklung der Plazenta. In: Die Plazenta des Menschen. V Becker, ThH Schiebler, F Kucli, eds. Stuttgart: Thieme, 1981; 13–50, with permission.)

interposed between the syncytium and the tropohoblastic basal lamina. Fetal capillaries are poorly developed. The reticular stroma may cause diagnostic problems as it has a weak affinity for conventional stains and may simulate villous edema. Starting at about the 8th week PM, the immature intermediate villi act as growth centers of the villous trees by forming new mesenchymal villi. This is accomplished by villous sprouting, as described above. Thus, new mesenchymal villi are formed from both old mesenchymal villi and immature intermediate villi.

Stem Villi

Stem villi are derived from immature intermediate villi by a gradual process (Figures 7.1 A, 7.4, 7.5). They begin to appear at about the eighth week PM. The large "trunks" and "branches" of the villous trees (trunci chorii, rami chorii, ramuli chorii) and the anchoring villi are all stem villi and differ only in caliber and position within the hierarchy

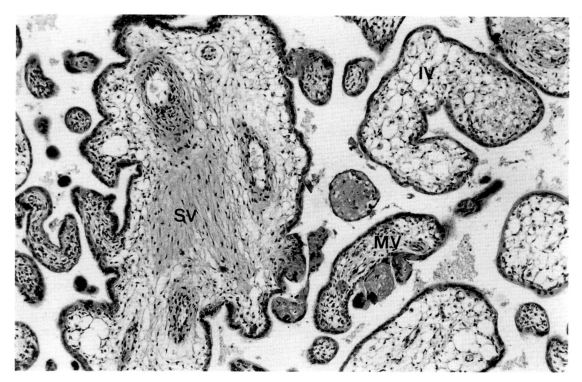

Figure 7.4. Immature intermediate villi and stem villi. Fifteenth week PM. The larger immature intermediate villi exhibit the first signs of central stromal fibrosis, originating from the larger fetal vessels, thus establishing the first stem villi (SV). Several typical immature intermediate villi (IV) and mesenchymal villi (MV) can be seen. As is typical for mesenchymal villi of the second and third trimester, they are associated with degenerating villi and are becoming transformed into intravillous fibrinoid. ×125.

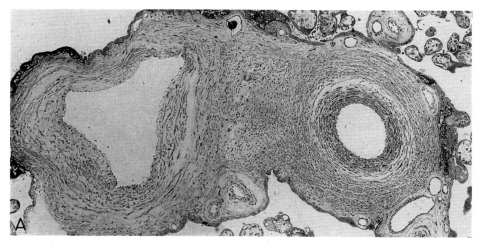

Figure 7.5. Cross section of a large stem villus. Note that the adventitias of the artery (right) and vein (left) directly continue into the surrounding dense fibrous stroma of the villus. Superficially, numerous smaller vessels of the paravascular capillary net are seen. As is typical for stem villi of the mature placenta, the trophoblastic covering has been replaced by fibrinoid in many places. ×115. (From Leiser R, Luckhardt M, Kaufmann P, Winterhager E, Bruns U. The fetal vascularisation of term human placental villi. I. Peripheral stem villi. Anat Embryol 1985;173:71–80, with permission.)

of villous branching. At term, they make up 20% to 25% of the placental volume but, because of the typical branching pattern, their "volumetric" share is highest in the central subchorionic area of the placenta. *Functionally, stem villi serve to mechanically support the structure of the villous trees.* Their share in the function of maternofetal exchange is negligible.

Histologically, stem villi have a *thick trophoblastic cover*. Cytotrophoblastic cells are easily identified below the syncytiotrophoblast on about 20% of the villous surfaces (Figure 7.1 A). In the mature placenta, the surfaces of the villi are often degenerative and partially replaced by fibrinoid. This is more prominent in large caliber stem villi. The stroma consists of *condensed bundles of collagen fibers with occasional fibroblasts and rare macrophages* (Figures 7.4, 7.5). Mast cells are occasionally seen. In the larger stem villi, there is a central artery and corresponding vein along with smaller arterioles, venules, and superficial paravascular capillaries (Figure 7.5). These structures are comparable to the vasa vasorum of large vessels in other organs. The adventitia of the vessels continues without sharp demarcation into the surrounding fibrous stroma. Centrally, the connective tissue cells are myofibroblasts, whereas peripherally they are noncontractile fibroblasts. The *central myofibroblasts around the stem vessels form the perivascular sheath.*

The transition from immature intermediate villi to stem villi is gradual. Initially, the vessels acquire a distinct media and adventitia, which expands to include the entire villus. Concurrently, an increase in the connective tissue leads to compression and finally disappearance of the stromal channels. In "immature" stem villi, there is a *superficial rim of reticular stroma separating the fibrous stroma from the trophoblastic cover*, which represents a differentiation gradient, the most central layer showing the highest degree of differentiation. Stem villi are established when the superficial reticular stroma beneath the trophoblast is thinner than the fibrous tissue surrounding the stem vessels.

Mature Intermediate Villi

In the third trimester, the mesenchymal villi switch from forming immature intermediate villi to forming **mature intermediate villi**, the precursors of the terminal villi. Mature intermediate villi are *long and slender*. When their surfaces bear developing terminal villi, they form a *zigzag configuration* as the terminal villi branch off. At 32 to 34 weeks gestation, there are many groups of mature intermediate villi with round to oval cross sections alternating with slender longitudinal sections (Figure 7.6). The stroma consists of *seemingly unoriented, loose bundles of connective tissue fibers and connective tissue cells* (Figure 7.1 E). Rudimentary narrow stromal channels may also be found. There are *numerous capillaries, small terminal arterioles, and collecting venules without a media*. Cross sections contain less than 50% vascular lumens and thus they participate significantly in fetomaternal exchange. Approximately 25% of the placental volume at term consists of this villous type.

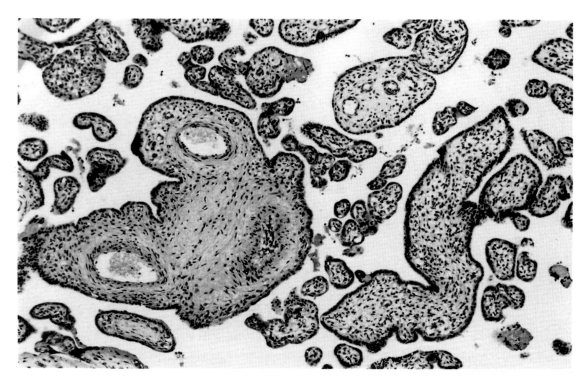

Figure 7.6. Mature intermediate villi. Twenty-ninth week PM. During this period, the mature intermediate villi and the stem villi (lower left) are the prevailing villous types. Immature intermediate villi with typical reticular stroma (lower right) are less common. ×125.

Terminal Villi

Terminal villi are the final ramifications of the villous tree. They are *grapelike outgrowths of the mature intermediate villi* and appear as single villi or poorly ramified side branches (see Figures 7.1 B, 7.6). The peripheral end of the mature intermediate villus normally branches into an aggregate of terminal villi and is connected to them by a narrow neck region. There are *scant connective tissue fibers and rare macrophages with a thin trophoblastic cover in intimate contact with sinusoidally dilated capillaries* (Figures 7.6, 7.7). Strictly speaking, terminal villi are those villi in which *the vascular lumens comprise at least 50% of the stromal volume and which contain no vessels other than capillaries and sinusoids.*

The **sinusoids** of terminal villi are not comparable to the sinusoids of the liver, spleen, and bone marrow as *they possess a continuous endothelium and complete basal lamina.* Contrary to the development of other villous types, the terminal villi are not formed by cellular outgrowths but rather are *formed passively by capillary growth and coiling.* This results in stretching of trophoblast and thinning of the vasculosyncytial membranes. Accordingly, maldevelopment of the terminal villi is a consequence of abnormal fetoplacental angiogenesis (see Chapter 18). These villi are the primary site of fetomaternal exchange

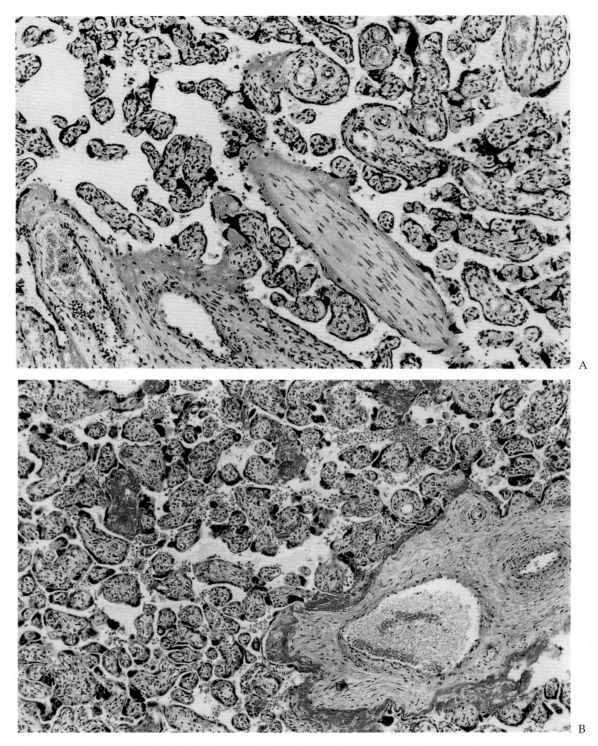

Figure 7.7. (A, B) Terminal villi. Thirty-eighth week PM. Dominating villous types are mature inter-mediate villi and terminal villi, both of small caliber. Several stem villi of varying caliber can also be seen in between. As is typical for term placentas, the trophoblastic cover of the stem villi is partly replaced by fibrinoid. The stromal core is completely fibrotic. Reticular stroma or cellular connective tissue (a typical sign of immaturity that is usually visible below the trophoblast in earlier stages) throughout the last few weeks is absent. ×125.

for the transfer of oxygen, carbon dioxide, and water. In the term placenta, they comprise 45% or more of the placental volume and approximately 60% of the cross section.

Anatomy of the Intervillous Space

After leaving the spiral arteries, maternal blood circulates through the
intervillous space, flowing directly around the villi outside the confines
of the maternal vascular system. At delivery, much of this blood is lost
and, therefore, on histologic examination the usual appearance of the
intervillous space is that of a system of narrow clefts. The inlets of the
spiral arteries are near the centers of the villous trees while the venous
outlets are arranged around the periphery. Therefore, *each fetomaternal
circulatory unit is composed of one villous tree with a corresponding, centrifugally perfused portion of the intervillous space* (Figure 7.8). This unit
has been called a "**placentone**." Most of the 40 to 60 placentones are in
contact with each other and overlap. The peripheral placentones are
more clearly separated from one another than the central units.

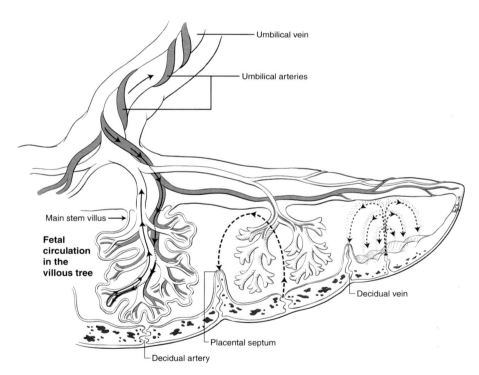

Figure 7.8. Typical spatial relations between villous trees and the maternal bloodstream. According to
the placentone theory, a placentone is one villous tree together with the related part of the intervillous
space. In the case of typical placentones, which prevail in the periphery of the placenta, the maternal
blood (arrows) enters the intervillous space near the center of the villous tree and leaves near the clefts
between neighboring villous trees. One or only a few villous trees occupy one placental lobule (cotyledon). In the central parts of the placenta, the villous trees, because of size and nearby location, may
partly overlap so that the zonal arrangement of the placentone disappears.

Maternal venous blood is collected in the *"perilobular zone," which is the portion of most densely packed terminal villi.* The remaining immature intermediate villi and sprouts of mesenchymal villi are concentrated in the center of the placentone. The placentone ranges in diameter from 1 to 4 cm, and therefore the entire unit may not be well represented in histologic sections. In addition, placentones from different locations may show varying degrees of maturation. Thus, even careful study of several sections from a given placenta may be difficult to interpret without knowledge of this anatomy.

Selected References

PHP4, Chapter 7, pages 116–154.

Castellucci M, Scheper M, Scheffen I, et al. The development of the human placental villous tree. Anat Embryol (Berl) 1990;181:117–128.

Demir R, Kosanke G, Kohnen G, et al. Classification of human placental stem villi: review of structural and functional aspects. Microsc Res Technique 1997;38:29–41.

Graf R, Schönfelder G, Mühlberger M, et al. The perivascular contractile sheath of human placental stem villi; its isolation and characterization. Placenta 1995;16:57–66.

Kaufmann P. Entwicklung der Plazenta. In: Becker V, Schiebler TH, Kubli F (eds) Die Plazenta des Menschen. Sturrgart: Thieme, 1981:13–50.

Kaufmann P. Basic morphology of the fetal and maternal circuits in the human placenta. Contrib Gynecol Obstet 1985;13:5–17.

Kaufmann P, Scheffen I. Placental development. In: Polin RA, Fox WW (eds) Neonatal and fetal medicine. Physiology and pathophysiology, vol I. Orlando: Saunders, 1992:47–55.

Kaufmann P, Sen DK, Schweikhart G. Classification of human placental villi. I. Histology and scanning electron microscopy. Cell Tissue Res 1979; 200:409–423.

Krantz KE, Parker JC. Contractile properties of the smooth muscle in the human placenta. Clin Obstet Gynecol 1963;6:26–38.

Leiser R, Luckhardt M, Kaufmann P, et al. The fetal vascularisation of term human placental villi. I. Peripheral stem villi Anat Embryol 1985;173:71–80.

Wigglesworth JS. Vascular organization of the human placenta. Nature (Lond) 1967;216:1120–1121.

Chapter 8

Development and Histology of the Nonvillous Portions of the Placenta

General Considerations

The nonvillous parts of the placenta include the **chorionic plate, cell islands, cell columns, placental septa, basal plate, marginal zone**, and **fibrinoid deposits** (Figure 8.1). These structures do not participate in maternofetal exchange, but have mechanical and metabolic functions. Irrespective of their location and structure, the nonvillous parts of the placenta have the same three basic components, which structurally and functionally do not vary from one area to the next:

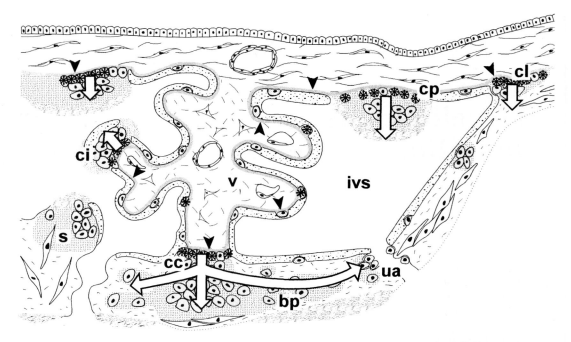

Figure 8.1. Schematic drawing of the distribution of the various trophoblast populations. Trophoblastic cells that rest on the trophoblastic basal lamina (arrowheads) of the membranes, chorionic plate, villi, cell columns, and cell islands represent the proliferating trophoblastic stem cells (Langhans' cells). Those close to the intervillous space (ivs) differentiate and fuse to form the syncytiotrophoblast, which usually takes place in the placental villi (v). Without contact to the intervillous space, the daughter cells of the proliferating stem cells (marked by asterisks) do not fuse syncytially but rather differentiate and become invasive extravillous trophoblastic cells. Their routes of invasion/migration are symbolized by arrows. Extravillous trophoblastic cells can be found in cell columns (cc), cell islands (ci), chorionic plate (cp), chorion laeve (cl), septa (s), basal plate (bp), and uteroplacental arteries (ua). Fibrinoid is point-shaded; fibrin is line-shaded.

- **Extravillous trophoblast,**
- **Fibrinoid**, and
- **Decidua** (in some locations).

Extravillous Trophoblast

Historically, the derivation of extravillous trophoblast was in dispute, and so the term "**X-cells**" was applied. When it was demonstrated that these cells were a type of trophoblast and thus of fetal origin, new designations were proposed including extravillous trophoblast, nonvillous trophoblast, trophoblastic giant cells, placental site trophoblast, trophocytes, spongiotrophoblast, and intermediate trophoblast. Among placental biologists, the term "**extravillous trophoblast**" is in general use, whereas among pathologists the term "**intermediate trophoblast**" is widely applied. Unfortunately, this latter term is misleading. It had originally been used to designate villous trophoblastic cells that were *transitional* between villous cytotrophoblast and syncytiotrophoblast, cells that were in the process of donating their nuclei to the syncytium. The implication was that "intermediate trophoblast" was intermediate between cytotrophoblast and syncytiotrophoblast and therefore a type of *villous trophoblast*. However, the term "intermediate trophoblast" is currently used by many pathologists to indicate those cells in extravillous sites such as the implantation site, chorion laeve, chorionic plate, and so on. Therefore, this use of intermediate trophoblast is roughly equivalent to the traditional term, **extravillous trophoblast**. The term "villous intermediate trophoblast" has also been recently introduced. If intermediate trophoblast are in fact equivalent to extravillous trophoblast, then by definition "villous intermediate trophoblast" do not exist. These distinctions are important in understanding the derivation and differentiation of trophoblastic tumors (see Chapters 25, 26).

Histologically, extravillous trophoblastic cells are *round to polygonal cells* that are present singly or in groups. They are usually associated with fibrinoid, a type of extracellular matrix material (see below). They tend to have *pleomorphic, hyperchromatic, or irregular nuclei* (Figure 8.2) and amphophilic cytoplasm. Occasionally more eosinophilic cytoplasm may be identified. The cells predominantly mononuclear, but binucleate, trinucleate, and multinucleate cells are also seen. Extravillous trophoblast in the chorionic plate and chorion laeve are often smaller and less pleomorphic than those present in the implantation site but have the same general characteristics.

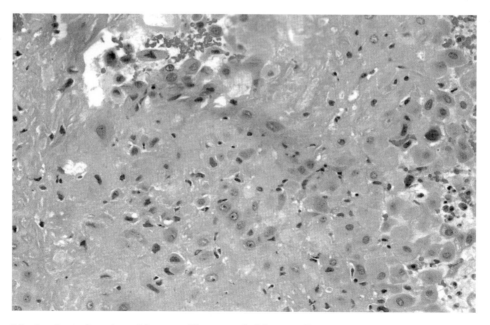

Figure 8.2. Implantation site with extravillous trophoblastic cells intermixed with decidual cells. H&E. ×200.

Trophoblastic Stem Cells

The vast majority of trophoblast from the previllous stages of placentation are consumed for the development of the placental villi. These trophoblast form the **villous cytotrophoblast**, the inner layer of the villous surface epithelium, and the **villous syncytiotrophoblast**, the syncytium that forms the superficial layer facing the intervillous space. The remaining trophoblastic cells, **the extravillous trophoblast**, are the basic material for the development of all *nonvillous parts of the placenta: the chorion laeve, marginal zone, chorionic plate, basal plate, cell columns, septa, and cell islands.* These trophoblastic cells are a relatively homogeneous population that differs predominantly in location and extent of differentiation.

The **proliferating trophoblastic stem cells** are those trophoblastic cells that *rest on the basal lamina of the fetoplacental stroma.* These stem cells differentiate into both extravillous and villous trophoblast (Figure 8.1). Populations of stem cells include the *villous cytotrophoblast, the basal layers of the cell columns, the cell islands, the chorionic plate, and the chorion laeve.* It can be seen that, although these cells are in different sites, they all are in contact with the basal lamina of the fetoplacental stroma. The future fate of these stem cells, whether they fuse to form syncytiotrophoblast and acquire a villous phenotype or whether they acquire an extravillous phenotype, depends on the surrounding environment, that is, contact with extracellular matrix molecules. *Transformation to extravillous trophoblast occurs on exposure to maternal blood or maternal extracellular matrix. Transformation to villous trophoblast occurs with contact to the syncytiotrophoblast.* Accordingly, the stem cells of the cell columns have a double function, contributing trophoblast for subsequent invasion *and* acting as a growth zone for villous trophoblast of the anchoring villi. Other populations of stem cells have the capacity to differentiate along both pathways but primarily contribute to either the villous or extravillous pathway.

Proliferative Phenotype

Although extravillous trophoblast is present in a variety of locations, its general structure and function are surprisingly homogeneous. First and second trimester extravillous trophoblast in the proximal portion of the cell columns are **proliferative** and will stain positively with proliferation markers such as MIB-1 or antibodies against PCNA. These proximal **proliferating extravillous trophoblastic cells** are either in *immediate contact with the basal lamina* or *separated from it by other proliferating trophoblastic cells.* These cells represent the *stem cells of the extravillous pathway of differentiation* (Figures 8.1, 8.3) and are said to have a proliferative phenotype.

Invasive Phenotype

Further differentiation of extravillous trophoblast results in a switch from a proliferative to an **invasive phenotype** (Figure 8.3). This is called the invasive pathway. In normal placentation, proliferation and

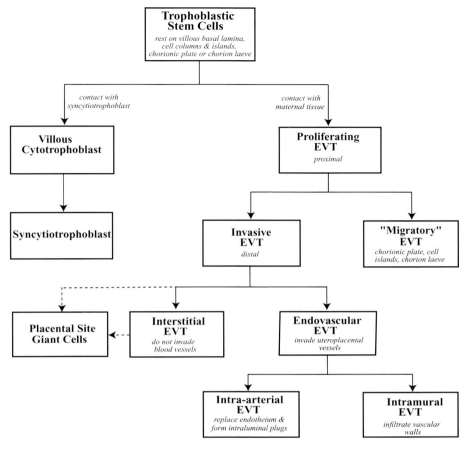

Figure 8.3. Diagram of trophoblastic differentiation. Dotted lines indicate possible routes. See text for discussion. EVT, extravillous trophoblastic cells.

invasion do not coexist in one and the same cell. *Thus, temporal and spatial separation of proliferation and invasiveness limits the depth of trophoblastic invasion.* This separation is thought to embody the major difference between "normal" trophoblastic invasion in pregnancy as compared to "malignant" invasion in tumors, the latter being characterized by temporal and spatial coincidence of proliferation and invasion. Differences between the proliferative and invasive phenotypes are shown in Table 8.1.

The extravillous trophoblast of the chorionic plate and cell islands, which are exposed to maternal blood but not maternal tissues, do not show true invasive behavior. This phenotype is often called "**migratory.**" Biologically, this may be a quantitative rather than a qualitative difference and a result of local environmental factors. Recent observations in tubal pregnancies have revealed proliferation in the deeply invasive extravillous trophoblastic cells. Here, the trophoblast is essentially normal, the only difference being the abnormal implantation site. This difference suggests that proliferation is downregulated by local

Table 8.1. Differences between the proliferative and invasive phenotype of extravillous trophoblast

	Proliferative phenotype	Invasive phenotype
Invasion	−	+
Proliferation	+	−
Contact on or near fetal stromal basal lamina	+	−
Expression of proliferation markers	MIB-1, c-erbB-1	c-erbB-2
Integrin expression	Epithelial types (α6β4, α3β1)	Interstitial types (α5β1, α1β1, αvβ3, αvβ5)
Secretion of extracellular matrix	Polar	Apolar

factors in the normal intrauterine milieu but not in the fallopian tube. Both tubal pregnancy and placenta accreta (see Chapter 12) have in common locally deficient decidualization, which leads to abnormally invasive implantation.

Interstitial Phenotype

After leaving the basal lamina that faces the chorionic or villous stroma, the invasive extravillous trophoblast further differentiates into either an **interstitial phenotype** or **endovascular phenotype** (Figure 8.3). *Interstitial trophoblast are those cells that do not invade blood vessels, while endovascular trophoblast invade the walls and lumens of uteroplacental vessels* (Figure 8.4).

Normal epithelia either secrete extracellular matrix in a polarized manner as a basal lamina or not at all, and this is also true for *villous trophoblast*. In contrast, the **interstitial extravillous trophoblast** secrete extracellular matrix in an **apolar** fashion, a feature usually only seen in mesenchymal cells. Matrix molecules accumulate extracellularly in large, three-dimensional patchy aggregates called **fibrinoid**, which completely embed the extravillous trophoblast. Typically, this apolar matrix is secreted in the direct vicinity of maternal tissues, namely facing the maternal blood (e.g., cell islands, intervillous surface of the chorionic plate, placental septa) or maternal decidua (basal plate with cell columns, chorion laeve). As a consequence, fibrin from maternal blood and decidual secretory products are added to the extracellular matrix.

The **endovascular extravillous** trophoblast further differentiates into **intramural extravillous trophoblast** and **intraarterial extravillous trophoblast**. The intramural trophoblast infiltrate the walls of uteroplacental vessels and therefore are essential to the conversion of decidual vessels into uteroplacental vessels. The intraarterial trophoblast replace the endothelium, and as they do, they undergo "pseudovasculogenesis," in which they achieve an endothelial phenotype. Early in gestation, intraluminal plugs of these cells may be present under normal conditions. However, later in pregnancy, they are considered an abnormal finding and are often associated with other abnormalities of implantation and the decidual vessels (see Chapter 18).

Multinucleated Extravillous Trophoblast

Giant multinucleated extravillous trophoblastic cells in the implantation site and superficial myometrium are called **placental site giant cells**. Placental site giant cells tend to be *vacuolated and degenerative* (Figure 8.5) and are occasionally found in association with fibrinoid deposits. They are likely to be highly differentiated extravillous trophoblastic cells that have *reached the end of the differentiation pathway*. Because surprising few invasive trophoblast undergo apoptosis, local syncytial fusion at the end of the invasive pathway is an alternative mechanism for reducing the number of invasive trophoblast.

Trophoblastic Invasion

Trophoblastic invasion in intrauterine pregnancies is a tightly controlled, complex process that is still poorly understood. There are mechanisms supporting and inhibiting invasion from both the trophoblastic and endometrial side, suggesting that promotion and inhibition of invasiveness cannot be allocated to the fetal and maternal tissues, respectively. *Rather, every cell type in the maternofetal junctional zone has developed mechanisms for both supporting and inhibiting invasion, resulting in an extremely complex but obviously well-balanced control system.*

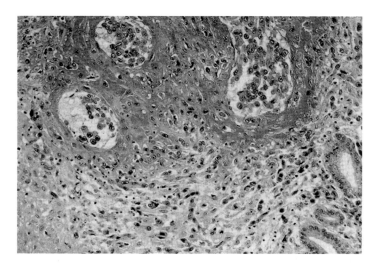

Figure 8.4. Extravillous trophoblastic cells invading a decidual vessel; physiologic conversion of the decidual vessel into a uteroplacental vessel. Note the fibrin in the wall, whose muscular coat is destroyed; the vessels are surrounded and thoroughly infiltrated by extravillous trophoblastic cells. The paler cells at the bottom are decidual stromal cells; endometrial glands are at bottom right. H&E. ×160.

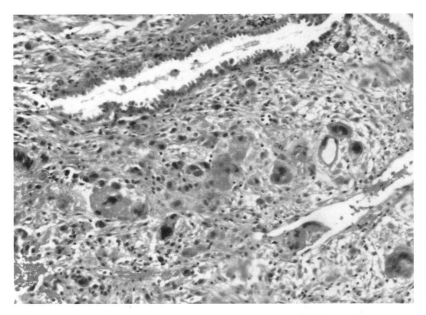

Figure 8.5. Multinucleated placental site giant cells present in the implantation site. H&E. ×200.

It is of particular interest to note that the immune response to malignant tumors shares many similarities to normal trophoblastic invasion.

Decidua

The changes that occur in the human endometrium in response to the physiological stimuli of pregnancy and implantation of the blastocyst are called *decidualization*. If the stimulus is a physiological one, the resulting tissue is the **decidua**, but if the stimulus is experimental or artificial, the tissue is called pseudodecidua. Decidualization is characterized by the enlargement of endometrial stromal cells, which eventually assume an epithelioid appearance. The cells are *round to polygonal, with sharply defined cell borders and a single nucleus containing a small but prominent nucleolus* (Figure 8.6 A). Up to three nuclei can occasionally occur. During decidualization, the endometrial glands initially enlarge and can often be observed in first trimester specimens. When pregnancy ensues, *the nuclei undergo endomitosis, become polyploid,* and acquire the morphologic features known as the **Arias–Stella change** (Figure 8.6 B). Ultimately, *the glands atrophy, although occasional remnants may be found in the basal plate and in the placental bed*. These disintegrating residual glands may lead to confusion with uterine vessels invaded by trophoblast and lined by intraarterial trophoblast.

Within the decidual tissue are also considerable numbers of bone marrow-derived cells including **macrophages, T lymphocytes, granulocytes**, and **large granular lymphocytes** (endometrial natural killer cells, endometrial NK cells, or "endometrial granular cells"). At term, increased numbers of granulocytes can be found at the maternofetal interface and at the maternal surface of the delivered placenta. These cells likely represent an inflammatory response to the mechanisms preceding separation of the placenta.

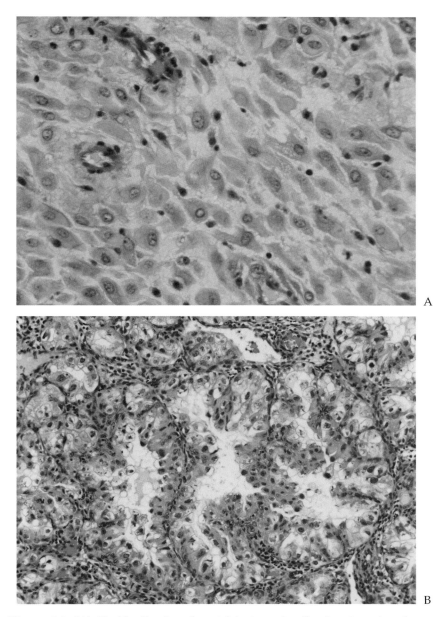

A

B

Figure 8.6. (A) Decidualized endometrial stromal cells showing abundant cytoplasm and vesicular nuclei H&E. ×200. (B) Arias–Stella reaction of the decidua. Note the marked nuclear atypia and pleomorphism. H&E. ×200.

Fibrinoid

Fibrinoid is one of the most prominent components of the human placenta. It is a nonfibrous, acellular, relatively homogeneous material *derived from cellular secretion, cellular degeneration*, and other sources as yet unknown. Its light microscopic appearance varies from *glossy and homogeneous to lamellar, fibrous, or reticular* (Figure 8.7). In routine sections, the color of fibrinoid varies from slightly pink to intense red. When Mallory's Trichrome stain is used, the color is a light blue but may vary from dark blue to lilac or even red. *Because fibrin, blood clot, and secretory products are usually deposited in proximity and cannot be easily discriminated, the general term fibrinoid, rather than fibrin, is used.*

Fibrinoid is typically found in the following locations:

- **Subchorionic region** (Langhans' stria) (Figures 8.1, 8.7),
- **Intervillous space** (perivillous) (Figure 4.1 H, page 46),
- **Chorionic villi** (intravillous) (Figure 4.1 F),
- **Placental septa** (Figure 4.1 K),
- **Cell islands** (Figure 4.1 J),
- **Cell columns** (Figure 4.1 I),
- **Basal plate** (Figure 4.1 A),
   - Superficial basal plate, facing the intervillous space (Rohr's stria) (Figure 4.1 I)
   - Deep basal plate, (uteroplacental fibrinoid, Nitabuch's stria) (Figure 4.1 L)

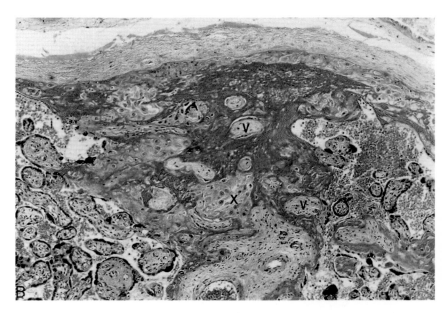

Figure 8.7. Section of the chorionic plate at the 40th week PM (after last menstrual period). There is deposition of Langhans' fibrinoid below the chorionic plate near term. Clusters of extravillous trophoblast cells (X) and residues of buried villi (V) are typically incorporated into mature Langhans' fibrinoid. ×85.

Table 8.2. Location of fibrinoid and composition of fibrinoid subtypes

Location	Composition
Subchorionic fibrinoid (Langhans' stria)	
Facing chorionic connective tissue	Fibrinoid
Facing intervillous space	Fibrin
Perivillous fibrinoid	Fibrin
Intravillous fibrinoid	Both
Placental septa	Both
Cell islands	
Superficial layers	Fibrin
Central	Fibrinoid
Cell columns	
Facing intervillous space	Fibrin
Embedding invasive trophoblast	Fibrinoid
Basal plate	
Superficial—facing the intervillous space	Fibrin
Deep—uteroplacental fibrinoid	Both, predominance of fibrin in superficial zone
Intramural in uteroplacental vessels	Mostly fibrin
Membranes (chorion laeve)	
Trophoblast layer	Fibrinoid
Trophoblast-decidual junction	Fibrin

- **Uteroplacental arteries and veins** (intramural) (Figure 1.6 L, page 9), and
- **Fetal membranes** (chorion laeve) (Figure 4.2, page 50).

Detailed histochemical, biochemical, immunohistochemical, ultrastructural, and experimental studies have revealed that fibrinoid is composed of two histologically similar types that differ in their origin and composition. **Fibrin-type fibrinoid** *is derived from the coagulation cascade and is mainly composed of fibrin.* **Matrix-type fibrinoid** *is a secretory product of extravillous trophoblastic cells and is mainly composed of collagen IV and glycoproteins of the extracellular matrix.* It may also contain fibrin and secretory products of decidual cells. Because the fibrin-type fibrinoid is generally composed of fibrin, we use the term **fibrin**, and for matrix-type fibrinoid, the term **fibrinoid**. Generally, both may be found in all the above-mentioned locations in varying proportions (Table 8.2).

Fibrin and Fibrinoid

As a general rule, **fibrin** *lines the intervillous space in all those locations where the syncytiotrophoblast layer is interrupted.* It is never directly in contact with cytotrophoblast but rather is separated from it by fibrinoid. *Fibrin is always interposed between fibrinoid and maternal blood.* The typical distribution of **fibrin** lining the intervillous space suggests *an origin from maternal blood*; however, one cannot exclude a contribution from fetal plasma. Immunohistochemically, **fibrin** shows intense reactivity with fibrin antibodies that *do not cross-react with fibrinogen*. It contains *plasma fibronectins* but not basal lamina molecules or interstitial matrix molecules and binds with Ulex Europaeus lectin (UEA-I), indicating it is partially composed of encased and disintegrated remnants of endothelial cells and blood cells.

Fibrinoid *embeds the postproliferative extravillous trophoblastic cells and is found where trophoblastic migration or invasion takes place.* Single or clustered extravillous trophoblastic cells are typically surrounded by ample glossy extracellular matrix. The extracellular matrix molecules found in fibrinoid are primarily *secretory products of the extravillous trophoblast.* Decidual cells secrete a similar extracellular matrix and so may also contribute to fibrinoid. Characteristically, fibrinoid is immunoreactive for the basal lamina molecules *collagen IV* and *laminin*, as well as for *cellular fibronectins.* Fibrinoid does not stain with UEA-I, but traces of fibrinogen may be found.

Intravillous fibrinoid present in the *subtrophoblastic space and villous stroma* may be seen in up to 3% of villous cross sections at term. Scattered villi may be partially or completely replaced by fibrinoid. Intravillous deposition of fibrinoid is increased in pregnancies complicated by *maternal diabetes, Rh incompatibility, preeclampsia, and other disorders.* The etiology of this deposition is not fully understood, but it may occur secondary to an immunologic attack against the villous cytotrophoblast, clotting of intervillous blood or may be due to villous degeneration. Usually, the deposits begin as small nodules under the syncytiotrophoblast that "grow" to finally replace the stroma. The originally intact syncytium may degenerate only secondarily, if at all. The question as to maternal or fetal derivation of intravillous fibrinoid is still open.

Functions of fibrin and fibrinoid include the following:

Fibrin
- Mechanical stability and support of the stem villi, chorionic plate, and basal plate
- Regulation of intervillous circulation by clotting of poorly perfused areas
- Barrier to trophoblastic invasion
- Alternative route of maternofetal transport after damage to syncytiotrophoblastic surfaces

Fibrinoid
- Adhesiveness of the placenta to the uterine wall
- Promotion of trophoblastic invasion
- Assistance with reepithelialization of damaged villous surfaces
- Immunoprotection to mask fetal antigens and act as an immunoabsorptive sponge

Uteroplacental Vessels

The **uteroplacental arteries** derive from the uterine spiral arterioles after physiologic conversion (see below). They are branches or continuations of the myometrial arteries, and follow a spiral course as they enter the basal plate. They cross the uterine wall almost perpendicularly up to the 8th week of gestation. With advancing gestation, as the placental area enlarges, their course becomes more oblique so that by 10 weeks, distal segments are almost parallel to the basal plate. *The most distal segments become converted, and this is associated with decidual necrosis.* The latter is a common finding at the periphery of the placental site between 8 and 14 weeks gestation. A single decidual spiral artery delivers its blood into the center of a cotyledon, and an occasional lateral vessel adds to the supply. The venous openings are peripheral in the cotyledon. This idealized arrangement is generally seen only at the placental periphery (see Figure 7.8).

Physiologic Conversion of the Decidual Arterioles

Trophoblastic invasion of the uteroplacental arteries and the subsequent alterations have been designated "**physiologic conversion**" to distinguish them from the changes seen in the placental bed vessels of patients with preeclampsia and other disorders (see Chapter 18). Trophoblastic infiltration of the arterial walls is accompanied by the *loss of elastic fibers and smooth muscle cells* due to proteolytic activities of the invasive endovascular trophoblastic cells. *Intramural fibrin and fibrinoid* replace the vessel walls. There is a considerable *increase in the luminal diameter* of the vessels, which may reach as much as five times their original diameter (see Figure 8.4). *Intraluminal thrombi* may also be present. These changes transform the originally flexible vessels into rigid channels, which are incapable of constricting. Thus, because of the absence of local regulatory mechanisms, the nutrient supply to the placenta will not be reduced despite changes in blood pressure in the mother.

   Intraarterial trophoblastic cells locally replace the maternal endothelium and form trophoblastic plugs, which very early in development may obstruct the lumen. The discrimination between **intraarterial trophoblastic cells** and maternal endothelial cells is not always easy because these trophoblastic cells essentially *achieve an endothelial phenotype.* The majority of cells lining the lumens of uteroplacental arteries in the endometrium and inner myometrium are intraarterial trophoblast, in contrast to the uteroplacental veins in which the maternal endothelium becomes replaced by trophoblast only rarely. However, the muscular coat of the **uteroplacental veins** is even more reduced than that of the arteries, and smooth muscle cells are usually absent near the venous openings. The endothelium of the veins is discontinuous and *may extend to cover the surrounding parts of the basal plate, parts of septa, cell islands, and sometimes even perivillous fibrinoid deposits.* The maternal endothelial lining of the intervillous space is particularly impressive in the marginal zone of the placenta.

   Physiologic conversion decreases uteroplacental flow resistance by widening of the arterial lumens. *Only a balance between the intervillous maternal blood pressure and the intravillous fetal blood pressure keeps the fetal vessels open and allows intravillous fetal blood flow.* Elevation of fetal blood pressure results in increased filtration through fetal vessels, villous edema, and reduced flow to the fetus. The physiologic changes of the spiral arteries that keep the intervillous blood pressure low are essential to maintain adequate maternofetal exchange. Lack of normal dilation will result in increased maternal flow impedance and, if the maternal blood pressure is kept constant, the increased impedance will cause reduced intervillous perfusion and will directly impair delivery of oxygen and nutrients into the placenta and the fetal circulation. On the other hand, if the maternal blood pressure is increased, such as in the case of preeclampsia, maternal perfusion of the placenta and delivery of oxygen and nutrients into the placenta may be kept constant. This situation, however, will result in increased intervillous blood pressure, increased fetoplacental impedance, reduced fetoplacental circulation, and reduced oxygen and nutrient transfer to the fetus. Therefore, depending on the maternal response to deficient vascular trophoblastic invasion, different clinical features may result, explaining the heterogeneity of clinical entities such as preeclampsia and growth restriction.

Calcification, Mineralization, and Pigment

The mature placenta often has fine deposits of calcium salts, which appear as *irregularly distributed, yellow, and stippled deposits on gross examination* (see Figure 3.7, page 30). They have a gritty sensation when a knife passes through the placenta on sectioning. Immature placentas rarely have any significant amount of calcifications, whereas they are quite common in postmature placentas. Calcium deposits are *blue in H&E preparations and occur most commonly in the fibrin and fibrinoid in the basal plate and the placental septa* (Figure 8.8). Calcifications detected by ultrasonography were formerly used in "placental grading," but as they are not a reliable sign of postmaturity this practice has largely been abandoned. Massive or excessive calcification of the placenta may occur but this is *not* considered to be associated with any significant clinical abnormalities in the mother or infant. However, at present we do not understand the normal mechanisms that lead to calcification of the placenta, let alone when it attains seemingly pathologic quantities.

   In addition to the typical, grossly identifiable, calcification, one may find microscopic granular purple deposits lining the *villous basement membranes* (see Figure 20.13, page 388). These **villous microcalcifications** are most common in abortion specimens. These deposits will stain with the von Kossa stain; however, phosphorus and carbonate salts of all sorts also stain with the von Kossa reaction. Therefore, such "calcified" basement membranes may actually represent deposits of other minerals. Indeed, pregnancies complicated by hydramnios have a high rate (67%) of mineralization of the trophoblastic basement membrane, which has been shown in some cases to be iron. This type of mineralization has been described in other conditions including *fetal*

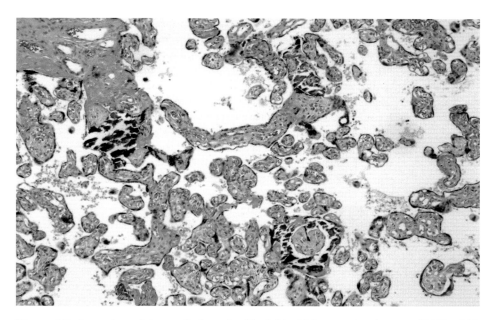

Figure 8.8. Irregular calcium salt deposits (dark black) in mature placenta. H&E. ×160.

vascular thrombosis, anencephaly, trisomy 21, Bartter syndrome, and congenital nephrotic syndrome. These deposits are likely caused by deficient transport through the trophoblast, which are not consumed by the fetus due to cessation of capillary flow.

Melanin has also been demonstrated in the basement membranes of villi and in Hofbauer cells. It is present as often in Caucasians as in African-Americans. These deposits occur more frequently in association with chronic skin lesions, and the condition has been called "dermatopathic melanosis of placenta." Melanin-containing macrophages in the amnion have also been found in cases of prolonged amnion rupture. **Lipofuscin**, or "aging pigment," has been also demonstrated in placentas beyond 32 weeks. However, it is generally accepted that only maturation, not aging, occurs in placental tissue.

Chorionic Plate

Development

On day 8 PC (post conception), the primary chorionic plate begins to form. The early chorionic plate is composed only of *syncytiotrophoblast* and *cytotrophoblast* and separates the lacunar system from the blastocyst cavity (see Figures 5.1 B,C, page 70). As soon as the mesenchyme spreads onto the cytotrophoblastic surface of the blastocyst cavity, after day 9 PC, the primary chorionic plate becomes triple layered, consisting of *mesenchyme, cytotrophoblast,* and *syncytiotrophoblast.* During the third week PC, *the exocoelomic cavity forms in the extraembryonic mesenchyme* (see Figure 5.4, day 18, page 77). The latter will ultimately become the chorionic mesoderm. Toward the exocoelomic cavity, the mesoderm is lined by a single layer of flat mesothelium. Toward the chorionic plate, the syncytiotrophoblastic layer is usually replaced by fibrinoid early in pregnancy. These fibrinoid deposits within and along the surface of the chorionic plate are called **Langhans' fibrinoid**. Toward the intervillous space, the plate is mostly covered by **fibrin**, derived from blood clotting in the intervillous space. The cytotrophoblastic layer degenerates focally, but in some places the trophoblast proliferates. The trophoblastic cells, which rest directly on the chorionic mesenchyme, retain their proliferative capacity as stem cells. Their daughter cells become **extravillous trophoblastic cells** as they lose contact with the mesenchymal layer.

With advancing gestation, villi become attached to the fibrinoid and become deeply incorporated into the Langhans' fibrinoid layer. *The syncytial layer of the incorporated villi degenerates, and the underlying trophoblastic cells transform into extravillous trophoblastic cells and migrate into the fibrinoid.* In areas of the chorionic plate that are devoid of such incorporated villi, the thickness of the chorionic plate rarely exceeds 200 μm, whereas adjacent foci with conglomerated, encased villi may measure up to several millimeters in thickness. In the second month of gestation, fetal blood vessels contact the chorionic plate (Figure 5.4, days 28 and 40, page 77) and enter the early stem villi. These vessels pass through the chorionic plate, connecting the villous trees with the umbilical cord. At 17 weeks of gestation, the amnion lines the amniotic cavity, and this "attachment" of the amnion to the primary chorionic plate transforms the latter into the definitive **chorionic plate**. Ample folding of the amnion on the chorionic plate is a common histologic finding.

Structure at Term

At term, the following layers of the chorionic plate can be distinguished (Figures 8.9, 8.10):

- **Amnion**
  - **Amnionic epithelium**
  - **Amnionic mesoderm**
- **Spongy layer, separating amnion and chorion**
- **Chorion**
  - **Chorionic mesoderm**
- **Extravillous trophoblast**
- **Langhans' fibrinoid layer encasing the extravillous cytotrophoblast**

The amnionic epithelium is usually a *single-layered columnar epithelium*. The **amnionic mesoderm** is composed of two layers. **The compact layer** is devoid of cells but contains a *condensed three-dimensional lattice of collagen fibers*. The **fibroblast layer**, in contrast, has a *loose, two-dimensional network of fibers that are arranged parallel to the amnionic epithelium*. Three to four thin layers of filaments alternate with layers

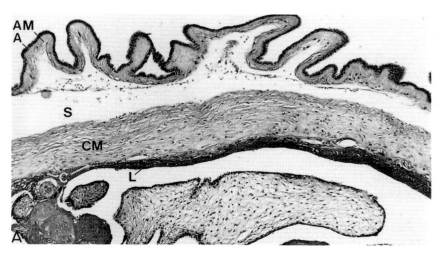

Figure 8.9. H&E-stained paraffin section of the chorionic plate at the 21st week PM. Amnionic epithelium (A), amnionic mesenchyme (AM), spongy layer (S), chorionic mesenchyme (CM), chorionic (extravillous) cytotrophoblast (C), Langhans' fibrinoid (L). ×85.

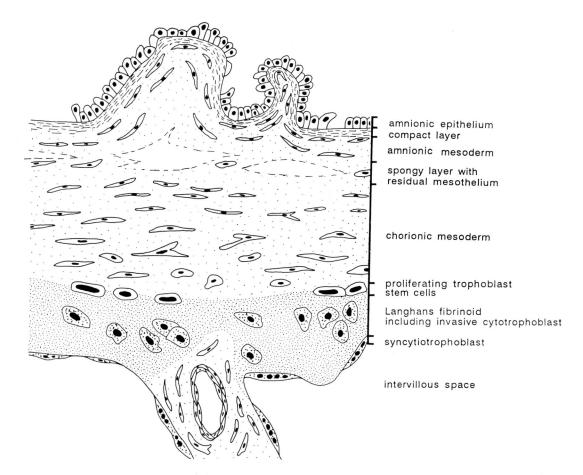

Figure 8.10. Diagram of the layering and cellular composition of the chorionic plate.

of loosely arranged fibroblasts, thus forming an incomplete irregular network.

The **spongy layer** is structurally similar to the corresponding layer of the free membranes and separates amnion and chorion. The next layer is the **chorionic mesoderm**, which contains small fibroblasts with long extensions and condensed nuclei and myofibroblasts. The chorionic vessels, which originate by branching from the umbilical vessels, run in the mesoderm. The chorionic mesoderm is followed by an **incomplete basal lamina**. A layer of **extravillous trophoblast** is found on its other side. Centrally, this layer is discontinuous, consisting of small groups of cells (Figure 8.10). The basal lamina is absent where the chorionic mesoderm is directly in contact with the Langhans' fibrinoid without interposed trophoblast. The deepest of these cells are the proliferative layer. Their accumulation near the margin of the placenta account for growth at the placental margin.

Langhans' fibrinoid layer is a constant feature, with a thickness and structure that increases continuously throughout pregnancy. *In its early stages, the intervillous surface of Langhans' layer is still mostly covered by syncytiotrophoblast, but this becomes completely replaced by additional fibrinoid during later pregnancy.* Abundant scattered or aggregated extravillous trophoblast cells can be seen in the fibrinoid, and these have been shown to be of an invasive phenotype (see above). *Subchorionic fibrinoid forms the "bosselations" and the laminated subchorionic plaques seen on the fetal surface of placentas.* These deposits vary markedly and result from eddying in the places where the intervillous blood is turned back toward the basal plate.

Basal Plate

Development

The **basal plate** is defined as the *maternal aspect of the intervillous space.* It is the most intimate and most important contact zone of maternal and fetal tissues (see Figure 4.1 L, page 46). The definitive basal plate is composed of various tissues including *extravillous trophoblast, decidua, fibrinoid, residues of degenerating villi, and maternal vessels.* The precursor of the basal plate is the **trophoblastic shell** (Figure 8.11), which early in development separates the lacunar system from the endometrium (Figures 5.1 B,C, page 70). Because of the intimate relationship between the trophoblastic shell and the surrounding endometrium, the first steps in the formation of the basal plate are coupled with the mechanisms of implantation. On day 13 PC, trophoblast begin to invade the stroma (Figures 5.1 E,F, page 70) and an exact border separating trophoblastic shell and endometrium can no longer be defined. *The trophoblast ultimately invades the entire thickness of the decidua, down to the superficial myometrium* where glands are absent. The necrotic residues of decidua and trophoblast are transformed into fibrinoid, which has a considerable admixture of fibrin.

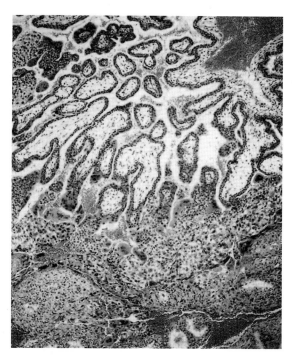

Figure 8.11. Trophoblastic shell of 13-day pregnancy. The cytotrophoblastic columns are covered with syncytium. Placental site giant cells are intermingled with decidua (right). H&E. ×300.

Two irregular layers of fibrinoid exist, **Rohr's fibrinoid** and **Nitabuch's fibrinoid**. From day 22 PC onward, the term **basal plate** is used. The basal plate generally includes the *base of the intervillous space together with all placental and maternal tissues that adhere to it after parturition* (Figure 8.12).

The basal plate grows laterally as well as in thickness. This change is largely a consequence of proliferation of the extravillous trophoblast originating from cell columns with migration of the daughter cells into the tissues of the basal plate. Focally, the lateral growth of the basal plate may not be accompanied by a corresponding distension of the uterine wall. Thus, in these areas, the basal plate folds over the uterine wall and pulls the basal plate tissues into the intervillous space. This is how the **placental septa** develop. Detached parts of the septa, which are connected to the villous trees only by some interposed fibrinoid, make up a subpopulation of the **cell islands** (see below).

Structure at Term

The mature basal plate is of variable thickness, ranging from 100 μm to 1.5 mm. At term, it has lost its typical earlier layering in most places

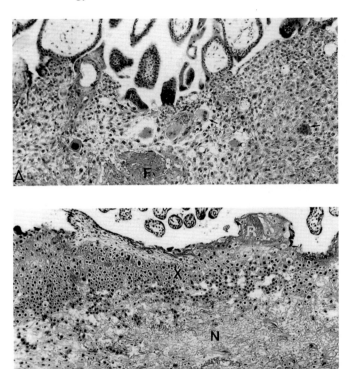

Figure 8.12. Developmental stages of the basal plate, paraffin sections. (A) At the 8th week PM. The basal plate is composed of a dense mixture of extravillous trophoblastic and decidual cells, intermingled with a few trophoblastic giant cells (arrows). There is little fibrinoid (F). ×75. (B) At the 23rd week of gestation the typical layering of the basal plate is evident. Facing the intervillous space, it is covered by an interrupted layer of Rohr's fibrinoid (R), followed by a nearly complete layer of extravillous cytotrophoblast (X). The latter is largely separated from the decidua cells (D) by a loose layer of Nitabuch's fibrinoid (N). ×85.

(Figure 8.13). The following layers make up the mature basal plate (from the superficial surface to the deep maternal surface), but only rarely can all the layers be identified in an undisturbed order.

- **Inner surface**
- **Rohr's fibrinoid**
- **Principal layer**
- **Nitabuch's fibrinoid**
- **Separation zone**

The **inner surface** of the basal plate faces the intervillous space. It shows *residual syncytiotrophoblastic lining* present only in small patches of degenerating syncytium with no underlying cytotrophoblast. *Maternal endothelium* lines the intervillous surface of the basal plate. Where syncytiotrophoblast and maternal endothelium are absent, the basal plate is covered by Rohr's fibrinoid. The superficial fibrinoid layer of the basal plate, **Rohr's fibrinoid** is an *incomplete and irregularly structured layer*, consisting of homogeneous or lamellar material (Figure 8.13) and is similar to Langhans' fibrinoid of the chorionic plate. In some areas, it engulfs attached villi and here it is continuous with perivillous fibrinoid. In most places, Rohr's fibrinoid consists of *fibrin*, but where it encases extravillous trophoblastic cells, usually near cell columns, patches of fibrinoid can also be found.

The **principal layer** is highly variable in composition and measures from 50 µm to 1 mm in thickness. It is composed of *extravillous cytotrophoblast, fibrinoid, loose connective tissue, decidual cells, remnants of encased anchoring villi, and "buried" cell columns*. Most of the connective tissue of this region is of maternal origin and is composed of *decidual cells, fibroblast-like cells, and some macrophages*. The extravillous trophoblastic cells arise from the cell columns and are largely of the nonproliferative, invasive phenotype. Cytotrophoblast and decidual cells may be intensively admixed but do not have direct contact as they are separated by fibrinoid, the external lamina of the decidual cells, or both.

Nitabuch's fibrinoid layer, also called *uteroplacental fibrinoid*, is a netlike or lamellar structure (see Figure 8.12). It consists of both fibrinoid and fibrin and is located in the immediate maternofetal "battle-

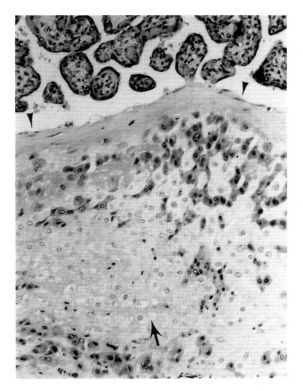

Figure 8.13. Extravillous trophoblastic cells (dark cells) in decidua basalis of a near-term placenta. The arrow indicates a decidual stromal cell. The endothelial cells that are believed to line the basal portion of the intervillous space, above Rohr's fibrin layer, are indicated by arrowheads. H&E. ×240.

field" of the junctional zone. This fibrinoid layer is a rather consistent, more or less uninterrupted layer that varies from 20 μm to more than 100 μm in thickness. In the most complete areas, Nitabuch's fibrinoid separates superficial trophoblastic cells from decidual cells and marks the *exact maternofetal border*. In many places, the layer may split and rejoin, with trophoblast, decidual cells, or endometrial connective tissue interposed. Mixed populations of the two cell types on one or both sides of this layer are the most typical finding.

The **separation zone** of the placenta from the placental bed is usually not located within Nitabuch's fibrinoid; rather, placental separation occurs in most cases somewhat deeper. Therefore, some additional tissues may be attached to the placental floor and form the deepest layer of the basal plate. Most cells in this layer are *decidual cells, endometrial stroma, and trophoblastic elements*. Multinucleated giant cells may also be present. The deeper tissue layers of the placental site, which remain in utero and are later discharged as lochia, show a similar admixture of maternal and placental tissues and are referred to as the **placental bed**. In situ, the placental bed and basal plate cannot be delimited from each other because the demarcation zone becomes visible only shortly before delivery. Therefore, they together comprise the "**junctional zone**" for in situ specimens and include all tissue of maternal, fetal, and mixed origin that lies basal to the intervillous space. The term *basal plate is applicable only to the delivered placenta*.

Placental separation depends on the existence of decidua at the placental site. Where a decidual layer is lacking, as with an extrauterine pregnancy or placenta accreta (see Chapter 12), the placenta cannot separate spontaneously. Placental separation occurs primarily on a mechanical basis, in that *the contracting uterus creates a shearing force, which separates it from the noncompressible placenta*. There are decidual changes before separation, including a reduction in collagen fibers, an accumulation of interstitial fluid, and degenerative changes and thinning of the decidual spongy zone. After placental separation, both surfaces, those of the placental bed and the basal plate, are covered by a thin layer of fibrin, which is thought to be deposited during or slightly after delivery of the placenta.

Marginal Zone

The marginal zone is not precisely defined and consists of the *transitional zone between the chorionic plate, the basal plate, and the membranes*. It has characteristics of all three regions. The internal margin, which by definition separates it from the chorionic plate, is the line connecting those points where the most peripheral branches of the chorionic plate vessels dive vertically into the placenta. The outer margin, which separates it from the membranes, is the grossly visible transition from placenta to membranes. At this point, the intervillous space is occluded by fusion of the chorionic plate with the basal plate.

Macroscopically, the marginal zone is often represented by a slightly prominent *opaque ring in the subchorionic region*, called the **subchorionic**

closing ring. It measures about 1 cm in width. The opacity of the sub-chorionic closing ring is due to an increased number of extravillous trophoblastic cells and decidual cells. The presence of the subchorionic closing ring nearer to the center of the placenta is referred to as a **circumvallate placenta** (see Chapter 13). In histologic preparations of the marginal zone, connective tissue trabeculae are continuous with the peripheral branches of the villous trees. The trabeculae extend into the membranes and end blindly in the decidua. They are thought to be important for the *mechanical stability of the marginal zone and for anchoring the membranes to the placenta.*

Large uteroplacental veins present near the placental margin open into the intervillous space and comprise the **marginal sinus**. They are *an area of venous outflow.* The border between the maternal veins and the intervillous space is difficult to define for two reasons. First, maternal endothelial cells spread from the venous lumina and line the intervillous surfaces of the basal and chorionic plates in the entire marginal zone. Second, the smooth muscle cells of the venous media also extend far into the placenta and form a muscular ring around the placental margin, extending to both the basal plate and chorionic plate. The initial part of the marginal uteroplacental veins is largely replaced by fibrinoid, and signs of cellular degeneration can be observed in the surrounding tissues. It is likely that the thin peripheral decidual cover is responsible for the occurrence of the so-called marginal sinus hemorrhage.

Placental Septa

Placental septa are found in nearly every mature placenta. Their absence is rare and is usually linked to pathologic conditions. They are *irregular protrusions of the basal plate* into the placenta composed of fibrinoid and various cells (Figure 8.14). Short basal plate protrusions into the intervillous space, precursors of future septa, are visible as early as in the sixth week post menstruation (PM) (Figure 8.15). These early septa consist of *cytotrophoblast with anchoring villi near their tips.* They further develop by traction on the anchoring villi combined with excessive proliferation of their cytotrophoblastic feet. Ultimately, there is buckling or folding of the basal decidua induced by the pressure of expanding villous lobules without distension of the uterine wall (Figure 8.14).

In the mature placenta, septa are shaped like irregular plates or pillars that *partially subdivide the intervillous space.* Their position normally corresponds to that of the grooves that are visible at the basal surface of the delivered placenta (see Figure 3.7, page 30), hence their designation "**intercotyledonary septa.**" Most often, they are shallow, measuring between 12 and 18 mm in height, originating from the floor of the placenta but rarely reaching the fetal surface. Because septa develop from the basal plate, their composition generally resembles that of the basal plate. Specifically, they are composed of **decidual cells** and **extravillous trophoblastic cells** embedded in **fibrinoid** and partly

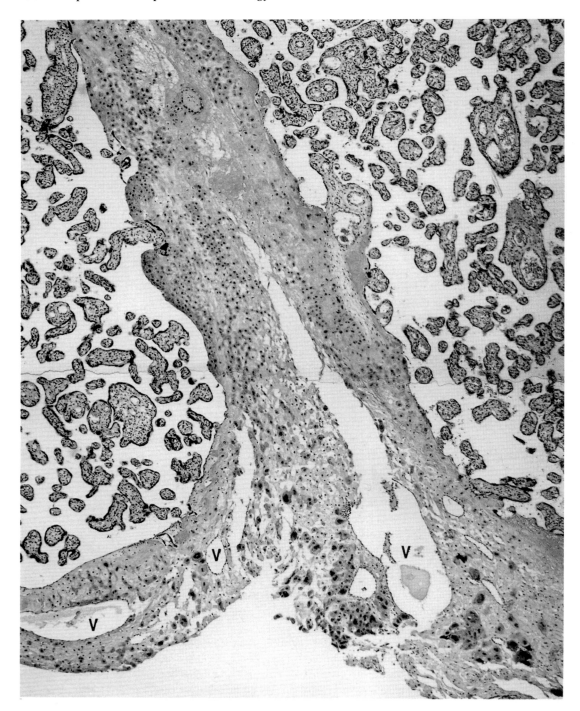

Figure 8.14. Paraffin section of a placental septum, 37th week PM. Note the numerous anchoring villi inserting at the septum. In its base several vessel cross sections (V) represent uteroplacental veins. ×65.

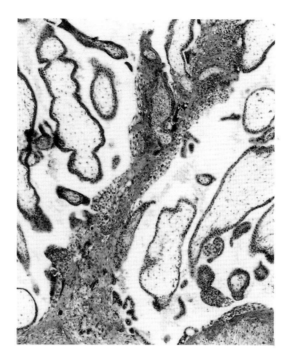

Figure 8.15. Paraffin section of an early placental septum (middle) during the eighth week PM. In this stage the septa have a cellular composition similar to that of the early basal plate. They are largely devoid of fibrinoid and can be interpreted as being extensions and folds of the early basal plate. ×90.

surrounded by **fibrin**. Anchoring villi are attached to the septa by means of cell columns, the latter representing the foci of extravillous trophoblastic proliferation. In addition, the septa may contain all other basal plate constituents such as endometrial glands and vessels. *In early pregnancy (Figure 8.15) the septa are composed mostly of cells; with advancing gestation fibrinoid is accumulated and embeds the extravillous trophoblastic cells.* From the intervillous space, fibrin is added. *At term, fibrin and fibrinoid are the predominant elements of septa.*

Septa are a frequent site of **placental cysts** (Figure 8.16). They may occasionally be grossly visible; microscopically they can be found in nearly every placenta. Septal cysts consist of trophoblastic cells surrounding a cystic space and are histologically similar to the cysts of the cell islands. They often show necrosis, and thus it has been suggested that they are degenerative in nature.

Cell Islands

Cell islands are round or irregularly shaped structures *connected to either the villous tree or the chorionic plate.* Their diameters vary from several hundred micrometers to 3 mm. They are composed primarily of *extravillous trophoblastic cells encased in fibrinoid without an admixture of decidual cells* (Figure 8.17). They resemble septa in structure and com-

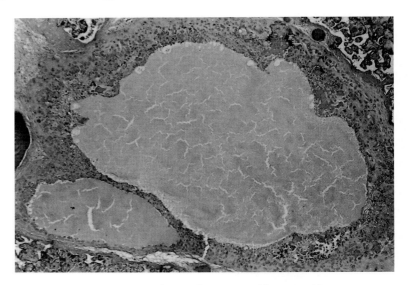

Figure 8.16. Placental septum with cyst. ×40.

position and, in histologic sections, often cannot be differentiated from them. Cell islands are comparable to the basal ends of the anchoring villi, the **cell columns** (see below). *The major difference between a cell island and a cell column is the topographic relation: Cell islands are freely floating cell columns; cell columns are anchored to the basal plate or to septa.* The extravillous trophoblast are not in contact with decidual tissues and so do not invade decidual tissues but rather migrate within

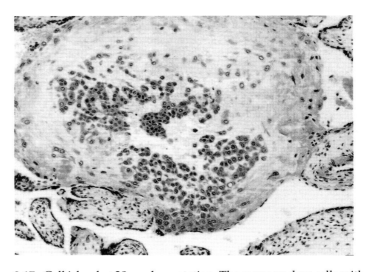

Figure 8.17. Cell island at 20 weeks gestation. The mononuclear cells with dark cytoplasm in the center are the extravillous trophoblastic cells. They are surrounded by "fibrinoid.". Note that there is no differentiation to syncytium among the extravillous trophoblast cells. Incorporated decidual cells are rare findings. The surrounding placental villi may be attached to the surface; sometimes they are incorporated into the fibrinoid. H&E. ×160.

their own extracellular matrix. They ultimately degenerate and form cysts.

Cell Columns

Cell columns are the *trophoblastic connections between the anchoring villi and basal plate or placental septa*. The development of cell columns starts around day 15 PC when the primary villi become invaded by extraembryonic mesenchyme and form tertiary villi. These processes spread from the chorionic plate peripherally but do not reach the basal plate. Instead, *the basal parts of the villous stems that are connected to the basal plate persist as primary villi. These massive trophoblastic segments of the anchoring villi are called the* **cell columns**. These developmental events are identical to those at some free-floating villous tips, leading to the formation of cell islands.

Cell columns are composed of a **multilayered core of cytotrophoblast** surrounded by an incomplete sleeve of **syncytiotrophoblast**. As soon as cell columns are surrounded by fibrinoid and buried in the basal plate, their syncytiotrophoblastic cover becomes replaced by **fibrin** (Figure 8.18). The cytotrophoblastic core continues without sharp demarcation into the anchoring villus. The cell columns represent the *proliferative zones of extravillous trophoblast,* and the various steps from trophoblastic proliferation via differentiation to invasion are present in these columns. The cell columns are an indispensable source of tro-

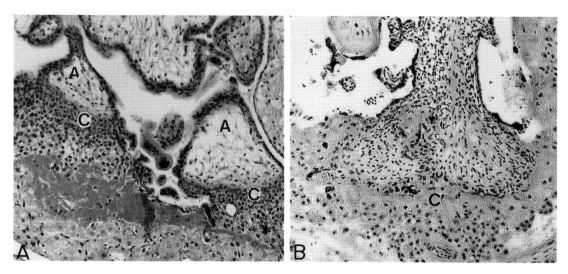

Figure 8.18. Histology of cell columns. (A) At the 15th week PM the anchoring villi (A) are connected to the basal plate (below) by broad or slender feet consisting of cytotrophoblast, the so-called cell columns (C). They are proliferative zones for the villous trophoblast and trophoblast of the basal plate. ×95. (B) At the 28th week PM, the cell columns are deeply incorporated into the basal plate by surrounding fibrinoid deposition. Also, its cytotrophoblast is progressively replaced by fibrinoid, indicating reduced proliferative activity of these growth zones. ×95.(From Kaufmann P, Entwicklung der Plazenta. In: Die Plazenta des Menschen. V Becker, ThH Schiebler, F. Kubli, eds. Stuttgart: Thieme, 1981, with permission.)

phoblastic proliferation, and *all extravillous trophoblastic cells invading the basal plate and the placental bed derive from this stem cell population* (see Figure 8.1). *Cells derived from this stem cell population migrate laterally into the villi as well as basally into the basal plate.* With advancing gestation, the number of cells is reduced by decreasing proliferation and continuous migration. In some places, there are almost no trophoblastic cells left so that anchoring villous stroma and the nearly naked basal lamina directly face basal plate fibrinoid. However, even at term, one can still can find largely intact cell columns.

Selected References

PHP4, Chapter 9, pages 171–188.

Arias-Stella J. Gestational endometrium. In: Norris HJ, Hertig AT, Abel AT, Abel MR (eds) The uterus. Baltimore: Williams & Wilkins, 1973:183–212.

Boyd JD, Hamilton WJ. Placental septa. Z Zellforsch 1966;69:613–634.

Boyd JD, Hamilton WJ. The human placenta. Cambridge: Heffer & Sons, 1970.

Brosens I, Robertson WB, Dixon HG. The physiological response of the vessels of the placental bed to normal pregnancy. J Pathol Bacteriol 1967;93:569–579.

Enders AC. Fine structure of anchoring villi of the human placenta. Am J Anat 1968;122:419–452.

Fisher SJ, Librac C, Zhou Y, et al. Regulation of human cytotrophoblast invasion. Placenta 1992;13:A.17.

Frank HG, Malekzadeh F, Kertschanska S, et al. Immunohistochemistry of two different types of placental fibrinoid. Acta Anat 1994;150:55–68.

Grünwald P. The lobular architecture of the human placenta. Bull Johns Hopkins Hosp 1966;119:172–190.

Hunt JS. Immunobiology of the maternal-fetal interface. Prenat Neonat Med 1998;3:72–75.

Kaufmann P, Castellucci M. Extravillous trophoblast in the human placenta. Trophoblast Res 1997;10:21–65.

Kaufmann P, Huppertz B, Frank HG. The fibrinoids of the human placenta: origin, composition and functional relevance. Ann Anat 1996;178:485–501.

Loke YW, King A. Human implantation: cell biology and immunology. Cambridge: Cambridge University Press, 1995.

Pijnenborg R, Dixon G, Robertson WB, et al. Trophoblastic invasion of human decidua from 8 to 18 weeks of pregnancy. Placenta 1980;1:3–19.

Wigglesworth JS. Vascular anatomy of the human placenta and its significance for placental pathology. J Obstet Gynaecol Br Commonw 1969;76:979–989.

Section III
Multiple Gestation

This section is concerned exclusively with the placentas of twins and multiple births. Chapter 9 covers basic issues in twin placentation such as incidence and zygosity, discusses the types and origins of twin placentation, and covers aspects of the gross examination that are particular to twin placentas. Diamnionic-dichorionic, diamnionic-monochorionic, and monoamnionic-monochorionic placentation are specifically addressed in this chapter. Chapter 10 continues with specifics of pathogenesis, pathology, and clinical features of twin variants such as fetus papyraceous, conjoined twins, and acardiac twins as well as twin-to-twin transfusion. Chimerism, mosaicism, sacrococcygeal teratoma, and epignathus are also discussed as these topics have significance in the study of multiple gestations.

Chapter 9

Multiple Gestation: General Aspects

General Considerations

There is no doubt that the complexity of human twinning cannot be understood without knowledge of placentation, and placental examination is vital to this endeavor. Examination of the placenta also contributes to the determination of zygosity as well as an understanding of abnormal events. With the advent of assisted reproductive technology, twins and higher multiple gestations are becoming more common. Because multiple gestations represent a disproportionate portion of complications with *higher rates of prematurity, perinatal morbidity, perinatal mortality, and malformations than singletons,* placental examination has become especially important.

Zygosity

With regard to zygosity, there are generally two types of twins, "fraternal" or **dizygotic (DZ) twins** and "identical" or **monozygotic (MZ) twins**. In higher multiple births, these types are often admixed. *MZ twins arise from fertilization of one ovum by one sperm with subsequent division of the zygote into two genetically identical individuals. DZ twins arise from fertilization of two ova by two sperm, resulting in two nonidentical individuals.* MZ twins by definition are identical genotypically and phenotypically and are of like sex. DZ twins often have significant phenotypic similarity due to their relationship as siblings and may be of different or like sex. An interesting, but as yet unexplained, observation is that among DZ twins there is an excess of like-sex pairs.

Incidence

The overall twinning rate has, for many years, been constant at a rate of 1 in 80 births. However, with the advent of assisted reproductive technology, the twinning rate has increased dramatically and is now approximately 1 in 30 births. The occurrence of higher multiple births, such as triplets, quadruplets, etc., has commonly been estimated by the "Hellin–Zeleny" hypothesis. This useful approximation says that if twins occur with a frequency of $1/N$, then triplets have a frequency of $(1/N)^2$, quadruplets have a frequency of $(1/N)^3$, and so on. The *DZ twinning rate varies with ethnicity, race, and geographic location* and is estimated to be 1.4 to 49.0 per 1000 births. This, of course, only applies to spontaneous conceptions. In contrast, *the MZ twinning rate is nearly constant* at about 3.5 per 1000 births. The sex proportion of all MZ twins is 0.487 while DZ twins have a proportion of 0.518. In other words, MZ twins are more commonly female. Conjoined twins and acardiac twins (see Chapter 10) are also more commonly female, while abortuses are more often male. Theories abound to explain these phenomena, but at present the cause is unknown.

Twin Placentation

There are three types of twin placentation: **diamnionic-dichorionic (DiDi)**, **diamnionic-monochorionic (DiMo)**, and **monoamnionic-monochorionic (MoMo)**. This nomenclature is based on which of the fetal membranes the twins share (Figure 9.1). In DiDi placentas, each twin has its own chorion and amnion; in DiMo placentas, twins share the chorion but have separate amnions; and in MoMo placentas, both amnion and chorion are shared and the twins reside in the same amniotic cavity. *Monochorionic placentas **always** come from MZ (identical) twins. Dichorionic placentas, however, may occur with both DZ and MZ twins.* About 20% of all twin placentas will be DiMo (and thus MZ), 35% will be DiDi twins of different sex and thus DZ, and 45% will be DiDi of the same sex. Of the latter, only 18% will be MZ. Therefore, overall, 72% of twins are DZ and 28% are MZ.

In MZ twins, different types of placentation and twinning occur depending on when the split occurs. They may be DiDi, DiMo, or MoMo, and the later the split, the more structures they share (Figure 9.2). If the split occurs before the formation of the blastocyst in the first 5 to 6 days after fertilization, two separate chorions will develop and the placentation will be DiDi. Even if they are dichorionic, the disks are *almost* always fused. This occurs in approximately 25% of MZ twins. If the split occurs after formation of the chorion but before formation of the amnion, 7 to 8 days after fertilization, the placenta will be DiMo. This is the most common type of MZ twins, occurring in approximately

Dizygotic Twins

Monozygotic Twins

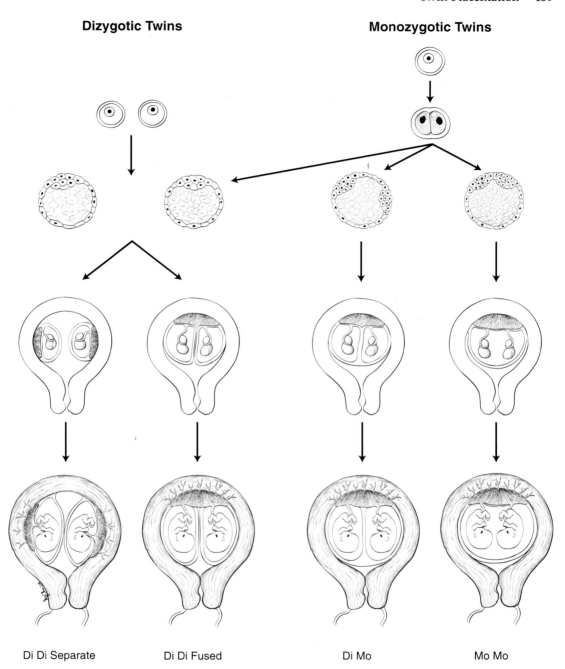

Di Di Separate   Di Di Fused   Di Mo   Mo Mo

Figure 9.1. Diagram of types of placentation in dizygotic and monozygotic twins. Dizygotic twinning results in two zygotes. If these implant close together, a fused placenta results, and if they implant far apart, separate placentas result. Depending on which the embryonic split occurs, monozygotic twinning may result in fused or separate diamnionic-dichorionic placentation (DiDi), diamnionic-monochorionic placentation (DiMo) or monoamnionic-monochorionic placentation (MoMo).

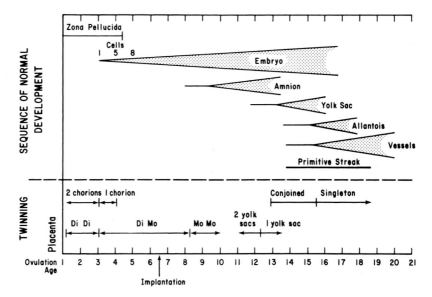

Figure 9.2. Interpretation of early events in monozygotic (MZ) twinning. Embryonic events are depicted in the upper portion. The bottom portion suggests that certain placental structures result if twinning occurs at certain times. It is also assumed that with later development (after day 8) MZ twinning becomes ever more difficult. Once the primitive streak is formed, conjoined twins may develop at first. Soon, however, the presumed twinning "impetus" is ineffective. DiDi, diamnionic-dichorionic; DiMo, diamnionic-monochorionic; MoMo, monoamnionic-monochorionic.

75%. If the split occurs after formation of the amnion, but before the formation of the embryonic axis, from 9 to 15 days after fertilization, there will be one amnion and one chorion and the placenta will be **MoMo**. Later splitting will result in varying degrees of **conjoined twins**. The MoMo placenta is rare, occurring in less than 1% of MZ twins. It is also associated with the highest perinatal morbidity and mortality in twins.

Twin placentas from DZ twins are always DiDi but may have different configurations, depending on where the two zygotes implant (see Figure 9.1). If the zygotes implant close together, the placental disks will become fused as they grow, forming a **fused DiDi placenta**. If they implant further from each other, they will became **separate DiDi placentas**. At times, the placental disks may be separate but the membranes may be "fused."

Pathogenesis
A fundamental difference exists in the respective etiologies of DZ and MZ twins. DZ twins (and higher multiples) are the result of *polyovulation, a process that is familial, likely hereditary, and related to ethnicity, race, and maternal age.* Polyovulation may be related to increased FSH production, increased GnRH production, or greater follicle sensitivity to FSH. Polyovulation can be induced by the administration of

gonadotropins and other hormones, as is evident from their use for stimulation of ovulation in infertility patients. Follicle-stimulating hormone (FSH), and to a lesser extent luteinizing hormone (LH) and estradiol, is elevated in twin-bearing mothers, suggesting that the genesis of DZ twins is at least partially caused by excess production of FSH. Genes responsible for higher FSH levels may explain the why DZ twins run in families and why racial differences in DZ twinning rates exist. There is a steady rise in DZ twinning up to the maternal age of 35 and then after that, a sharp decline.

Although DZ twinning is familial, it is not so for MZ twinning. The incidence of *MZ twinning* is nearly the same throughout the world and appears to be a *sporadic event, unrelated to heredity*. The actual cause of MZ twinning is not fully understood, but it appears that *MZ twins originate from the spontaneous separation of the blastomeres occurring at random during the early embryonic period*. Interestingly, although multiple births after gonadotropin stimulation are generally multizygotic, there is often an admixture of DZ and MZ infants. In vitro fertilization has 12 times the expected MZ twinning rate compared to single sperm injection fertilization.

Clinical Features and Implications

The incidence of **congenital anomalies** in twins is higher than in singleton gestations. *Anomalies occur with a frequency of approximately 10% in twins, 3 times the singleton rate*. Discordance for anomalies between twins is common, and the discordance is higher in MZ compared to DZ twins, reaching 80%. Triplets and higher multiples share this discordance as well. Certain anomalies are much more common in twins; for instance, sirenomelia is increased 100 fold in twins versus singletons. Some anomalies, such as anencephaly, occur in DZ twins with the same frequency as in singletons but are increased in MZ twins. Other anomalies such as porencephaly and visceral ischemic lesions are much more commonly seen in MZ as they are *related to the vascular anastomoses in the placentas* of these twins (see Chapter 10). Most anomalies in twins have no evidence of a genetic component even though anomalies with a strong genetic etiology, such as cleft lip and cleft palate, are frequently discordant in MZ twins. Possible explanations for the increased incidence of anomalies and the discordance include adverse placentation [e.g., velamentous insertion of cord or single umbilical artery (SUA)] or unequal splitting.

Umbilical cord abnormalities are much more common in multiple gestations, and this includes **velamentous cord insertion, marginal cord insertion, SUA**, and **hypocoiled umbilical cords** (see Chapter 15). Velamentous insertion is nine times more common in twins than in singletons. Marginal insertions are found twice as often in twins, and both velamentous and marginal insertions are found twice as frequently in monochorionic placentas compared to dichorionic placentas. Membranous umbilical vessels are susceptible to *compression, thrombosis, and rupture*, and if membranous vessels are present over the cervical os (vasa previa), they may rupture during delivery and lead to fetal exsanguinations. Cord prolapse may also occur. Abnormal cord insertions and SUA in turn are often associated with *preterm delivery, premature rupture of membranes, fetal anomalies, and fetal growth restriction*. Growth discrepancies are seen quite commonly in monochorionic twins with velamentous insertions.

The mortality of twins is also much greater than that of singletons, being approximately 10%. Prematurity is one of the most important factors in determining outcome, and this is significantly increased in multiple gestations. In addition, monochorionic twins generally deliver earlier than dichorionic twins. *Monochorionic twins have a higher mortality rate than that of dichorionic twins and the mortality of monoamnionic twins is the highest.* This difference is predominantly due to the consequences of vascular anastomoses. Perinatal mortality increases exponentially with each higher multiple offspring, being approximately 16% in triplets, 21% in quadruplets, and 41% in quintuplets. This is one of the prime motivators for the practice of "fetal reduction" during early pregnancy in which triplets are "reduced" to twins.

Numerous maternal complications are associated with multiple gestation as well. These include *premature delivery, preeclampsia, polyhydramnios, placenta previa, abruptio placentae, uterine inertia, and postpartum hemorrhage*. Placental abnormalities often mirror these events. Hydramnios in twin pregnancies is most commonly due to the transfusion syndrome but may also be secondary to fetal or placental anomalies. Uterine atony and postpartum hemorrhage are most likely caused by increased uterine distension from multiple pregnancy.

Examination of the Placenta in Multiple Gestation

Gross Examination

Examination of the placenta in multiple gestations involves all the aspects of examination of the singleton placenta. There is then the added complexity of the relationship between the placentas and the fetuses. To derive benefit from the study of twin or multiple births, it is mandatory that the umbilical cords be labeled in the order as they are delivered for identification of the infants with their respective placentas. This of course must be done in the delivery room, and a standard protocol for identification of multiples should be used. For example, ties or clamps may be placed around the placental cut ends of the cords and optimally around individual cord fragments. The first placenta and infant, "A," should be labeled with one tie or clamp, "B" with two ties or clamps, "C" with three, and so on. The labeling should be explained on the requisition, e.g. A = 1 clamp, etc.

In twins there are several additional features than need to be evaluated:

- The relationship of the placental disks:
  ○ If separate, the placentation is **DiDi separate**
  ○ If separate, but connected by membranes, the placentation is **DiDi separate**
  ○ If fused, the placentation is **DiDi fused** or **DiMo**.

- Examination of the nature of the dividing membranes:
  - Sections should be taken of the dividing membranes, either by excising and rolling a square of these dividing membranes, or by taking a section from the site where the membranes insert on the surface, the so-called "T zone" or "T section."

The experienced examiner may make the diagnosis of DiMo versus DiDi twin placentation by macroscopic inspection using the following criteria:

- The dividing membranes of DiMo placentas, with only **two amnions**, are usually *translucent, thin, and contain no blood vessel remnants* (Figure 9.3).

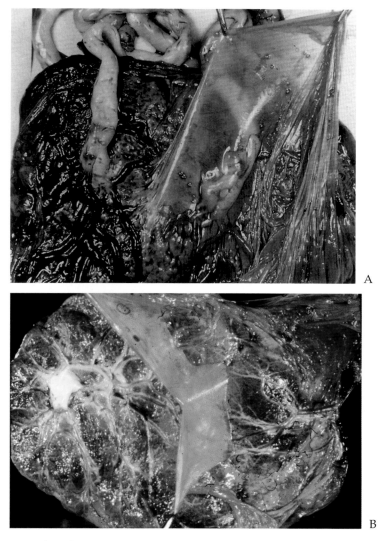

A

B

Figure 9.3. (A, B) Diamnionic-monochorionic twin placenta. The "dividing membranes" are held up to disclose their transparency. (See Figure 9.4 for contrast with DiDi placenta.)

- DiDi membrane partitions, with **two amnions and chorions**, are more *opaque, containing remnants of vessels* that are grossly visible as fine branching streaks (Figure 9.4).
- The fetal surface of DiDi placentas show a white, slightly elevated *ridge of fibrin* not present in DiMo placentas (Figure 9.4). This is the **twin peak** sign seen by sonography.
- The area of fusion between the two placentas, the **vascular equator**, will show an abrupt termination of the surface vessels from each placenta in a DiDi placenta, while in the DiMo placenta, vessels will cross, intermingle, and anastomose (Figures 9.3, 9.4).

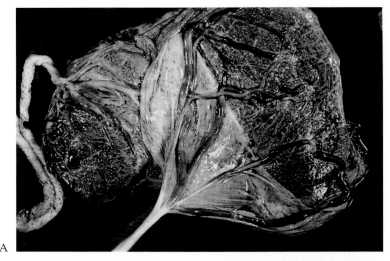

A

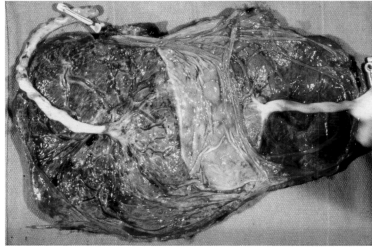

B

Figure 9.4. (A, B) DiDi fused twin placenta with visible ridge on the fetal surface at the dividing membranes. The latter appear opaque and thicker than those seen in Figure 9.3.

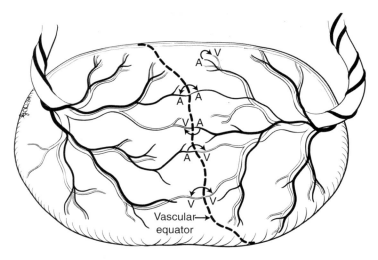

Figure 9.5. Diagram of the vascular equator of a DiMo twin placenta to show A-A, V-V and A-V anastomoses. The normal pairing of artery and vein derived from one twin is also depicted (top). A = artery, V = vein.

Examination of Vascular Anastomoses

Monochorionic placentas virtually always have blood vessel connections or anastomoses between the two placentas. Vascular anastomoses may be arteriovenous (either from A to B or from B to A), vein to vein, or artery to artery (Figure 9.5). Injecting fluid in one vessel and documenting its appearance in the circulation of the other placenta facilitates examination of the vascular anatomy. *General examination of the placenta should be completed first, but samples for histological study should only be removed after injection has been done.* **Milk, water, any colored liquid**, or even **air** may be used for injection. The following procedure is recommended:

- The umbilical cords should be cut near the placental surface to reduce vascular resistance.
- The amnion should be stripped from the chorionic surface to better expose the vessels.
  - Arteries and veins can be distinguished by the fact that **arteries cross over veins**. A ratio of 1:1 is usually found in the final vascular ramifications.
- The major vessels may be followed to their ends visually, and it is usually quite clear which vessels are likely to have communications between the two fetal circulations.
- A-A and V-V anastomoses will appear as direct connections between vessels from one placenta to the other. A-A are the most common type and V-V are the least common type. *To demonstrate these anastomoses, it is often sufficient to stroke the blood back and forth through the vessels.*
- A-V anastomoses are more difficult to demonstrate. Normally, the fetal arteries terminate in the periphery, dip into the villous tissue, and emerge as nearby veins, which then course back toward the

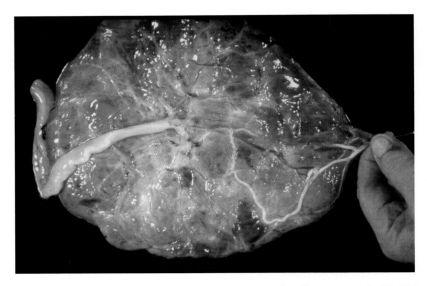

Figure 9.6. Injection technique for demonstration of A-V anastomosis. Fluid is injected while holding the vessel around the needle to prevent leakage.

umbilical cord. Injection is suggested to conclusively demonstrate these anastomoses (Figures 9.5, 9.6).

○ Injection of deep A-V anastomoses:
  ▪ These perfuse a shared cotyledon.
  ▪ A needle is inserted into a vessel near the point of presumed anastomosis and then, holding to the needle to prevent back-pressure, the liquid is gently injected (Figure 9.6). Alternatively, an umbilical vessel may be injected.
  ▪ One cotyledon will distend as the fluid is accumulated. After a short time, the fluid will emerge from a vessel in the other placenta.

• It is suggested that the vascular relationships be *recorded in a drawing*, if complicated.

Following examination of anastomoses and examination and sectioning of the dividing membranes, the remaining routine sections of each placenta should be taken (see Chapter 3).

Diamnionic-Dichorionic Twin Placenta

The DiDi twin placenta is the most common type of twin placenta. Sections of the dividing membranes in fused DiDi placentas will easily demonstrate the presence of two amnions and two chorions (Figures 9.7, 9.8). DiDi placentas share with the other types of twins an *increased frequency of marginal and velamentous insertion of the umbilical cord and single umbilical artery*. With rare exception, DiDi placentas have no vascular anastomoses. A very common feature of DiDi twin placentas is the phenomenon of **irregular chorionic fusion** (Figure 9.9). Here, the membranes do not meet over the areas perfused by the individual fetuses, and a portion of one may be covered by the membranes of the

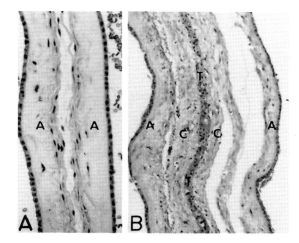

Figure 9.7. (A) Diamnionic (monochorionic) "dividing membranes" of identical (MZ) twins. There is always a space between the two amnions. The amnion usually consists of single layer of cuboidal epithelial cells and scant connective tissue. (B) Diamnionic-dichorionic "dividing membranes." The right amnion is dislodged from the underlying chorion, a frequent artifact. The trophoblastic remnants in between the membranes have fused. A, amnion; C, chorion; T, trophoblast. H&E. ×100.

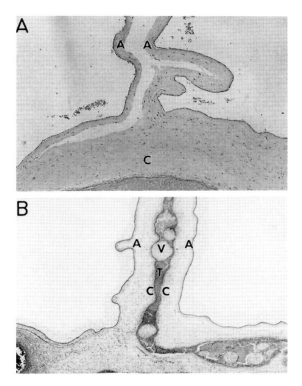

Figure 9.8. (A) T section of dividing membranes of monochorionic diamnionic twins. Note the contiguity of the chorion over the surface of the placenta at bottom. (B) T section of diamnionic-dichorionic twin placenta. There are atrophic villi and trophoblastic remnants between the two chorionic membranes. Again, the two chorions appear to have fused. A, amnion; C, chorion; T, trophoblast; V, atrophic villi. H&E. ×40.

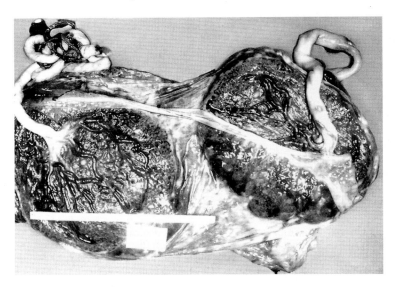

Figure 9.9. DiDi twin placenta with "irregular chorionic fusion." The chorion laeve of the left placenta overlaps one-third of the placenta at right. There is no vascular fusion.

other. This condition develops when the intraamniotic fluid pressure of one cavity expands its sac and pushes the other away. It is not unlike the process of lifting the marginal chorion in cases of circumvallate placentation (see Chapter 13). As a result, the "vascular equator" is usually **not** in the same location as the dividing membranes. This is particularly important in the determination of the weights of the respective placentas. *One must always separate twin placentas along the vascular equator and **not** along the dividing membranes.* The irregular fusion has no influence on fetal well-being, and no vascular fusion takes place in the areas of overlap.

Diamnionic-Monochorionic Twin Placenta

The DiMo twin placenta is the most common placentation in MZ twins. Both twins reside in the same chorionic sac, but each twin is enclosed in its own amniotic sac. The "dividing membranes" are composed of two amnions only (see Figures 9.7, 9.8). Similar to DiDi twins, the membranes may move over the surface before birth, and the dividing membranes are often at a place that does not correspond with the vascular equator (see above). The cord insertion is often marginal or velamentous, and single umbilical artery in one or both twins is much more common than in singletons.

Monoamnionic-Monochorionic Twin Placenta

The MoMo twin placenta is the least common type and occurs only once in 10,000 to 16,000 pregnancies or once in 100 sets of twins. The fetal surface of MoMo twin placentas usually has a continuous sheet of amnion without ridges or folds between the cord insertions. By definition, there are no dividing membrane. The umbilical cords usually *insert close to each other on the placental surface* (Figures 9.10, 9.11). There may also be a *single fused cord or a forked cord* (Figure 9.12). Since the yolk sac develops around day 11, MoMo twin placentas may have a partially divided yolk sac or two yolk sacs. Anastomoses of fetal blood vessels are even more common in MoMo placentas than in DiMo twin placentas and are often large, this perhaps being the reason for the rarity of the twin-to-twin transfusion syndrome in MoMo twins (see Chapter 10).

When examining the apparent MoMo placenta, one must be mindful of artifacts causing a **"pseudomonoamnionic" placenta**. Disruption of the membranes during delivery may cause the dividing membranes to be pulled away from the fetal surface, giving the erroneous impression of a MoMo placenta. The intertwin membranes may spontaneously rupture prenatally, or there may be intentional rupture of the membrane for therapeutic purposes such as amniocentesis, funipucture, or treatment for twin-to-twin transfusion syndrome (see Chapter 10). These events may make it impossible to differentiate a DiMo from a MoMo placenta. Clinical history and the position of the cords may be helpful. If the dividing membranes are disrupted before delivery, morbidity and mortality may occur from cord entanglements just as with true MoMo twins.

The perinatal mortality of MoMo twins reaches 40%. Fetal death most commonly occurs due to entanglement of the umbilical cords from fetal movement resulting in venous obstruction (see Figure 9.11). Knotting of the cords is unpredictable and is often found in very young

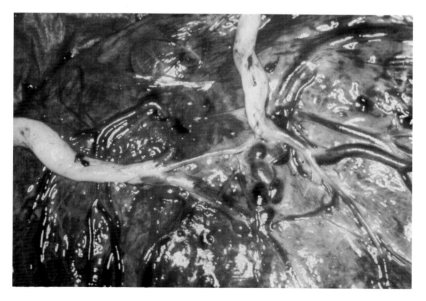

Figure 9.10. MoMo twin placenta with amnions removed. The cords insert next to each other, adjacent to major anastomoses visible on the surface.

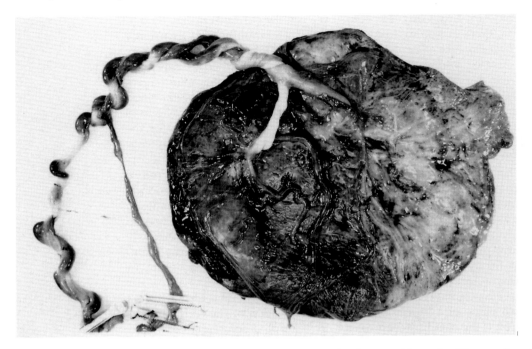

Figure 9.11. MoMo twins at 38 weeks gestation with fetal death of one at 23 weeks. The survivor is alive and well. Note the entangling and knotting of cords, the thin cord of the dead twin, and the extensive infarction of the right placental half.

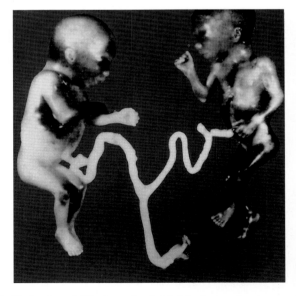

Figure 9.12. Forked umbilical cord of MoMo twin abortuses at 17 weeks gestation. The smaller twin (right) had a single umbilical artery but no other anomalies. (Courtesy Dr. Marilyn Jones, San Diego, CA.)

pregnancies with early abortion ensuing. Fetal demise usually occurs before 24 weeks, when enough room for fetal motions and entanglement is still possible. After 30 to 32 weeks, few deaths occur.

Suggestions for Examination and Report: Twin Placenta

Gross Examination: In DiMo twins, vascular anastomoses should be documented. In all twins with fused placental disks, the dividing membranes should be submitted for microscopic examination. The disks should be separated along the *vascular equator* and then weighed and examined separately. See section above on gross examination for additional details.

Comment: Possible diagnoses are diamnionic-dichorionic (fused or separate) twin placenta(s), diamnionic-monochorionic twin placenta, or monoamnionic-monochorionic twin placenta. A comment on the nature of the vascular anastomoses should also be included. For example, when a single dominant A-V anastomosis is present, the possibility of twin-to-twin transfusion syndrome should be entertained. If multiple anastomoses of various types are present, a comment to that effect should be made. As previously stated, a drawing of the vascular connections can be helpful in many cases.

Selected References

PHP4, Chapter 25, pages 790–796, 801, 804–826, 862–864, 876–878.

Baldwin VJ. Pathology of multiple pregnancy. New York: Springer-Verlag, 1994.

Benirschke K. Twin placenta in perinatal mortality. NY State J Med 1961;61: 1499–1508.

Bleker OP, Breur W, Huidekoper BL. A study of birth weight, placental weight and mortality of twins as compared to singletons. Br J Obstet Gynaecol 1979; 86:111–118.

Bulmer MG. The biology of twinning in man. London: Oxford University Press, 1970.

Cameron AH. The Birmingham twin survey. Proc R Soc Med 1968;61:229–234.

Carr SR, Aronson MP, Coustan DR. Survival rates of monoamniotic twins do not decrease after 30 weeks' gestation. Am J Obstet Gynecol 1990;163: 719–722.

Coulton D, Hertig AT, Long WN. Monoamniotic twins. Am J Obstet Gynecol 1947;54:119–123.

Eberle AM, Levesque D, Vintzileos AM, et al. Placental pathology in discordant twins. Am J Obstet Gynecol 1993;169:931–935.

James WH. Twinning rates. Lancet 1983;1:934–935.

MacGillivray I, Campbell DM, Thompson B (eds) Twinning and twins. Chichester: Wiley, 1988.

Naeye RL, Tafari N, Judge D, et al. Twins: causes of perinatal death in 12 United States cities and one African city. Am J Obstet Gynecol 1978;131: 267–272.

Ramos-Arroyo MA, Ulbright TM, Christian JC. Twin study: relationship between birth weight, zygosity, placentation, and pathologic placental changes. Acta Genet Med Gemellol 1988;37:229–238.

Robertson JG. Twin pregnancy: morbidity and fetal mortality. Obstet Gynecol 1964;23:330–337.

Spellacy WN, Handler A, Ferre CD. A case-control study of 1253 twin pregnancies from 1982–1987 perinatal data base. Obstet Gynecol 1990;75:168–171.

Chapter 10

Multiple Gestation: Twin Variants and Related Conditions

Vanishing Twin and Fetus Papyraceous

Clinical Features and Implications

The phenomenon of a "**vanishing twin**" occurs when a *multiple pregnancy is identified sonographically during the first 15 weeks of pregnancy, but the outcome is a single fetus*. When the diagnosis of twins is made before 10 weeks, the rate of disappearance is 71%. When the diagnosis is made between 10 and 15 weeks, the disappearance rate is 62%. Twins first diagnosed after 15 weeks more often develop a fetus papyraceous when one twin dies. A clue to the presence of a vanished twin or fetus papyraceous may be an elevation in maternal α-fetoprotein (AFP) or acetylcholinesterase, which occasionally may pose clinical problems.

Pathogenesis

If one twin dies in gestation and the pregnancy continues undisturbed, the fetus may become a **fetus compressus** or **fetus papyraceous**. If the fetus is large, it may macerate, lose much of its fluid, and become *flattened, misshapened, and paper-like*, hence the name. This is most common when death occurs during the second trimester. The fetus papyraceous has become quite common due to the practice of "fetal reduction" used after fertilization via assisted reproductive technology.

Pathologic Features

A fetus papyraceous may be so small and compressed that it is difficult to identify on gross inspection. It may appear as a *flattened disk of macerated tissue in the membranes* of the remaining twin (Figure 10.1). Occasionally, a pigmented macule representing the eye is the only clue to the diagnosis (Figure 10.2) and radiographs or histologic sections may be necessary to document their nature (Figure 10.3). The associated placenta, which is usually completely infarcted, may also be difficult to identify, as it often persists as only a crescent of atrophied tissue at the periphery of its twin. When maceration is advanced, the fetus may become a **lithopedion**. This feature is more common when a fetus is retained for months beyond the expected gestation and need not be a twin.

Suggestions for Examination and Report: Fetus Papyraceous

Gross Examination: Careful examination of membranes is sometimes necessary to identify a fetus papyraceous. Dissection of the dividing membranes between the fetus papyraceous and the other placenta(s) should also be undertaken. Histologic sections of the fetus papyraceous and the associated placenta should be submitted to document their presence.

Comment: The final report should contain a comment about the placentation and zygosity (if possible) along with the diagnosis of a fetus papyraceous.

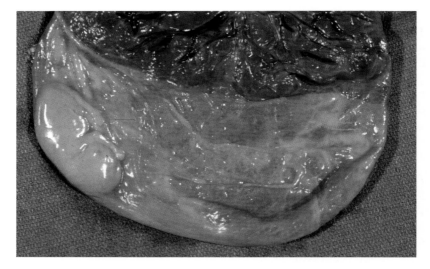

Figure 10.1. Fetus papyraceous (on the left) in the membranes of a twin placenta. Its dichorionic placenta was a flattened mass of atrophied tissue.

Figure 10.2. Term placenta with a separate embryo in the membranes (arrow), a fetus papyraceous. The ocular pigment is readily seen. No placental remains could be identified.

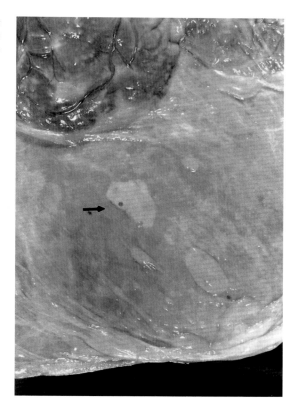

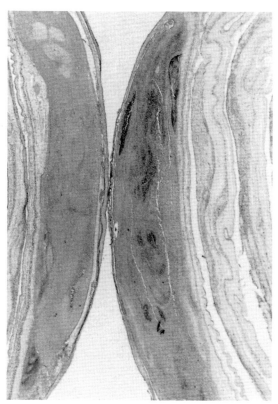

Figure 10.3. Membrane roll of fetus papyraceous with macerated embryonic structures. H&E. ×16.

Acardiac Twins

An **acardiac** fetus is one of *monozygotic (MZ) twins or higher multiples that has absence of the heart or a severely malformed heart.* **Acardiac twins** are the most severely malformed fetuses that one can imagine. They range from a small, teratoma-like mass to large fetuses with a great variety of anomalies. The incidence of acardiac pregnancies is difficult to ascertain, as most are not reported, but an estimation is 1 in 35,000 to 48,000 births. Acardiacs are more common in higher multiple births than in twins. Well over 600 cases have been reported.

Pathogenesis
The acardiac develops due to the presence of *two dominant anastomoses in the monochorial placenta. An artery-to-artery anastomosis brings blood from a usually normal co-twin to the monster, and a vein-to-vein anastomosis returns the blood* (Figure 10.4). The normal twin provides the cardiac flow to the monster but in a reversed fashion. The reversal of blood flow has been proved to exist with the use of Doppler sonography. The presence of the placental anastomoses is the fundamental cause of the acardiac dysmorphism, and therefore dichorionic (and dizygotic, DZ) human twins cannot develop into acardiacs as they lack these communications. The fact that *vascular reversal nourishes the acardiac is without question and this vascular reversal can lead to suppression of cardiac development.* In fact, much of the failure of organ system development is from the deficient circulation, because blood arrives deoxygenated

Acardiac Placenta
Anastomoses in Placenta

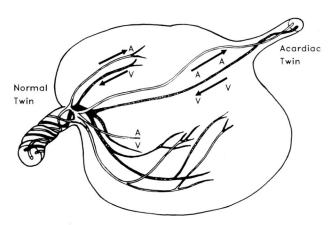

Figure 10.4. Usual pattern of vascular anastomoses in acardiac twins. A = artery; V = vein.

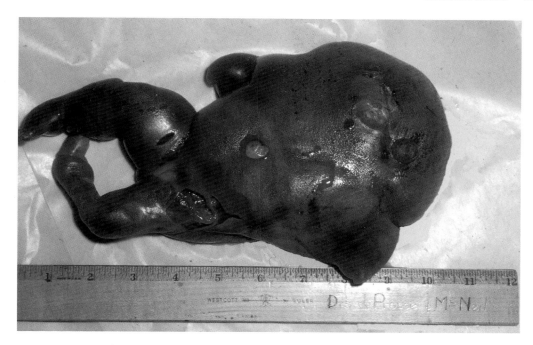

Figure 10.5. Acardiac twin with typical plethoric appearance.

and at a reduced pressure. The fact that the lower limbs of acardiacs are usually better formed than the arms has been considered to result from preferential perfusion of the legs, as they are closest to incoming reversed arterial flow. The term **TRAP (twin reversed arterial perfusion)** has been applied to this syndrome. We believe that many of the previously described placental teratomas are really acardiac fetuses that lacked the development of a defined or recognizable umbilical cord. The presence of a cord is usually considered a prerequisite for the diagnosis of "acardiac fetus" but the presence of axial skeleton as a criterion is preferred.

Pathologic Features

There is a *wide spectrum of appearance of acardiacs*, ranging from a total absence of most organs to the presence of well-formed organs including gonads (Figures 10.5, 10.6). They may appear similar to an inside-out teratoma with little resemblance to a fetus. They may have a relatively well-formed lower trunk and legs with a misshapen upper body or they may even have remnants of a face and arms. The only organ that has not been described in acardiacs is the liver. For the study and diagnosis of acardiacs, it is usually best to obtain a radiograph of the specimen before dissection, as it gives some idea of the complexity of the abnormality, enables better classification, and delineates if a skull

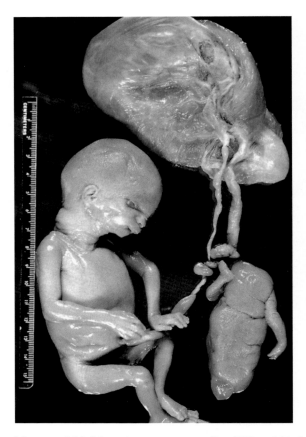

Figure 10.6. Macerated MoMo twins, one an acardiac (150 and 20 g). The twins died because of entangling of cords. The acardiac had a remnant of heart with calcification in the remaining muscle fibers. H&E. ×160. (Courtesy Dr. S. Kassel, Fresno, California.)

is present. *Most acardiacs have a monoamnionic-monochorionic (MoMo) placenta, although some with diamnionic-monochorionic (DiMo) placentas have also been described.* Most, but not all, acardiac fetuses have a *single umbilical artery.*

Clinical Features and Implications

Acardiacs occasionally have great mobility, and may die of cord entanglement (Figure 10.6). In cases of a DiMo placenta, *amnion nodosum is usually present in the acardiac* because of its deficient or absent urine production. Acardiacs often develop *hydrops*, and the pregnancy is thus frequently complicated by polyhydramnios. This problem may result from hypoproteinemia or heart failure of the donor twin. Plethora is also frequently observed in acardiacs and probably represents stagnation of blood, transfused by the pale, normal co-twin (Figure 10.5). This is often reflected in the placenta as well.

Conjoined Twins

Pathogenesis

Incompletely separated or **conjoined twins** (Siamese, x-pagi, double monsters) take their origin after day 13 of embryogenesis. The precise manner of the formation of conjoined twins is uncertain, with theories of incomplete splitting and partial fusion of embryonic precursors being the most popular. Conjoined twins occur in approximately 1 of 50,000 births, or in 1 of 600 twins. They are much more common in the Japanese population, in Nigeria, and in South Africa. For unknown reasons, 70% of conjoined twins are female. Most fused twins are joined at the chest, thoracopagus, and thoracoomphalopagus, representing 28% of the total, but they may be joined in an infinite number of configurations (Figure 10.7). Conjoined siblings in higher gestations have also been reported.

Pathologic Features

The placenta of conjoined twins is MoMo; however, separate placental disks have been reported. *The structure of the umbilical cords varies widely.* Approximately 6% have two cords. When the cord is fused, it has a variable number of umbilical vessels (Figure 10.8). As few as three and up to eight vessels have been reported; the latter case had six arteries and two veins. *Single umbilical artery (SUA) is also found quite commonly in conjoined twins.* Some cords are separate in their insertion onto the placental surface but fuse along their length. There is no association of cord vasculature and structure with the type of conjoined twin.

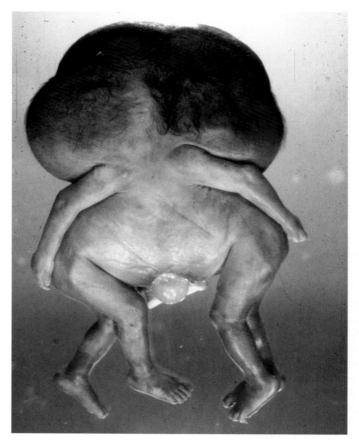

Figure 10.7. Conjoined twins with fusion of anterior portion of the head, chest and upper abdomen.

Twin Variants

DZ and MZ twinning are the most common types of twinning, but other unusual variants have been described. In what has been called the **third type of twin**, *the ovum and polar body are fertilized separately by two different sperm*. Thus, the twins have the same maternal genetic contribution but two different paternal contributions. Therefore, the twins are intermediate in their genetic configuration between MZ and DZ twins. This type of twinning occurs in less than 1% of twins and likely develops in situations when the polar body is of similar size to the oocyte. It has been recognized by the finding of one corpus luteum in cases of presumed DZ twins. *The placentation is diamnionic-dichorionic (DiDi) and the placentas will usually be fused.* Another unusual variant of twinning occurs in **superfecundation** where two ova are fertilized by sperm from two different fathers. **Superfetation**, on the other hand, is when fertilization occurs at different times, resulting in twins of different gestational ages.

Triplets and Higher Multiple Births

Multiple births are becoming more common and presently nonatuplets hold the record. Triplets and higher plural births are not only *smaller than expected for their gestational age; they also commonly deliver much earlier than twins or singletons.* Triplets may be any combination of MZ and DZ twins and chorionicity, that is, TriTri (triamnionic-trichorionic), TriDi (triamnionic-dichorionic), TriMo (triamnionic-monochorionic), DiMo, and MoMo. Terminology for the chorionicity of triplets and higher multiples (Figure 10.9) is usually based first on the total number of chorions and amnions. For example, quadramnionic-trichorionic describes quadruplets with four chorions and three amnions. The diagnosis would then read *Quadramnionic-trichorionic quadruplet placenta, diamnionic-monochorionic for quadruplets B and C*, for example. Otherwise, examination and reporting are similar to that for twins.

Uneven numbers of monozygotic multiples (such as triplets or quintuplets) may be explained by assuming that, on occasion, one embryo

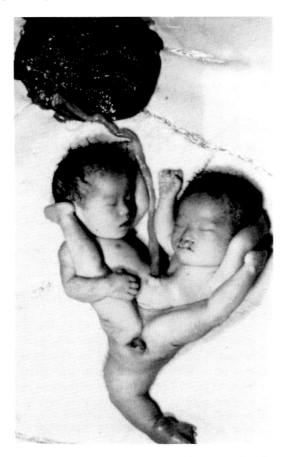

Figure 10.8. Conjoined twins (ischiopagi) with a MoMo placenta, a single velamentous umbilical cord, and single umbilical artery (SUA). They were delivered at 40 weeks gestation. One had a cleft face and microcardia. There were two female genital tracts. (Courtesy Dr. S. Sekiya, Tokyo.)

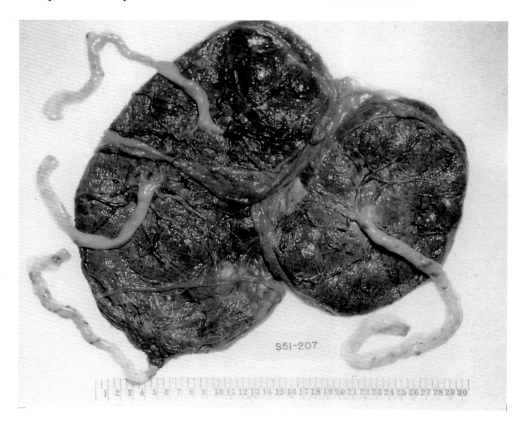

Figure 10.9. Quadruplet placenta (QuaTri), with DiMo MZ twins at bottom left, one having marginal insertion of the umbilical cord (35 weeks, 920 g).

may not have survived. Alternatively, there may be one division initially and then a secondary division occurs, or three or more embryonic centers might arise simultaneously instead of two. Because plural gestations generally have poor outcomes, their early diagnosis and "selective reduction" of some is relatively common.

Suggestions for Examination and Report: Triplets and Higher-Order Multiples

Gross Examination: Examination should be along the same lines as that for twins, that is, documentation of the vascular anastomoses, separation of fused disks along the vascular equator, and separate examination of each placenta. In complex arrangements, a drawing of the relationships may be helpful.

Comment: As noted above, the number of amnions and chorions should be included in the diagnosis. The specifics of individual relationships may be added as in the following example, "Triamnionic-dichorionic triplet placenta (diamnionic-monochorionic for triplets A and B)."

Twin-to-Twin Transfusion

Chronic Twin-to-Twin Transfusion Syndrome

Pathogenesis

The **twin-to-twin transfusion syndrome (TTTS)** is a specific entity caused by the *unidirectional, prenatal transfusion of blood through arteriovenous (A-V) anastomoses in the monochorionic twin placenta* (Figure 10.10). Thus, one twin is a **donor**, and the other is the **recipient**. Usually, there is a *discrepancy in size and development of the twins, particularly with respect to amniotic fluid and fetal fluid status*. The syndrome is variable in its consequences because the A-V anastomoses may be single or multiple, of varying size, and may or may not be associated with artery-artery (A-A) and/or vein-vein (V-V) anastomoses. When a simultaneous large anastomosis coexists, the most severe aspect of the syndrome is prevented due to equalization of blood flow between the twins. The twins reach greater gestational maturity or may not even develop TTTS. Prenatal diagnosis is usually made when one monochorionic twin shows oligohydramnios and the other shows polyhydramnios. The twins may also show a significant weight discrepancy. This has led to use of the term TOPS for "twin oligohydramnios polyhydramnios sequence," a practice with which we strongly disagree.

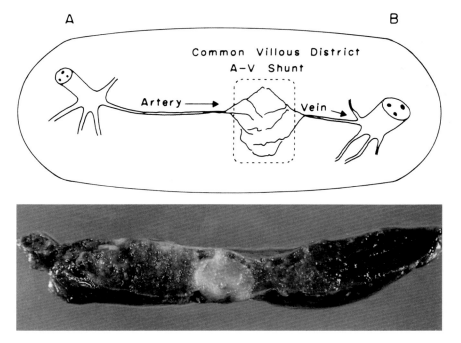

Figure 10.10. Vascular anastomoses in chronic twin-to-twin transfusion syndrome (top). The predominant anastomosis is an artery-to-vein anastomosis from the donor (A, left) to the recipient (B, right). Cross section of a monozygotic placenta after injection of shared cotyledon has been injected with water (bottom). Note that the placenta of the donor (A, left) is paler than the placenta on the right.

Use of this term ignores the etiology, which lies in the placental anastomoses.

Pathologic Features

The prenatal unidirectional exchange of blood results in deprivation of nutrients from the **donor** twin and excessive development of the **recipient**. The twins may be remarkably discordant (Figure 10.11), and there is a high degree of brain-sparing growth restriction in the smaller twin. *Typically, one twin is dehydrated and anemic, possessing organs much smaller than expected. The recipient is often plethoric and has enlarged organs.* The discrepancy is particularly striking in the hearts, and this is one of the most important means for the diagnosis of the transfusion syndrome. After birth or demise of one twin, rapid blood shifts may occur between the twins, which negate the usefulness of hematologic values. The remarkable pallor of the donor twin's placental portion and congestion of the recipient's placenta may be quite striking (Figure 10.12). The histologic structure of the villi can differ substantially as well

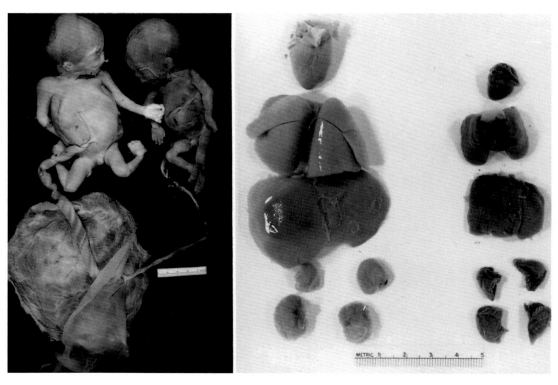

Figure 10.11. Macerated DiMo twins with chronic transfusion syndrome at 28 weeks gestation. The donor (left) is plethoric; the recipient (right) is edematous and pale. Recipient (twin A) 285 g; 15 cm CR length; heart 3 g; lungs 10 g; liver 17.5 g; kidneys 1.5 g. Donor (twin B) 189 g; 13 cm CR length; heart 0.7 g; lungs 3 g; liver 4 g; kidneys 1 g. The plethora of twin B is thought to be due to this twin's earlier death, with exsanguination of A into B (acute twin–twin transfusion).

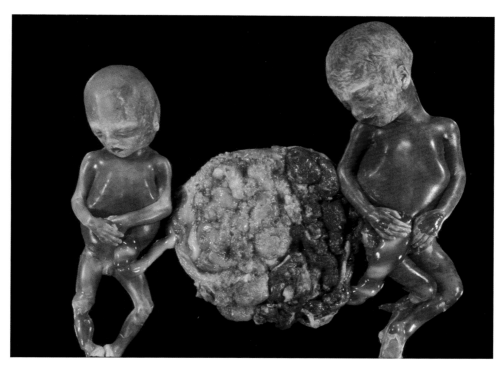

Figure 10.12. DiMo placenta at 26 weeks with chronic TTTS (twin-to-twin transfusion syndrome). Both fetuses died in utero. The recipient's placenta (right) is markedly congested, while the donor's (left) is markedly pale.

(Figure 10.13), with enlarged, edematous villi in the donor and congested villi in the recipient. Both usually contain markedly increased nucleated red blood cells.

Clinical Features and Implications

The frequency of the transfusion syndrome is difficult to determine but it is estimated to occur in *5% to 30% of monochorionic twins*. Observations suggest that it may be more common. There is a wide spectrum of severity and so assigning a precise frequency and assessing therapeutic efficacy is difficult. For unknown reasons the syndrome is much more common in female twins. Typically, the transfusion syndrome is first recognized by the finding of *polyhydramnios*. It usually develops around midgestation, but has been diagnosed as early as 12 weeks. The donor twin has oligohydramnios and may move much less than the recipient, so the term "stuck twin" has been applied to this feature. Clinical diagnosis of TTTS is often difficult. In general, the earlier clinical manifestations are present, the poorer the prognosis, although overall the prognosis is poor, particularly if untreated. When the condition is diagnosed before 28 weeks of gestation, the overall survival rate is as low as 21%.

The hydramnios often leads to preterm labor and premature rupture of the membranes, and delivery often occurs before the 30th week of gestation. Alternatively, one twin may die, in which case the hydram-

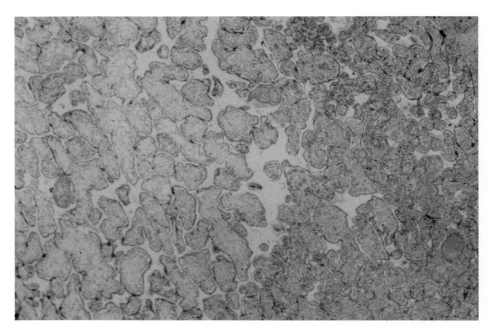

Figure 10.13. Histologic appearance of DiMo placenta depicted in Figure 10.12. The section has been taken through the vascular equator of the two placental portions. The donor's placenta is on the left and the recipient's on the right. Note that the chorionic villi of the donor are larger and more immature appearing with somewhat edematous stroma. The recipient's villi are smaller, more mature, and much more congested with blood.

nios ceases nearly immediately and the pregnancy may reach term. If one or both of the twins are liveborn, *neonatal morbidity and mortality are significant*. The donor often succumbs from hypovolemia and heart failure while the recipient may succumb from congestive heart failure. Other pathophysiologic consequences of the syndrome include *poor fetal growth, periventricular encephalomalacia, intracranial hemorrhage, intraventricular hemorrhage, polycythemia in the recipient, anemia in the donor, hypoglycemia, hyperbilirubinemia, skin necrosis resembling aplasia cutis, cardiac dysfunction, cardiac hypertrophy, and thrombosis.*

Treatment Considerations

It has now become possible to *obliterate the interfetal vascular connections by prenatal laser treatment*. This is hoped to result in improved outcome and normalization of the pregnancy. Other modes of treatment include *septostomy* (of the dividing membranes) and *amniocentesis* of the twin with polyhydramnios. In the future, mapping not only the anastomoses but also the character and location of ablated vessels is likely to be important in planning future treatment options.

Acute Twin-to-Twin Transfusion

Pathogenesis

Acute twin-to-twin transfusion may occur *with or without* chronic TTTS. It occurs to some degree in *all DiMo twins when one twin dies in* *utero.* If placental anastomoses are small, the placenta of the dead fetus gradually atrophies and becomes completely infarcted. If, on the other hand, there are large interfetal vascular communications, the placental half belonging to the dead fetus will continue to be perfused by the survivor. The vascular bed of the dead twin is devoid of counterpressure and becomes a "sink." The surviving twin may then literally exsanguinate into the dead twin. Therefore, *when one twin of a DiMo pair dies, the survivor experiences some degree of acute blood loss into the dead twin's circulation through superficial large interplacental anastomoses.* These acute hypotensive events occur in the surviving twin immediately after one twin dies. Sonographically, reversal of blood flow in the umbilical cord has been observed after death of one twin.

Clinical Features and Implications

Cerebral palsy is five times more common in twins than in singletons and mostly affects MZ twins. When there is intrauterine fetal demise of one twin, cerebral palsy is particularly common in the surviving twin. Death of the surviving twin is also quite common. The presence of cerebral lesions, such as porencephaly, correlates well with the presence of vascular anastomoses in MZ twins. This is thought, in many cases, to be the result of irregular flow through placental anastomoses, particularly V-V anastomoses.

Suggestions for Examination and Report: Twin-to-Twin Transfusion

Gross Examination: Documentation of vascular anastomoses is essential to the diagnosis of twin transfusion syndromes (see Chapter 9). In addition, careful attention to the color of the villous tissue (pallor of the donor and congestion of the recipient) is recommended.

Comment: The presence of a monochorionic placenta with a dominant artery-to-vein anastomosis is consistent with the diagnosis of chronic TTTS. With fetal demise of one twin, acute twin-to-twin transfusion should be considered as it occurs even in the absence of chronic TTTS. Both may lead to significant morbidity and mortality.

Chimerism and Mosaicism

Chimerism and mosaicism are related but different phenomena. **Whole-body chimerism** is when an *individual is composed of two populations of cells, the origin of which is two genetically different fertilization products.* It may develop in very early stages of development, when dizygotic twin embryos fuse to form a single individual. When *two spermatozoa fertilize an ovum and a polar body and then form a single embryo,* such individuals represent, genetically speaking, fraternal twins fused into one body. This is a variant of the **third type of twin** (see above).

These chimeras are not necessarily clinically manifest. Most are discovered when the two populations of cells have different sex chromosomes (XX/XY), resulting in gonadal abnormalities, most common among which is **true hermaphroditism**. Whole-body chimeras may also be discovered during routine blood grouping tests, because of unusual phenotypic features, such as heterochromia (eyes of different color) or abnormal patches of the skin resulting from the irregular distribution of melanocyte precursors derived from different genotypes.

It is important to distinguish two pathogenetically different types of chimeras: blood chimeras and whole-body chimeras. **Blood chimeras** *develop from fused placentas with connections between the fetal vessels enabling blood exchange between DZ twins.* This has long been described in animals, but vascular connections between the placentas of human DZ twins are rare. *Study of these individuals shows that they are blood chimeras but not whole-body chimeras.*

Mosaics are different from chimeras as they are *individuals composed of different cell lines but derived from a single fertilization product.* Because of "lyonization" and X chromosome inactivation, all human females are mosaics. Not only may mosaics have different cell lines with different chromosome numbers but, because of mutations, they may also have cell lines with different phenotypic expression.

Heterokaryotypic Monozygotic Twins

Heterokaryotypic MZ twins begin as MZ twins, and then nondisjunction of chromosomes in one twin gives them a different genetic makeup. Most commonly, this occurs with a sex chromosome resulting in karyotypes of 45XO and 46XY and MZ twins of different sex. Nondisjunction of autosomes may also occur, however. *These twins show mosaicism resulting from the simultaneous occurrence of twinning and somatic nondisjunction of chromosomes.* If the Y chromosome of a 46 XY embryo is lost by nondisjunction during early development, male and female (45 X0 and 46 XY) MZ twins may be the outcome. Heterokaryotypic MZ twins may have varying degrees and types of mosaicism. Mosaicism may be present in certain cell types only, such as lymphocytes, and in this case is directly due to the presence of placental anastomoses. Mosaicism of fibroblasts suggests the loss of a chromosome in one twin after splitting has occurred.

Sacrococcygeal Teratoma and Epignathus

Sacrococcygeal teratoma and **epignathus** (a tumorous mass affixed to the jaw) are, in our opinion, *malformed twins that are part of the spectrum of MZ twinning.* Some may take exception to this concept. Nevertheless, findings of perfectly formed extremities, digits, and other structures favor this view. At times, however, an apparently benign sacrococcygeal teratoma eventuates in a malignancy. An alternate etiologic point of view is that sacrococcygeal tumors and epignathi derive from misplaced germ cells.

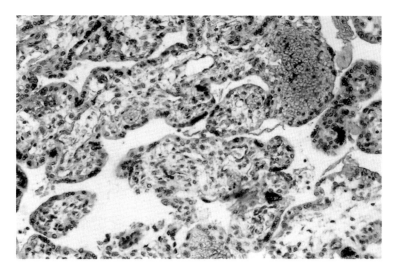

Figure 10.14. Villi of immature placenta in a patient with a large sacrococcygeal teratoma. Placenta weighed 880g at 31 weeks. The neonate died with extensive cerebral necrosis. The villi are irregular and patchily edematous, and have distended fetal capillaries. There is focal hemorrhage, and numerous nucleated red blood cells are present. The cytotrophoblast is more prominent than expected at this age. H&E. ×160.

Placentomegaly has often been described to be a complication of sacrococcygeal teratomas and the same is true of the placenta in epignathi. Other teratomas and acardiac twins may also be associated with hydramnios and fetal hydrops. These placental changes are likely the result of high output failure. In effect, the teratoma acts as an arteriovenous fistula. If there is hydrops, the placenta will be *exceptionally pale.* There may be *severe villous edema, and the villi may show increased cellularity and vascular congestion.* Numerous Hofbauer cells may be present as well as many nucleated red blood cells (Figure 10.14).

Selected References

PHP4, Chapter 25, pages 801, 804, 827–875.

Bajoria R, Wigglesworth J, Fisk NM. Angioarchitecture of monochorionic placentas in relation to the twin-twin transfusion syndrome. Am J Obstet Gynecol 1995;172:856–863.

Bejar R, Vigliocco G, Gramajo H, et al. Antenatal origin of neurologic damage in newborn infants. Part II. Multiple gestations. Am J Obstet Gynecol 1990; 162:1230–1236.

Bendon RW. Twin transfusion syndrome: pathological studies of the monochorionic placenta in liveborn twins and of the perinatal autopsy in monochorionic twin pairs. Pediatr Pathol Lab Med 1995;15:363–376.

Benirschke K. Chimerism, mosaicism and hybrids. In: Human genetics. Proceedings, Fourth International Congress Human Genetics, Paris. Amsterdam: Excerpta Medica, 1971:212–231.

Benirschke K. Intrauterine death of a twin: mechanisms, implications for surviving twin, and placental pathology. Semin Diagn Pathol 1993;10:222–231.

Bieber FR, Nance WE, Morton CC, et al. Genetic studies of an acardiac monster: evidence of polar body twinning in man. Science 1981;213:775–777.

Costa T, Lambert M, Teshima I, et al. Monozygotic twins with 45X,46,XY mosaicism discordant for phenotypic sex. Am J Med Genet 1998;75:40–44.

De Lia JE. Surgery of the placenta and umbilical cord. Clin Obstet Gynecol 1996;39:607–625.

Dimmick JE, Kalousek DK. Developmental pathology of the embryo and fetus. Philadelphia: Lippincott, 1992.

Jauniaux E, Elkazen N, Leroy F, et al. Clinical and morphologic aspects of the vanishing twin phenomenon. Obstet Gynecol 1988;72:577–581.

Kaplan C, Perlmutter S, Molinoff S. Epignathus with placental hydrops. Arch Pathol Lab Med 1980;104:374–375.

Liu S, Benirschke K, Scioscia AL, et al. Intrauterine death in multiple gestation. Acta Genet Med Gemellol 1992;41:5–26.

Machin GA. Some causes of genotypic and phenotypic discordance in monozygotic twin pairs. Am J Med Genet 1996;61:216–228.

Moore TR, Gale SA, Benirschke K. Perinatal outcome of forty-nine pregnancies complicated by acardiac twinning. Am J Obstet Gynecol 1990;163:907–912.

Scheller JM, Nelson KB. Twinning and neurologic morbidity. Am J Dis Child 1992;146:110–113.

Spencer R. Conjoined twins: theoretical embryological basis. Teratology 1992;45:591–602.

Section IV
Abnormalities of the Placenta

This section covers abnormalities and lesions of the placenta. The first chapter, Chapter 11, discusses abnormalities encountered in the early abortion specimen and the pathologic changes associated with chromosomal anomalies. Chapter 12 deals primarily with the abnormalities of the implantation site and uterus that occur in the postpartum period, including uterine atony, endometritis, retained placental tissue, and placenta accreta. Chapter 13 concerns itself with aberrations in placental shape, and as these aberrations are associated with abnormal implantation, theories of pathogenesis are briefly discussed. Placenta previa, as an abnormality in the location of implantation, has characteristics in common with these variants and so is discussed as well. Finally, pathologic lesions of the fetal membranes are presented in Chapter 14 and those of the umbilical cord in Chapter 15.

Chapter 11

Abortion and the Placenta in Chromosomal Anomalies

General Considerations

Abortions may be of several types, which are defined as follows:

- **Induced** or voluntary, which include
  - **Therapeutic**—electively terminated
  - **Criminal**—illegally instrumented
- **Spontaneous** or involuntary, which include
  - **Threatened**—uterine bleeding without cervical dilatation
  - **Inevitable**—uterine bleeding with cervical dilatation or effacement
  - **Incomplete**—all tissue has not yet passed
  - **Missed**—intrauterine retention after embryonic death
- **Habitual/recurrent**—three or more consecutive spontaneous miscarriages

Induced, spontaneous, and habitual abortion specimens are approached slightly differently, and each of these is discussed below. However, there are several goals in examination that should be addressed in all abortion specimens:

- To document the presence of a **pregnancy**
- To rule out an **ectopic pregnancy**
- To identify suspected or unsuspected **abnormalities of the placenta or fetus**
- To rule out **gestational trophoblastic disease**

Induced Abortions

Clinical Features and Implications

Pregnancies may be terminated legally or illegally, and both are termed **induced abortions**. There is little difference between the two from a pathologist's point of view, except that the latter type is more frequently followed by complications such as uterine infection and perforation. Induced abortions are performed by *dilatation and curettage (D&C), prostaglandins (with or without cervical laminaria), intraamnionic injection of hypertonic saline or urea solutions, and other means.* Some induced abortions are performed because of the prenatal diagnosis of fetal anomalies whereas others are presumably normal, but "unwanted," pregnancies. Although in the latter case the likelihood of anomalies is slight, occasionally abnormalities are identified on examination.

Complications of abortions, particularly "criminal" abortions, include *pulmonary embolism, uterine perforation, uterine hemorrhage, disseminated intravascular coagulation, life-threatening infections, septic abortions, and other minor complications.* These occur in up to 13% of induced abortions. In **septic abortions**, microscopic examination often reveals *acute villitis, acute intervillositis, and bacterial colonies filling the fetal villous capillaries.* Depending on the organism, some cases may show little inflammatory reaction. With the exception of infections, the various complications do not usually reveal specific pathologic lesions.

Pathologic Features

To document the presence of an intrauterine pregnancy, one must identify *implantation site, trophoblastic cells, or chorionic villi.* Occasionally, no chorionic villi may be found. In this case, the presence of *decidua with infiltration by extravillous trophoblast and physiologic conversion of decidual arterioles, that is, the implantation site,* is definitive proof of an intrauterine pregnancy (see Figure 1.7, page 13). A few chorionic villi may be present without an identifiable implantation site. In these cases, caution is advised because, under rare conditions, a few chorionic villi may be transported from the fallopian tube in an ectopic pregnancy. Thus, the presence of chorionic villi alone does not always document an **intrauterine** pregnancy. The same can be said for the presence of scattered trophoblastic cells without chorionic villi or implantation site. For these cases, a cautionary comment in the report and communication with the clinician is suggested.

At times, it may be difficult to differentiate decidual cells from extravillous trophoblast, a necessary task if one wants to identify the implantation site. *Decidual cells have distinct cell membranes with lightly eosinophilic cytoplasm containing oval nuclei with dispersed chromatin. In* contrast, *extravillous trophoblast are polygonal cells without distinct cell borders, which contain abundant amphophilic cytoplasm and irregular, mildly pleomorphic, hyperchromatic nuclei* (see Figure 8.4, page 113). Another clue to the presence of extravillous trophoblast and the implantation site is the characteristic *fibrinoid deposition*, typically seen in the vicinity of extravillous trophoblast. If after histologic examination doubt still remains, immunohistochemistry may be used. As trophoblast is epithelial in origin, *all trophoblastic cells stain strongly positive for cytokeratins, while decidual cells are always negative.* Cytokeratin staining is very sensitive for trophoblast but not specific and so care should be taken when using this stain for other purposes.

Although most tissue is normal in induced abortions, occasionally some abnormalities may be found. For instance, fetal death has been reported in approximately 2% of induced abortions, macroscopic anomalies in approximately 1%, and chromosomal abnormalities in 5% to 6%. Rarely, unsuspected gestational trophoblastic disease may be diagnosed in an induced abortion (see Chapter 23). Normal implantation is associated with a *mild decidual necrosis and inflammation.* However, extensive inflammation or necrosis is an abnormal finding that should be reported. Although these findings may indicate an imminent pregnancy loss or an underlying problem, they are relatively nonspecific. Finally, abnormalities in the decidual vessels and implantation site may be present in early abortion specimens. These include *lack of normal physiologic conversion, thrombosis, and marked vascular inflammation.* They are often associated with disorders of placental malperfusion (see Chapter 18).

When D&C or suction curettage is performed, instrumentation of the cervix and uterus has occasionally led to misplacement of fetal tissues. Paracervical or endometrial masses consisting of **fetal skeletal parts** have been identified months to many years after the last preceding pregnancy (Figure 11.1). Incompletely removed fetal tissues may cause unexplained bleeding and have been incriminated in *causing infertility* because they may act similarly to an intrauterine contraceptive device.

When abortions are induced by introduction of different substances into the amniotic cavity, certain pathologic changes may occur. Injection of **hypertonic saline** solution results in extensive fetal ion fluxes. This results in *hemorrhage and necrosis under the chorionic plate, intervillous thrombosis, amnion necrosis,* and occasional chorionic vascular obliteration (Figures 11.2, 11.3). In addition, the villous tissue is often pale secondary to hemolysis. This type of abortion is now rarely performed. Introduction of hypertonic urea gives similar changes, although not so severe.

Spontaneous Abortions

A **spontaneous abortion** or "miscarriage" is often defined as a conceptus expelled before the 20th week of gestation. Because the definition varies from state to state, a more usable definition is the *spontaneous delivery of a fetus prior to viability.* This is important to state

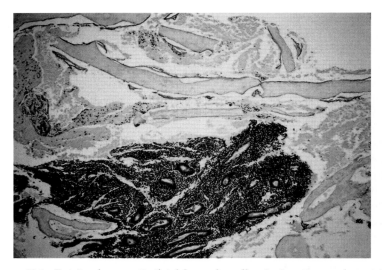

Figure 11.1. Retained, necrotic fetal bony lamellae in inactive endometrium that also shows mild chronic endometritis. They are remains of an abortion that took place several years ago. H&E. ×60. (Courtesy Dr. W. Tench, San Diego, California.)

at the outset, as the pathologic features of failed pregnancies differ markedly from those specimens obtained later in gestation, which are considered **preterm** deliveries. In addition, a pregnancy of less than 20 or so weeks gestation is usually considered an "embryo" and treated as a surgical specimen. Later it is considered a "fetus," whose examination constitutes an autopsy.

Pathogenesis

Most spontaneous abortions occur before 12 weeks of gestation, and many are due to **chromosomal errors**. Chromosomal anomalies are present in 50% of all spontaneous abortions and in 70% of those occurring during the first 6 weeks. Increasing maternal age considerably increases the risk of spontaneous abortion, especially after the age of 35, and this correlates with an enhanced risk of fetal trisomies. However, the exact mechanism of the abortion in this situation is still

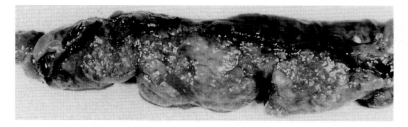

Figure 11.2. Macroscopic appearance of an immature placenta from a saline-induced abortion. Note the subchorionic hemorrhage, fibrinoid deposition, and pallor of the placenta.

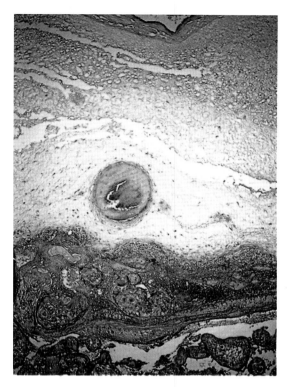

Figure 11.3. Placental surface in urea termination at 19 weeks gestation. The large chorionic fetal vessel is thrombosed and there is abundant edema in the overlying membranes. The chorionic plate shows a dense accumulation of fibrin, blood clot, and neutrophils. H&E. ×40.

disputed. Other less well delineated *genetic defects* also make up a proportion of spontaneous abortion.

Endocrine disorders are a cause of a certain percentage of spontaneous abortions, and these include *luteal phase defects, polycystic ovary syndrome*, and *poorly controlled maternal diabetes*. Numerous physical factors have been associated with an increased incidence of abortions. *Uterine anomalies*, particularly *septate uteri*, have been implicated, and in the latter case, abortion likely ensues when implantation occurs on the septum. *Submucosal leiomyomas* and *trauma* have also been reported to increase spontaneous abortion as well. *Cervical incompetence* (see Chapter 16) is associated with preterm labor, preterm delivery, and pregnancy loss. Other causes of spontaneous abortion are *multiple gestation* (Chapters 9 and 10), *antiphospholipid antibodies* (Chapter 18), *drugs* (Chapter 17), and *congenital malformations*. Relatively few spontaneous abortions occur in the period from 12 to 20 weeks gestation. Between 20 and 30 weeks, spontaneous termination is primarily due to **ascending infection** (see Chapter 16). *Placental and fetal infections* that may lead to fetal infection and death in the first trimester are less common but include *Listeria, cytomegalovirus, Toxoplasma, herpes simplex virus*, and *Coxsackie virus.*

Clinical Features and Implications

The incidence of spontaneous abortions is actually quite high. When prospective studies of complete populations are done on all pregnancies, including those that give few or no clinical symptoms of pregnancy, nearly 50% of conceptions terminate in abortion spontaneously. There are also conceptuses that vanish even before implantation. Clinically recognized gestations end in abortion in approximately 15% of cases. Spontaneous abortions are usually accompanied by uterine bleeding and cramping with subsequent spontaneous passage of tissue. Often the embryo or fetus will pass first, followed by the placenta. Therefore, curettages done on women who have previously passed tissue often contain only decidualized endometrium and fragments of involuting implantation site.

Pathologic Features

Specimens will consist of embryonic tissue, decidua, and placental tissue, and each should be examined in turn. Specimens may have a *complete or incomplete embryo, have no embryo, or may contain an intact gestational sac.* If the embryo is present, it may be *grossly disorganized*, presenting as a nodular, cylindrical, stunted, or barely recognizable embryo (Figure 11.4), it may show *focal, specific defects* such as spina bifida, cleft palate, etc., or it may be *without gross abnormalities*. The embryo may be macerated to a variable extent, and noting this may be helpful is assigning an estimation of intrauterine retention. Examination of abnormal fetuses is beyond the scope of this text; however, it is understood that with an abnormal embryo, as complete an examina-

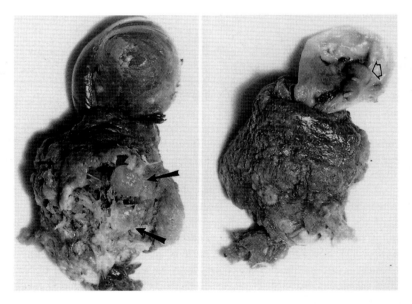

Figure 11.4. Spontaneous abortus at approximately 8 weeks gestation. Note the opened sac at right with the nodular embryo at the open arrow. The hypoplastic placenta with hydropic degeneration is seen at the arrows (left). The decidua basalis is hemorrhagic.

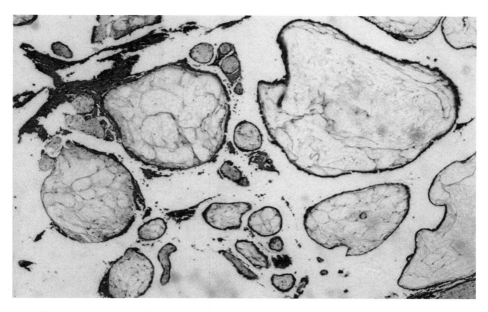

Figure 11.5. Early spontaneous abortion at about 6 weeks with prominent hydropic villi and no apparent red blood cells. H&E. ×40.

tion as possible should be done. The reader is referred to the references for several excellent monographs on the subject of evaluation and examination of fetal anomalies.

Pathologic changes in the villous tissue may also be present. Unfortunately, in early abortion specimens, these changes often do not provide information on the cause of the pregnancy loss. The few exceptions noted above include abnormalities of the implantation site vessels and excessive inflammation and necrosis. However, the pathologic changes in abortion specimens *are more often related to the timing of embryonic death and the age of the conceptus at the time of death than to the cause of the pregnancy failure.* The following is a list of the changes that generally occur after embryonic death:

- Early embryonic death–menstrual age less than 7 weeks (Figure 11.5)
  - Hydropic villi
  - Thinned trophoblastic cover
  - Lack of red blood cells and villous capillaries
- Embryonic death–menstrual age approximately 7 to 8 weeks (Figure 11.6)
  - Focal villous hydrops
  - Focal villous stromal sclerosis
  - Villous capillaries with varying degrees of vascular obliteration
  - Nucleated red blood cells, which may be "naked" in the stroma
  - Increased syncytial knots
  - Thickened trophoblastic basement membrane
- Embryonic death—menstrual age approximately 8 to 12 weeks
  - Increasing villous fibrosis with collagenous stroma

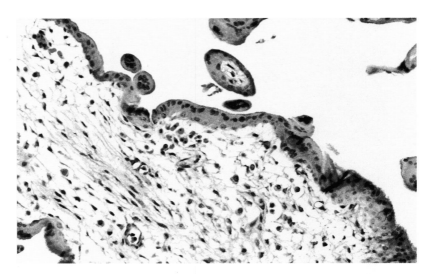

Figure 11.6. Early spontaneous abortion at about 7 to 8 weeks. This villus shows edema at the periphery and early fibrosis in the central region (at the left). Nucleated red blood cells are present "naked" in the villous stroma. H&E. ×40.

- Obliteration of villous vessels
- Ratio of nucleated to nonnucleated red blood cells changes from 100% to 10%
- Fine mineralization of trophoblastic basement membrane and villous stroma (see Figure 20.13, page 388)
- Perivillous fibrinoid deposition

The reason for the preponderance of hydropic change in aborted specimens is not fully understood. It is generally believed that, following fetal death, the trophoblast continues to transport water from the intervillous space into the villi, where it cannot be removed by an absent fetal circulation; hence, the villi enlarge. Villous vascularization occurs at about 6.5 weeks menstrual age and so conceptuses reaching that age will show the presence of villous capillaries and nucleated red blood cells and will show less hydropic change.

Recurrent or Habitual Abortion

Habitual abortion is usually defined as a condition in which a woman has had *three or more consecutive spontaneous abortions*. Three consecutive losses is the preferred definition because, after two consecutive spontaneous abortions, the chance of successful pregnancy is 80%. Known etiologies vary widely. There are many infectious causes (see Chapter 16) and a number of chronic debilitating diseases such as *lupus erythematosus, maternal heart disease, and endocrine disorders* (Chapter 17). *Recurrent villitis of unknown etiology, massive repetitive chronic intervillositis* (Chapter 16), and *maternal floor infarction* (Chapter 19) constitute another group. The relation of *substance abuse* to spontaneous abortion and to abruptio placentae is difficult to evaluate, especially the possible contribution of *maternal smoking*. Many patients who smoke or use various toxic substances additionally consume alcohol, have various infections, and are prone to suffer misuse and trauma (Chapter 17).

Parental chromosome aberrations and some *immunologic errors associated with placentation* are other well-studied causes of recurrent abortion. Some recurrent abortions are due to increasing maternal age with its increased chance of aneuploidy. Rarely, *balanced chromosomal translocations* of one parent have been the cause of habitual abortion. Therefore, it is suggested that in couples with recurrent abortions, the mother *and* the father be examined cytogenetically. The pathologist can contribute to a better understanding of the etiology by requesting cytogenetic evaluation of aborted specimens from recurrent aborters.

Chromosomal Anomalies

Some investigators have gone so far as to suggest that pathologic changes in chromosomally abnormal abortions are so characteristic that they enable chromosomal diagnosis from the morphologic findings of the villous tissue alone. When tested, experts and diagnostic pathologists are consistently unable to specifically label a given microscopic appearance with confidence. In general, *karyotyping is necessary to confirm the diagnosis.* The exception is the karyotypic abnormalities associated with hydatidiform moles (see Chapter 23). That being said, there are certain pathologic features that are commonly seen in aneuploid conceptuses. One of the hallmarks of a **chromosomal anomaly** is the presence of *growth restriction of the fetus* and an *abnormally small and thin placenta*. Other histologic features that are often associated with chromosomal defects in general are *increased villous size, villous edema, trophoblastic inclusions or invaginations, irregular villous contour, and cytotrophoblastic "giant" cells*.

Trisomies

There are few specific findings that characterize a placenta with **trisomy**, but many abnormalities have been found sporadically. First, the incidence of *single umbilical artery* (SUA) is higher. Placentas also tend to show *deficient vascularization* with a reduction in the number of small muscular arteries, decreased small muscular artery/villus ratio, and decreased capillaries. The villi are frequently *dysmature* with *trophoblastic inclusions or invaginations* (Figure 11.7). Occasionally, *increased syncytial knots* and *increased cellularity of the villous stroma* are also found.

Trisomy 16 is one of the *commonest cytogenetic anomalies found in spontaneous abortion material*. The embryo is generally absent with a small, empty chorionic cavity. Histologically, the *villi and trophoblast are hypoplastic with decreased vascularization*. Some villi may be *hydropic* (see Figure 11.5). Enlarged *"cytotrophoblastic giant cells"* are found in the stroma of up to 30% of villi (Figure 11.8). The origin of these cells is unclear but they may be edematous stromal cells, enlarged Hofbauer cells, or cells derived from "delaminating" cytotrophoblast. In **trisomy**

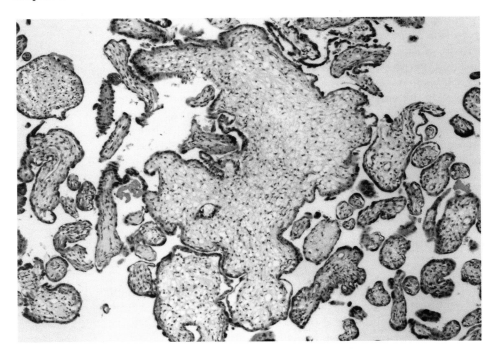

Figure 11.7. Spontaneous abortus with trisomy 13. There is scalloping of villi and trophoblastic "inclusions" most visible in the large villus in the center of the figure. H&E. ×40.

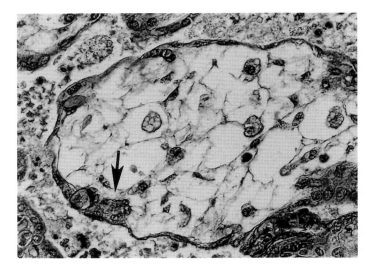

Figure 11.8. Villus with cytotrophoblastic giant cells in a spontaneous abortion. The much enlarged cells in the villous core represent enlarged Hofbauer cells (arrow). Cystic lacunae are developing in the villus. H&E. ×400.

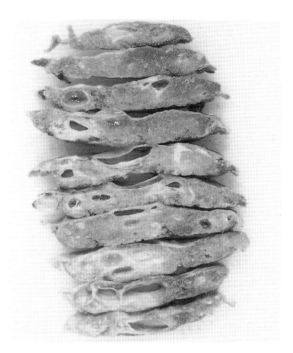

Figure 11.9. Cross sections through the placenta from a trisomy 18 stillbirth. The cysts are composed of enlarged villi.

18, *the chorionic villi are cystic and dilated, showing typical hydropic change.* Cysts may be large enough to be identified grossly (Figure 11.9). There may also be *increased syncytial knots* (Figure 11.10) or *increased cellularity of the villous stroma* (Figure 11.11).

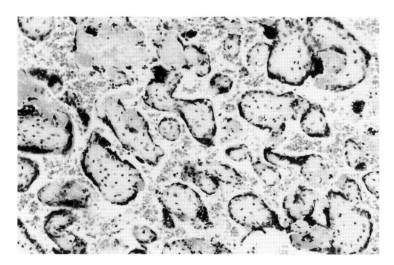

Figure 11.10. Villi of immature placenta (28 weeks gestation) of a stillborn fetus with trisomy 18. There is increased syncytial knotting despite the absence of preeclampsia. Villi lack fetal vessels because of fetal demise, but many have hyalinized centers. H&E. ×64.

The abortions of **trisomies 6 to 12** have a variable morphology. The placenta is *less mature* than expected for gestational age. *Giant cytotrophoblastic cells* are found in 40% of villi (see Figure 11.8). In **trisomies 13, 14, and 15** there is *variable placental maturation, decreased villous vascularity, and giant cytotrophoblast* in 50% of villi. Occasionally, *hydropic villi, scalloping, and trophoblastic inclusions may occur*. **Trisomy 21** is not accompanied by characteristic placental changes. Increased placental weight and size have, however, frequently been observed. There are even fewer characteristic patterns of the placentas of other trisomies, but *hydropic change is common and there is occasional atypical trophoblastic proliferation*.

Other Chromosomal Anomalies

Triploid conceptuses may be either *dygynic* or *diandric*, with the extra chromosome set deriving from the mother and father, respectively. Diandry results in partial hydatidiform moles. Triploidy due to dygyny is much more common in older women in whom nondisjunction of chromosomes occurs more commonly. The fetus is usually *small for the expected age* and often has characteristic anomalous features such as *digital fusion; frequently the embryos are nodular and degenerating. Single umbilical artery* is also common. Macroscopically, the placentas of triploids frequently show some degree of *hydropic change*, although not so prominent as seen with partial moles. Microscopically, some villi have *cavities or lacunae* within the villi, which are smaller than the cisterns seen in molar pregnancies (see Figure 23.4, page 421). Other villi may be disrupted or *compacted with increased cellularity* (see Figure 11.12), *and the trophoblast is variably hypoplastic*. There is characteristic *"infolding" or scalloping of trophoblast* into the villi, with trophoblastic nests occurring seemingly isolated in the villous stroma. A Breus' mole is occasionally found with triploid abortuses as well, although this is more common in monosomy X (see Chapter 14).

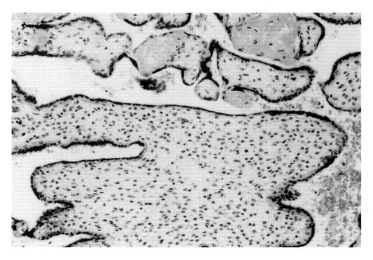

Figure 11.11. Trisomy 18 placenta with a marked increase in villous stromal cells. H&E. ×160.

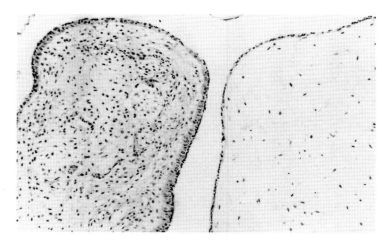

Figure 11.12. Two enlarged villi in a triploid abortus. One (left) is hypercellular, with faintly visible remnants of former fetal vessels; the other is hydropic. H&E. ×160.

Tetraploid abortuses usually have an *empty cavity and voluminous, poorly vascularized villi.* They frequently have *severe decidual and villous hemorrhages*, and their villi are invariably somewhat cystic. Occasionally, massive hydropic change may be seen. The embryos and placentas of **monosomy X** often appear relatively normal with only *villous fibrosis* present. Frequently, only a cord remnant is found in a cavity that is small for gestational age. In some cases there are *intervillous thrombi* of the so-called Breus' mole type (see Chapter 14). The embryo may have nuchal hygroma and severe hydrops.

Ancillary Testing

In abortion specimens, the chromosomal errors are composed of trisomy in 50% to 60%, triploidy in 18%, and monosomy X in 15%, and the remainder are double trisomies, tetraploidies, and individual chromosomal errors, such as rings, translocations, and mosaicism. The pathologist is occasionally asked to provide material for **cytogenetic study**. This is *best done from embryonic tissue* or from the chorionic surface when an embryo is not available or is macerated. In some cases, because of lack of viable embryonic tissue, placental tissue may be the only tissue able to grow in culture. Caution is advised when only placental tissue is obtained due to confined placental mosaicism (see below). Therefore, *if possible it is optimal to obtain both embryonic and placental tissue.* When sampling the placenta, it is best to cleanse the fetal surface, peel the amnion away, and to then obtain chorionic tissue with sterile instruments.

Chorionic villus sampling (CVS) is the procedure by which a small *sample of villous tissue is obtained early in gestation for the purpose of chromosomal or DNA testing.* CVS is usually done at about 11 weeks gestation. It has been suggested that chorionic villus sampling (CVS) is a significant cause of fetal loss and/or limb reduction defects. However, only a 0.8% increase of fetal loss in CVS patients has been documented. The relationship between limb defects and CVS exists principally in the gestationally earlier CVS and not when CVS is done after 9 weeks.

Because hydropic villi are such a frequent finding in many placentas of spontaneous abortions, the differentiation from moles and partial moles may present difficulty. Therefore, use of **flow cytometry** is advocated as a *rapid means for the delineation of diploidy and triploidy*. Thus, triploid "partial moles" may be differentiated from "complete" diploid hydatidiform moles, and diploid abortuses may be distinguished from triploid partial moles (see Chapter 23).

The sera of pregnant women are often tested with the **triple screen** and more recently the **quadruple screen** or **quad test**. The triple screen includes measurements of *beta-hCG, unconjugated estriol,* and *alpha fetoprotein* in the maternal serum. The quadruple screen adds *dimeric inhibin A*. Abnormalities in one or more of these markers are associated with increased risk of neural tube defects and chromosomal anomalies, particularly trisomy 21 and 18. The abnormalities and their associated test results are summarized in Table 11.1.

New methodology is evolving that will make it feasible to describe the genetic defects more accurately, such as the **polymerase chain reaction (PCR)**, **fluorescence in situ hybridization (FISH)** of whole cells, and delineation of translocations by spectral color staining of chromosomes. Some of these tests are feasible even using fixed tissue and individual, selected cells from paraffin-embedded tissues. Placental material, of course, also lends itself for *paternity diagnosis*.

Suggestions for Examination and Report: Abortions

Gross Examination: If villi are grossly identified, one section in an induced abortion is sufficient, while two to three sections should be submitted in a spontaneous abortion. It is also suggested a fragment of decidual tissue be submitted as it often contains a portion of the implantation site. If villi are not grossly seen, consideration should be given to submission of the entire specimen, particularly if an ectopic pregnancy is suspected. If the clinical history indicates a habitual abortion, tissue should be sent for chromosome analysis. Embryonic tissue should be submitted to document its presence and to further clarify gross abnormalities.

Comment: The tissues that are present, including implantation site, decidua, and chorionic villi, should be listed in the diagnosis if all are normal. Abnormalities such as lack of physiologic conversion and excessive inflammation should be listed separately. If features of chromosomal abnormalities are present, those should be listed, and a comment may be made that the findings are suggestive of a chromosomal anomaly or, if clinical history is given, that the findings are consistent with the clinical history of an anomaly.

Table 11.1. Maternal serum markers and risk of anomalies

Abnormality	AFP	hCG	UE3	DIA
NTD	↑	—	—	—
Trisomy 21	↓	↑	↓	↑
Trisomy 18	↓	↓	↓	—

Arrows indicate increase or decrease compared to normal results at that gestational age; results are reported as multiples of the median.
AFP, alphafetoprotein; hCG, human chorionic gonadotropin; UE3, unconjugated estriol; DIA, dimeric alpha inhibin; NTD, neural tube defect.

Confined Placental Mosaicism, Uniparental Disomy, and Imprinting

To understand the concepts of confined placental mosaicism and uniparental disomy, a few definitions are necessary.

- **Mosaicism** is present when an organism has two genetically distinct cell lines derived from a single fertilization product or genotype.
- **Chimerism** is present when an organism has two genetically distinct cell lines derived from two different fertilization products or genotypes.
- **Confined placental mosaicism** is present when the placenta has a different cell line than the fetus, both deriving from the same fertilization product or genotype.
- **Uniparental disomy** is the presence of two chromosomes from one parent.
- **Imprinting** is the transcriptional silencing of a portion (paternal or maternal) of one parental genome.

The presence of confined placental mosaicism, uniparental disomy, mosaicism, and chimerism has caused discrepancies in chromosomal findings between results obtained via CVS, amniocentesis, and fetal lymphocyte culture. Although some of the discrepancy may be due to contamination with maternal tissue, other discrepancies may be the result of the above-described conditions. The finding of mosaic cell lines may also reflect the differing origin of cells from the **inner cell mass (fetus)**, its **shell (placental trophoblast)**, the **amnion, chorion**, or from **connective tissue of the villi**. One must know which cells are found to be chromosomally abnormal to infer probable fetal genotype.

Confined Placental Mosaicism

Confined placental mosaicism (CPM) may manifest in different ways. An abnormal karyotype such as trisomy 18 might be found in the placenta while the fetus has a normal karyotype. The placenta will often be *grossly and histologically normal (although sometimes small)* while the fetus is *growth restricted*. It is postulated that an *aneuploid placenta functions less efficiently than a normal organ* and therefore produces fetal growth restriction. CPM may also present as a trisomic fetus with a euploid placenta. *Fetuses with trisomy 13 and 18 who survive turn out to* *have placental karyotype mosaicism.* In these cases, the mosaicism appears to be confined to cytotrophoblast and not found in villous stroma, chorion, or amnion. The suggestion is that *trisomics with mosaic (aneuploid/diploid) placentas have a better chance of reaching maturity than those with truly trisomic placentas.*

CPM is also found more frequently in *unexplained stillbirths and unexplained growth restriction.* It is found three times more commonly in placentas with intrauterine growth restriction (IUGR) fetuses than normal fetuses. Moreover, 10% of gestations with CPM have fetal cytogenetic abnormalities. Regrettably, there is not yet much direct correlation with placental pathologic features in CPM. For the pathologist, it is important to realize that CPM occurs in the setting of unexplained fetal growth restriction or demise and that *to document CPM, samples from multiple placental sites are necessary to make the diagnosis.* If resources allow, the placenta may be evaluated for CPM in cases of IUGR that have no other apparent cause.

Uniparental Disomy

In **uniparental disomy** (UPD), there are *two chromosomes from one parent* rather than one from each parent. It is an occasional finding in *growth-restricted newborns* and *stillborns* and appears to be linked to confined placental mosaicism. It is postulated to take its origin from a *trisomic conceptus with the loss of one trisomic chromosome, leaving the fetus with a normal chromosome complement.* Depending on which chromosome is lost, the fetus may end up with two chromosomes from the same parent, or UPD. There are several ways in which UPD may complicate CPM. A trisomic fetus that loses its extra chromosome becomes diploid and may have UPD. If the corresponding placenta remains trisomic, CPM results. On the other hand, the placenta may lose the extra chromosome and develop UPD.

Imprinting

A final aspect of this complex array of potential genetic events is the concept of **imprinting**. It is a reality affecting fetal and placental tissues as well as many disease states and is presumably accomplished via DNA methylation of specific genes. There is good evidence that some *paternal genes are silenced during embryonic development (maternal imprinting), whereas some maternal genes are silenced during placental development (paternal imprinting).* Imprinting is important in understanding how different types of triploidy may result in the development of partial hydatidiform moles. Partial moles are generally triploid with one set of maternal genes and two sets of paternal genes. The excess of paternal genes acts similar to silence of maternal genes and leads to preferential development of trophoblastic tissues over fetal tissues.

Selected References

PHP4, Chapter 21, pages 685–717.
Bennett P, Vaughan J, Henderson D, et al. Association between confined placental trisomy, fetal uniparental disomy, and early intrauterine growth retardation. Lancet 1992;340:1284–1285.

Honoré LH, Dill FJ, Poland BJ. Placental morphology in spontaneous human abortuses with normal and abnormal karyotypes. Teratology 1976;14: 151–166.

Kalousek DK, Barrett, I. Confined placental mosaicism and stillbirth. Pediatr Pathol 1994;14:151–159.

Kalousek DK, Barrett IJ, McGillivray BC. Placental mosaicism and intrauterine survival of trisomies 13 and 18. Am J Hum Genet 1989;44:338–343.

Moore GE, Ali Z, Khan RU, et al. The incidence of uniparental disomy associated with intrauterine growth retardation in a cohort of thirty-five severely affected babies. Am J Obstet Gynecol 1997;176:294–299.

Redline RW, Hassold T, Zaragoza M. Determinants of villous trophoblastic hyperplasia in spontaneous abortions. Mod Pathol 1998;11:762–768.

Salafia CM, Burns JP. The correlation of placental and decidual histology with karyotype and fetal viability. Teratology 1989;39:478 (P37).

Stirrat GM. Recurrent miscarriage. I: Definition and epidemiology. Lancet 1990;336:673–675.

Stirrat GM. Recurrent miscarriage. II: Clinical associations, causes, and management. Lancet 1990;336:728–733.

Tycko B. Genomic imprinting: mechanism and role in human pathology. Am J Pathol 1994;144:431–443.

Warburton D, Stein Z, Kline J, et al. Chromosomal abnormalities in spontaneous abortions: data from the New York City study. In: Porter IH, Hook EB (eds) Human embryonic and fetal death. New York: Academic Press, 1980: 261–287.

Chapter 12

Postpartum Hemorrhage, Subinvolution of the Placental Site, and Placenta Accreta

General Considerations

Postpartum hemorrhage is a major obstetric emergency, which, if not treated promptly, may result in rapid exsanguination of the mother through the large uterine vessels. The type of specimens submitted to the pathology laboratory depends on the clinical situation and may include the *placenta, retroplacental curettings, other sampling from the endometrial cavity or the uterus, or, in some cases, no specimen at all.* Pathologic examination is facilitated by knowledge of the clinical situations leading to postpartum hemorrhage, such as:

- **Injury from cervical lacerations or uterine rupture,**
- **Coagulation defects,**
- **Uterine atony,**
- **Retained placental tissue,**
- **Subinvolution of the placental site,**
- **Postpartum endometritis,**
- **Placenta accreta,** and
- **Placental polyps.**

In the case of injury or coagulation defects, specimens are rarely submitted. If they are, nonspecific alterations such as hemorrhage are usually the only findings. Therefore, these are not discussed further.

The remaining causes of postpartum hemorrhage usually result in pathologic lesions, and therefore are discussed in the following sections.

Uterine Atony

Pathogenesis
After delivery of the placenta, cessation of blood flow through the endometrial vessels is largely accomplished by *contraction of the uterus.* **Uterine atony** is defined as the absence of normal uterine contraction. The most common causes of uterine atony are:

- **Over-distension** from a large fetus, multiple pregnancy, or polyhydramnios,
- **Anesthetic agents,**
- **Prolonged, augmented, or rapid labor**, and
- **High parity.**

When the myometrium loses the ability to contract, the uterine vessels may bleed extensively and present a life-threatening situation necessitating hysterectomy.

Pathologic Features
In normal circumstances, the postpartum uterus is *enlarged from myometrial hyperplasia and hypertrophy.* The uterine wall is usually markedly thickened, but firm due to the contraction of the myometrium. If **atony** is present, the uterus will be *edematous and boggy,* and hemorrhage may be grossly evident. Microscopically, the findings are relatively non-specific and consist of typical hypertrophied myometrium with *diffuse, recent hemorrhage,* often in the vicinity of large, open, dilated vessels. Groups of myometrial fibers may be *separated by edema fluid* (Figure 12.1), but the findings can often be subtle.

Suggestions for Examination and Report: Uterine Atony

Gross Examination: Representative sections of the uterus should be submitted including the implantation site. The latter is usually a roughened, hemorrhagic area on the endometrial surface. Sections of the lower uterine segment and cervix, if present, should also be submitted. Attention should be given to the presence of lacerations, perforation, or evidence of other injury, particularly in the cervix.

Comment: Edema and hemorrhage are usually present, consistent with the clinical history of uterine atony. A comment may be made about the absence of other pathologic findings, specifically addressing any clinical differential diagnoses.

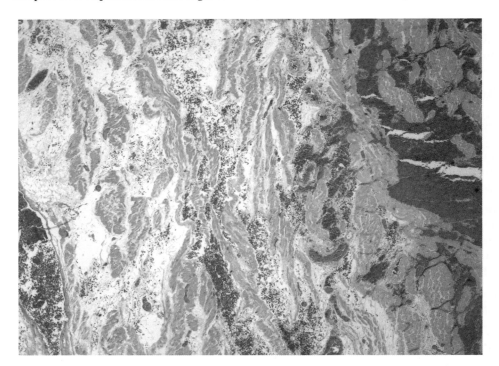

Figure 12.1. Microscopic appearance of the myometrium in a case of uterine atony. Muscle fibers are separated by edema fluid (at left) and there is focal recent hemorrhage. H&E. ×20.

Retained Placental Tissue and Involution of the Placental Site

It is often assumed that evaluation of the completeness of the maternal surface of the placenta will uncover the presence of missing placenta tissue that has been retained in the uterus. It is therefore quite interesting that many cases exist in which the placenta was described by experienced observers as "intact" and retained placental tissue was later found to be present. Thus, one cannot be reassured by the integrity of the placenta postpartum. On the other hand, when the maternal surface of the placenta is **not** intact, the likelihood of retention of placental tissue is heightened. Placental tissue may be retained for a number of reasons. It may be merely due to *inadequate removal of the entire placenta at delivery.* However, when there is associated **postpartum hemorrhage**, particularly delayed postpartum hemorrhage, it is more likely to be associated with a pathologic process. Delayed postpartum hemorrhage may occur days, weeks, or even months after delivery.

Normal Involution of the Placental Site

To understand subinvolution, one must first understand the complex process of normal placental site involution. Unfortunately, pathologists rarely receive normal postpartum uteri that would enable detailed study of the involutional changes at the former site of implantation. The following is an overview of the events at the placental site following normal delivery. They are also summarized in Table 12.1.

The separation of the placenta from the uterus takes place *within the decidua basalis*, largely as a result of the *shearing action of the myometrium as it contracts against the uncompressible placenta*. **Immediately following delivery**, contraction of the uterus clamps the arteries, stopping uterine bleeding. The endometrial surface becomes covered with *blood clot and fibrin*. **Within the first postpartum day**, the walls of the arteries and veins in the implantation site *become hyalinized. Fibrinoid necrosis and inflammation* develop in the arteries. *The implantation site decreases in size,* from about 18 cm, the approximate diameter of a term placenta, to 9 cm. From **postpartum day 1 to day 3**, the *veins thrombose* and the *arteries develop obliterative endarteritis*. There is early decidual necrosis and a modest neutrophilic and mononuclear infiltrate. From **day 3 to day 5**, *inflammation and necrosis* increase and reactive regenerating endometrial glands begin to appear. The thrombosed veins begin to organize, and the arteries show early intimal proliferation and continuing hyalinization. From **postpartum day 5 to day 8**, there is a *clear demarcation* of the necrotic decidua (which will be subsequently sloughed as the "lochia") from the remaining endometrium. *Endometrial glands show pronounced reactive changes and are increased in number.* They regenerate by regrowth and extension of the adjacent endometrial glands and stroma. *Arteries are nearly occluded* by endarteritis by this time. *Placental site giant cells are prominent* early in the involuting implantation site in the endometrium and superficial myometrium but their numbers decrease over the ensuing weeks. **Three to four weeks** after delivery, *the endometrium at the implantation site is regenerated and inactive with scattered hemosiderophages.* Veins have mostly been recanalized, but *some residual vessels show hyalinization,* which may persist for many weeks even under normal circumstances (Figure 12.2).

The rapidity of the **involution of myometrial muscle mass** postpartum remains a mystery. *The average postpartum uterus weighs about 1000 g and shrinks to less than 100 g in about 2 months.* The histologic changes are relatively minimal. Degenerative changes of the muscle occur within hours of delivery, and a mild chronic inflammatory infiltrate develops within the first 4 days and persists for up to 17 weeks. It is important to note that virtually *no myometrium repairs the incisional defect from cesarean sections and only a thin fibrous scar approximates the muscle layers.* Thus, in subsequent pregnancies the probability of dehiscence exists with possible **uterine rupture** and/or **placenta accreta** (see below).

Subinvolution of the Placental Site

Pathogenesis

When the uterus does not undergo normal involution, **subinvolution of the placental site** is said to occur. Here, there is *failure of the normal,*

Table 12.1. Histologic changes of normal placental site involution

Time postpartum	Gross size (cm)	"Slough"	Glands
Less than 1 day	From 18 to 9	Hemorrhage	Few, inactive
1–3 days	8 to 7	Early necrosis	Mild reactive change
3–5 days	6	Necrosis with inflammation	Regenerating glands, moderate reactive change
5–8 days	4.5	Well demarcated	Marked reactive change, increased numbers of glands, placental site giant cells
4–20 weeks	2.0	None	Inactive glands, hemosiderophages

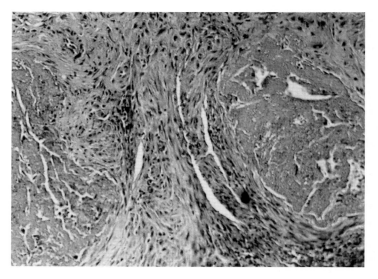

Figure 12.2. Normal involution of the placental site with thrombosed uterine vessels approximately 2 weeks after delivery. H&E. ×20.

Decidua	Veins	Arteries
Viable	Hyalinized	Fibrinoid necrosis, minimal inflammation
Necrosis and inflammation	Thrombosed	Obliterative endarteritis
Increased necrosis and inflammation	Organizing	Hyalinization, intimal proliferation
Necrosis and inflammation	Organizing thrombi	Hyalinization
None	Recanalized, hyalinized	Remnants of hyalinized vessels

physiologic obliteration of the blood vessels in the placental site as well as delayed myometrial involution. The uterus is somewhat boggy and edematous, but not to the degree that is seen in uterine atony. There may be delayed postpartum hemorrhage, which typically occurs 1 to 2 weeks after delivery, but occasionally occurs several months postpartum. This is in contrast to uterine atony in which hemorrhage occurs immediately after delivery and is much more severe. Subinvolution is, in fact, the most common cause of "delayed" postpartum hemorrhage. It is more common in *multiparous women and tends to recur in subsequent pregnancies.* Causes include *retained placental tissue, infection, placenta accreta, and idiopathic causes.*

Pathologic Features

Most patients with subinvolution have normal placentas at delivery. Later, bleeding occurs and usually uterine curettings are submitted to pathology. On histologic examination of the endometrial tissue, large *dilated arteries filled with blood and partially organized thrombi* are seen. The arteries are often found in groups of three or four, adjacent to normally involuting vessels (Figure 12.3). The histologic picture may be similar to normal involution, but the changes are delayed. Furthermore, in contrast to normal involution, where extravillous trophoblast is inconspicuous or absent, subinvolution is characterized by the *persistence of extravillous trophoblast*, particularly in a perivascular location. *Persistence of endovascular extravillous trophoblast* is also occasionally seen.

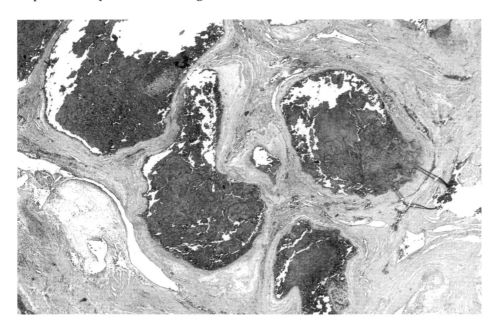

Figure 12.3. Subinvolution of the placental site. Note the enlarged, patent vessels with evidence of bleeding. H&E. ×40.

> *Suggestions for Examination and Report: Subinvolution of the Placental Site*
>
> **Gross Examination:** Subinvolution is most commonly seen in patients who present with postpartum bleeding. There are no specific issues relating to the gross specimen.
>
> **Comment:** Subinvolution of the placental site is a common cause of postpartum hemorrhage, particularly delayed postpartum hemorrhage.

Postpartum Endometritis

Postpartum endometritis is an intrauterine infection that is classically caused by group A streptococci, but many other organisms, including anaerobes, have been implicated. It is an **acute endometritis** characterized by *pronounced acute inflammatory infiltrates within endometrial stroma and gland lumens* (Figure 12.4) and may be associated with colonies of bacterial organisms. Phlebothrombosis and a plasma cell infiltrate may also be present. Endometritis is often associated with subinvolution, and in this case, the histologic features of subinvolution will also be present. Postpartum endometritis may lead to serious complications such as *sepsis, pulmonary embolism, and even death*.

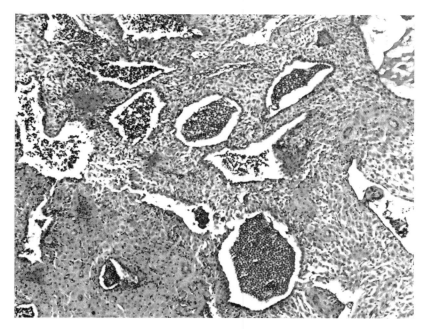

Figure 12.4. Postpartum endometritis showing an inflammatory infiltrate consisting predominantly of acute inflammatory cells within both the stroma and gland lumens. H&E. ×40.

Suggestions for Examination and Report:
Postpartum Endometritis

Gross Examination: There is no specific gross appearance.

Comment: The diagnosis of acute endometritis postpartum, particularly if bacteria are present, may have serious clinical sequelae.

Placenta Accreta, Placenta Increta, and Placenta Percreta

In normal implantation, the extravillous trophoblast invades the decidua in a controlled fashion and converts the spiral arterioles of the endometrium to uteroplacental vessels (see Chapter 8). In **placenta accreta**, there is a *failure of the normal decidua to form*, at least locally, because the endometrium is deficient and cannot decidualize. The trophoblast does not stop invading when it should and penetrates more deeply into the myometrium. Traditionally, placenta accreta has been divided into **placenta accreta**, **placenta increta**, and **placenta percreta** based on how deeply the trophoblastic tissues invade. In **placenta accreta**, *the chorionic villi are implanted on the myometrium without intervening decidua*, in **placenta increta** *the myometrium is invaded by the* *placental villous tissue*, and in **placenta percreta**, *the villi penetrate the entire uterine wall.* The underlying pathogenetic mechanisms and etiologies are likely to be the same, the only difference being a quantitative one, which, however, may be of considerable clinical importance, particularly in the case of placenta percreta.

Clinical Features and Implications

Placenta accreta is relatively rare with an incidence of around 1 in 7000 pregnancies. The incidence is higher in the setting of placenta previa, where it is estimated to be 1.18%. The occurrence of placenta accreta has been steadily rising, and this is thought to be secondary to the increased cesarean section rate (see below). It is often detected after delivery *when the placenta fails to separate or is incompletely delivered.* Incretas and percretas more frequently manifest antepartum and earlier in gestation because of hemorrhage or uterine rupture. In 45% of cases, there is an elevation of maternal serum alpha fetoprotein levels. Diagnosis by ultrasonography and magnetic resonance imaging (MRI) is possible, and cases have been reported as early as 14 weeks. Sonography of placenta accreta often displays *irregular lucencies in the villous tissue.* These "lakes" presumably derive from the abnormal implantation and an abnormal disposition of maternal spiral arterioles relative to the intervillous space.

Placenta accreta may be associated with *life-threatening hemorrhage that can lead to maternal and/or fetal death.* Maternal deaths occur in approximately 9.5% of cases and fetal deaths in a similar percentage. Placenta percreta may lead to *uterine rupture,* or it may invade the bladder causing hematuria. Massive hemorrhage from perforation has also been described. Thus, when a placenta percreta or a deep placenta increta is identified by radiologic studies, delivery by cesarean section with hysterectomy is usually undertaken, even in cases where the fetus is significantly premature. Although the usual treatment is hysterectomy, microembolization through the internal iliac arteries has been used to treat placenta accreta. Embolization is performed and the placenta is often left within the uterus, to be followed by spontaneous expulsion several days later. Pathologic changes of uterine retention of the placenta are discussed below.

Pathogenesis

In **placenta accreta**, the villous tissues are anchored to the uterus without intervening decidual cells due to a *deficiency of decidua.* Normally, the placenta separates from the uterine musculature in a plane just peripheral to Nitabuch's fibrinoid layer, within the decidua basalis. It is accomplished by the *shearing action of contracting myometrium against the stationary, noncontracting placenta and occurs in an irregular plane of friable decidual cells.* Without this layer, uterine contractions do not dislodge the placenta and portions of the placenta, or the entire placenta is retained. Sometimes, the area of adherence may be quite small and retention of placental tissue in the uterus may not be immediately noticed.

Placenta accreta is a nice example of the *importance of endometrial decidualization for proper control of trophoblast invasion.* This correlation is further underlined by the fact that *absence of decidualization in tubal pregnancy also coincides with increased trophoblastic invasiveness* and thus ectopic pregnancies are essentially tubal placenta accretas. They usually perforate the wall, becoming placenta percretas. A similar situation arises in the lower uterine segment and endocervix as decidualization is often not fully developed in these areas. At present, the specific decidual characteristics responsible for control of invasiveness are still unknown.

Any condition that leads to the development of **deficient decidua** predisposes the patient to placenta accreta. *The most frequent predisposing condition is a history of previous cesarean section and/or curettage.* The risk for development of placenta accreta increases with a history of multiple cesarean sections and multiple surgeries. Other predisposing conditions include *placenta previa (see Chapter 13), submucosal leiomyoma, cornual implantation, placenta membranacea (Chapter 13),* and *uterine anomalies.* In all these cases, there is the potential for deficient decidualization. Placenta accretas and particularly percretas are said to be increasing in frequency, and this undoubtedly relates to the greater frequency of cesarean sections. In a surgical incision, reconstitution of a *normal* uterine wall is not possible. Therefore, in the subsequent pregnancy, the expanding uterus may dehisce at the former incision site. If the placenta implants over this previous scar, uterine expansion will cause the placenta to be implanted on very thin scar tissue and/or peritoneum resulting in placenta accreta.

Pathologic Features

In placenta accreta, the placenta is often disrupted during delivery and there may be *missing cotyledons*. However, completeness of the maternal surface cannot always be accurately evaluated. If the placenta is relatively intact, a **focal placenta accreta** may still be present. When histologic sections of such a placenta are made, the deficiency of endometrium that underlies placenta accreta is generally not evident. It may be possible to make the diagnosis of placenta accreta if curettings are done that include the myometrium, but it is very difficult as the tissue is often impossible to orient. If portions of the myometrium are removed with the placenta and remain attached to the floor (Figure 12.5), the diagnosis may also be made. However, in the case of a placental specimen or curettings, the diagnosis of accreta can certainly not be ruled out. The diagnosis is much easier to accomplish when the entire uterus is available, which of course is the less acceptable outcome for the patient. Nevertheless, hysterectomy is a frequent sequela of placenta accreta.

The cesarean-hysterectomy specimen is often quite remarkable on gross examination (Figure 12.6). If the diagnosis is known before delivery, the placenta may be left "in situ" in the uterus. Then, the true relationship of the placenta to the implantation site may be studied. The serosal surface of the uterus is often *congested, hemorrhagic, and may show nodular protrusions representing a thinned myometrium overlying placental tissue* (Figure 12.6). Examination of the uterine cavity will show placenta implanted over *myometrium that is markedly thinned or even absent* (Figure 12.6). At times, only a thin covering of peritoneum is present over the placenta. If the placenta is not left intact, retained placental

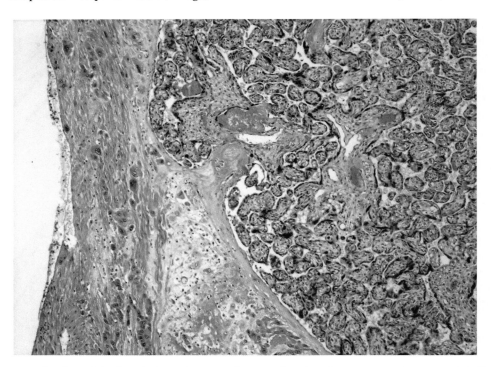

Figure 12.5. Section of the basal plate of a term placenta showing the presence of myometrial fibers to which chorionic villi are firmly attached (upper left). H&E. ×40.

tissue may still be visible firmly attached to the endometrium. In placenta percreta (Figure 12.7), placental tissue may be visible perforating through the uterine serosa. Care must be taken to ensure that loss of integrity of the serosa is not due to rough handling of the specimen before examination. Correlation with clinical history may be helpful in these cases. On microscopic examination, one sees *villous tissue that has grown onto or into the myometrium without intervening decidua*. It is important to note that it is the **lack of decidua** that is diagnostic of this entity (Figure 12.8). This point is discussed more fully in the next section.

There are several associated pathologic findings seen with placenta accreta. First, the normal *physiologic conversion of maternal vessels may be focally deficient*. This may be related to the abnormal invasiveness of trophoblast and/or to the general lack of availability of decidual vessels for implantation. There is also usually a *deficiency of placental septum formation*. When septa are present in a placenta accreta, they are composed of uterine muscle rather than decidua, extravillous trophoblast, and fibrinoid. This leads to abnormal flow patterns in the intervillous space, which may be appreciated on antepartum imaging.

Pitfalls in Diagnosis
There are several important pitfalls in the diagnosis of placenta accreta, partly caused by confusion in distinguishing the populations of cells that make up the placental floor. The first difficulty lies in the fact that in placenta accreta *rarely are the chorionic villi present **directly** on the*

myometrium. Villi implanted on the myometrium are really a fortuitous finding and are not required for diagnosis. Most often, there is *fibrinoid and extravillous trophoblast in between* the myometrium and the villous tissue (Figure 12.9 A). The crucial point here is that the diagnostic feature of placenta accreta is the **lack of decidua and not implantation onto the myometrium.** Therefore, if villi are present adjacent to fibrinoid or extravillous trophoblast, which is **then** adjacent to myometrium, and there is no intervening decidua, the diagnosis of placenta accreta is made. Insistence on the demonstration of villous implantation on the myometrium will result in *underdiagnosis.*

The second cause of underdiagnosis is confusion of extravillous trophoblast with decidua. Extravillous trophoblast are always present in the implantation site and are normally present adjacent to the myometrium and villous tissue. *If these trophoblastic cells are misinterpreted as decidual cells, the diagnosis will be missed* (Figure 12.9 A). If there is doubt about the true nature of cells in the implantation site, immunohistochemistry for cytokeratin can be extremely helpful as

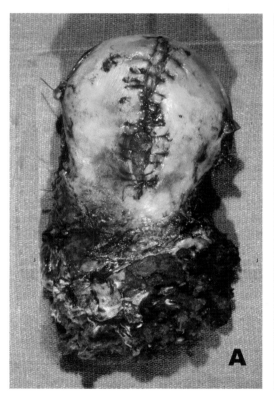
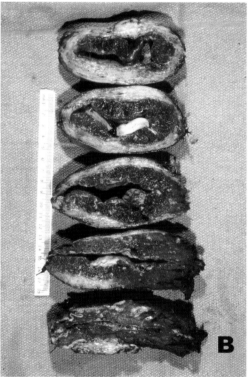

Figure 12.6. Cesarean-hysterectomy specimen with placental implantation over the cervical os leading to a placenta previa accreta. (A) Note the protrusion of hemorrhagic placental tissue in the lower uterine segment. A vertical scar represents the incision made during delivery. (B) Same specimen as part A. Serial transverse sections have been made with the most superior at the top and the most inferior at the bottom. Note that the myometrium becomes thinned to invisibility in the lower uterine segment.

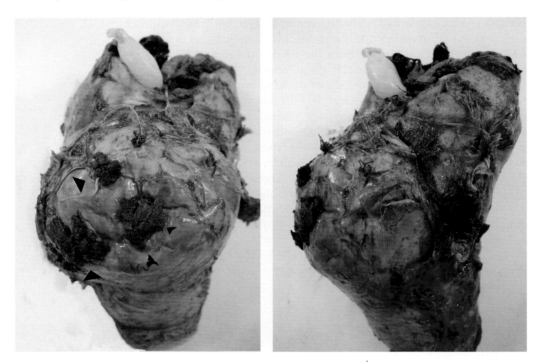

Figure 12.7. Photograph of cesarean-hysterectomy specimen with placenta percreta in which placental tissue can be seen protruding through the serosal surface (arrowheads at left).

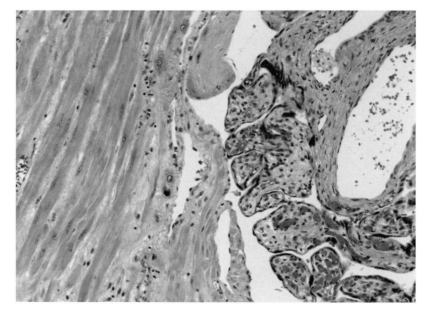

Figure 12.8. Placenta accreta showing "classic" picture with chorionic villi attached directly to the myometrium. H&E. ×200.

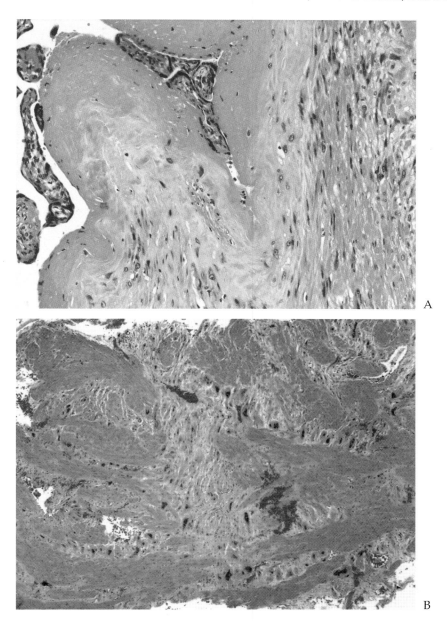

Figure 12.9. (A) Placenta accreta. Here, the chorionic villi implant on fibrinoid and extravillous trophoblast and not directly on myometrium, but with the absence of decidua is still diagnostic of placenta accreta. H&E ×100. (B) Placental site giant cells present within myometrium, a normal finding that is not diagnostic of placenta accreta. H&E. ×20.

trophoblastic cells are epithelial and are strongly positive for cytokeratins, while decidual cells are not.

Overdiagnosis of placenta accreta may also occur. In the normal implantation site, extravillous trophoblast and placental site giant cells (see Chapter 8) are present in the basal portion of the placenta, the decidua, *and the myometrium*. Often, the presence of placental site giant cells within the myometrium is interpreted as evidence of placenta accreta. However, the presence of these trophoblastic cells within the myometrium is *a normal finding and is not diagnostic of placenta accreta* (Figure 12.9 B).

Suggestions for Examination and Report: Placenta Accreta, Placenta Increta, and Placenta Percreta

Gross Examination: If only the placenta is submitted, examination should involve careful inspection of the maternal surface for completeness and the presence of firm white tissue, which may represent attached myometrium. Retroplacental curettings should be completely submitted for microscopic examination. In a hysterectomy specimen, the area of accreta is often obvious, particularly if the placenta is left in situ. Sections should be taken to include placenta and myometrium in areas where *the myometrium is thinned or where there is firm placental attachment.* The anterior lower uterine segment is the most common place for placenta accretas associated with previous cesarean section. If the site of accreta is not obvious, or the placenta is not included, multiple sections should be submitted from the most likely areas to show accreta, the lower uterine segment and cervix. The most hemorrhagic, roughened areas are the most likely to represent implantation site and/or retained placental tissue.

Comment: Comments should be directed to the location where the accreta was found and the extent of the accreta, for example, depth and breadth. Other pathology that may be associated with increased risk of accretas should also be commented on, such as uterine scar, bicornuate uterus, etc.

Placental Polyp

Placental polyps are polypoid fragments of tissue consisting of degenerated chorionic villi that have become encased in fibrinoid and layered clot. They represent **focal placentas accretas.** Because of the degenerative changes associated with intrauterine retention of this tissue, the diagnosis may be difficult to verify. At times, however, some myometrial tissue is also present and one finds *villi directly attached to myometrium.* Placental polyps may be *seen in endometrial curettings for postpartum bleeding or may be spontaneously passed weeks or months after delivery* (Figure 12.10). They are seen in up to 45% of women who present with delayed postpartum hemorrhage. When they are removed or spontaneously passed, the symptoms of bleeding usually abate. Rarely, failure to remove placental polyps has resulted in potentially life-threatening hemorrhage.

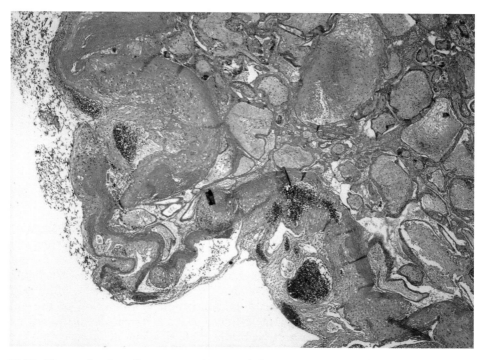

Figure 12.10. Placental polyp. Spontaneously passed tissue consisting predominantly of degenerating chorionic villi enmeshed in fibrinoid and extravillous trophoblast. Although the implantation of this placental fragment is not present, the diagnosis of placenta accreta is presumed. H&E. ×20.

Suggestions for Examination and Report: Placental Polyp

Gross Examination: Placental polyps are usually submitted as curettings or as an endometrial polyp in women with delayed postpartum bleeding. Unless unusually large, the specimen should be entirely submitted.

Comment: Placental polyps are usually indicative of a focal placenta accreta.

Squamous Epithelial Masses

Somewhat related to placental polyps are the rare pathologic findings of **squamous epithelial masses**. These are found in postpartum endometrial specimens and consist of collections of squamous *epithelial cells embedded in the endomyometrium and maternal vessels associated with an intense inflammatory response*. They undoubtedly arise from *vernix caseosa*. It is likely they occur secondary to *previous membrane rupture and subsequent reaction to amniotic fluid content*. They have minimal clinical impact.

Suggestions for Examination and Report:
Squamous Epithelial Masses

Gross Examination: There is no specific gross appearance of this lesion.

Comment: Inflamed masses of squamous epithelium postpartum are likely associated with a reaction to vernix caseosa after membrane rupture and have no clinical significance.

Involution of a Retained Placenta

Placentas may be retained in utero after a fetal demise, when only one of a set of twins survives, or when the placenta is not removed after delivery because of a placenta accreta. Because there is continued perfusion by maternal blood, the placental *tissue remains structurally intact for a long time*, particularly the trophoblastic cells. Initially there is *increased syncytial knotting*, followed by involution of the fetal vasculature resulting in *avascular villi. Fibrinoid also accumulates in the intervillous space.* Eventually, the placenta atrophies and comes to resemble an infarct with marked calcification and villous hyalinization (Figure 12.11). The more remote the fetal demise, the more likely the degenerative changes are to mask any other pathologic lesions present.

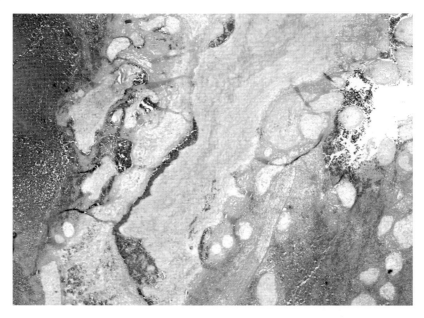

Figure 12.11. Involuting placenta in case of intrauterine fetal demise many weeks previously. Note the avascular, hyaline villi and the presence of increased fibrinoid in the intervillous space. H&E. ×20.

Suggestions for Examination and Report:
Involution of a Retained Placenta

Gross Examination: The placenta may appear grossly infarcted and is usually quite firm. The cord and membranes often are discolored red due to hemolysis. Routine sections should be submitted.

Comment: Increased syncytial knots, fibrinoid deposition, calcification, and degenerative changes are consistent with retention of placental tissue after delivery or fetal death.

Selected References

PHP4, Chapter 9, pages 229–236 (Trophoblastic Invasion), and Chapter 10, pages 273–280 (Implantation Site and Retained Placenta).

Anderson WR, Davis J. Placental site involution. Am J Obstet Gynecol 1968; 102:23–33.

Clark SL, Koonings PP, Phelan JP. Placenta previa/accreta and prior cesarean section. Obstet Gynecol 1985;66:89–92.

Cox SM, Carpenter RJ, Cotton DB. Placenta percreta: ultrasound diagnosis and conservative surgical management. Obstet Gynecol 1988;71:454–456.

Fox H. Morphological changes in the human placenta following fetal death. J Obstet Gynaecol Br Commonw 1968;75:839–843.

Fox H. Placenta accreta, 1945–1969. Obstet Gynecol Surv 1972;27:475–490.

Irving FC, Hertig AT. A study of placenta accreta. Surg Gynecol Obstet 1937; 64:178–200.

Jacques SM, Qureshi F, Trent VS, et al. Placenta accreta: mild cases diagnosed by placental examination. Int J Gynecol Pathol 1996;15:28–33.

Khong TY, Robertson WB. Placenta creta and placenta praevia creta. Placenta 1987;8:399–409.

Khong TY, Khong TK. Delayed postpartum hemorrhage: a morphologic study of causes and their relation to other pregnancy disorders Obstet Gynecol 1993; 82:17–22.

Lawrence WD, Qureshi F, Bonakdar MI. "Placental polyp": light microscopic and immunohistochemical observations. Hum Pathol 1988;19:1467–1470.

Rutherford RN, Hertig AT. Noninvolution of the placental site. Am J Obstet Gynecol 1945;49:378–384.

Williams JW. Regeneration of the uterine mucosa after delivery, with especial reference to the placental site. Am J Obstet Gynecol 1931;22:664–696, 793–796.

Chapter 13

Placental Shape Aberrations

General Considerations

Round or oval placentas are the predominant human placental form, but many other shapes exist (Figure 13.1). When the placenta is irregular, its shape is presumably determined by location, atrophy, and perhaps the manner of original implantation. Anomalies may develop from abnormal fetal genes expressed by the placenta, an abnormal maternal environment, or an abnormal fetal–maternal interaction. Interestingly, for each aberrant placental shape in humans, there is a counterpart in animals. Thus, the placenta membranacea is similar to the normally diffuse placenta in equines; the zonary placenta is typical of carnivores, and so on.

Multilobed Placentas

Bilobed Placenta

Pathologic Features

One of the most striking abnormalities is the **bilobed placenta** (placenta bilobata), in which *two roughly equal sized lobes are separated by a segment of membranes* (Figures 13.1, 13.2). It is present in 2% to 8% of placentas. The umbilical cord may insert in either of the lobes or in a velamentous fashion (see Chapter 15), in between the lobes, the latter

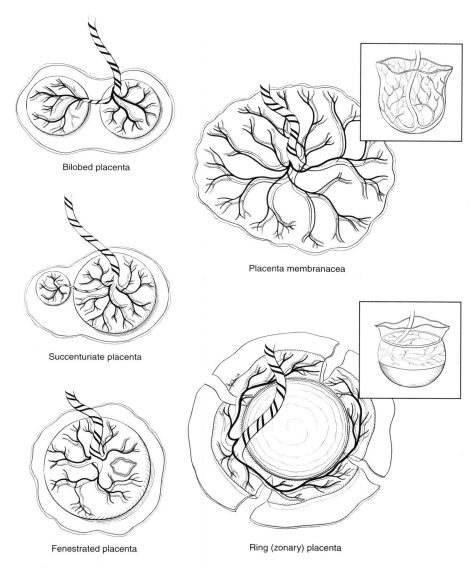

Bilobed placenta

Placenta membranacea

Succenturiate placenta

Fenestrated placenta

Ring (zonary) placenta

Figure 13.1. Diagram depicting placental shape abnormalities including multilobation (bilobed placenta and succenturiate placenta), placenta fenestrata, placenta membranacea, and ring or zonary placenta.

being the most common arrangement. Even if the cord insertion is not velamentous, there *are always membranous vessels connecting the two lobes*. If one lobe is much smaller than the other, then the placenta is said to have a **succenturiate** or **accessory lobe** (see below).

Pathogenesis
Multilobed placentas are thought to arise due to implantation in areas of decreased uterine perfusion. An example is lateral implantation in between the anterior and posterior walls of the uterus with one lobe on the anterior and one on the posterior wall. Other local factors leading to multilobation are implantation over *leiomyomas, in areas of*

previous surgery, in the cornu, or over the cervical os. After implantation, there is preferential growth in areas of superior perfusion and atrophy in areas of poor perfusion. This is called **trophotropism**. Indeed, intermediate forms exist in which there are two lobes, with partial or complete infarction of residual villous tissue between the lobes. This finding suggests that normal discoidal placentation was originally present but local factors led to atrophy or infarction, resulting in multilobation.

Clinical Features and Implications

The membranous vessels connecting the two lobes occasionally *thrombose, rupture, become compressed*, or present clinically as *vasa previa* with bleeding. Vasa previa occurs when the membranous vessels present "previous" to the delivering part of the baby (see Chapter 15). Both bilobed placentas and succenturiate lobes are associated with *multiparity, antenatal bleeding, placenta previa, and retained placental tissue.*

Succenturiate Lobes (Accessory Lobes, Placenta Succenturiata)

Succenturiate lobes have an incidence of approximately 5% to 6%. They may be single or multiple and differ from bilobed placentas only in the size and number of accessory lobes (Figures 13.1, 13.3). *Approximately half are associated with infarction or atrophy of the succenturiate lobes,* much higher than the overall incidence of infarction, which is esti-

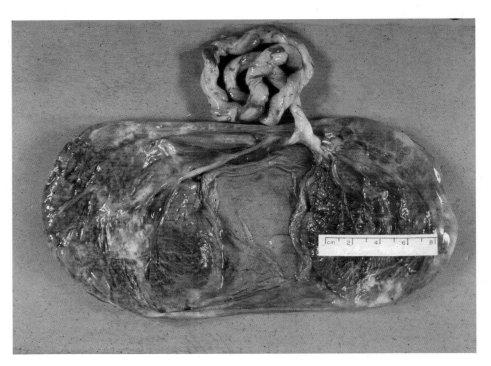

Figure 13.2. Bilobed placenta. Membranous vessels course from the velamentous cord insertion in between the two lobes.

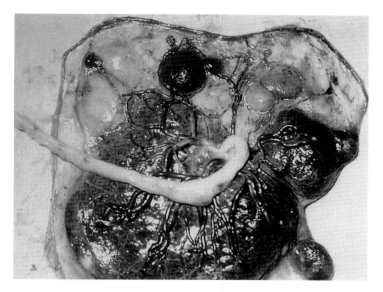

Figure 13.3. Succenturiate lobes in an immature placenta, with infarction of some of the lobes.

mated to be 13%. As with bilobed placentas, membranous vessels are always present connecting each lobe and thus may be susceptible to damage. The umbilical cord most commonly inserts into the dominant lobe.

> ### Suggestions for Examination and Report: Bilobed Placenta and Placenta with Succenturiate Lobes
>
> **Gross Examination:** Each lobe should be measured and weighed individually. The integrity of the membranous vessels connecting the lobes should be evaluated, and it is recommended that sections be taken of the vessels if they are ruptured, show gross thrombosis, or there is hemorrhage into the adjacent membranes. The vessels may be included in a separate membrane roll.
>
> **Comment:** If membranous vessels are present and associated with thrombosis, rupture, or hemorrhage into the membranes, the possibility of fetal hemorrhage should be considered.

Circumvallate and Circummarginate Placentas

Pathologic Features

In **circumvallate** placentas, the membranes of the chorion laeve do not insert at the edge of the placenta but rather at some inward distance from the margin, toward the umbilical cord (Figure 13.4). At the margin, one usually finds variable amounts of fibrin, recent clot, and

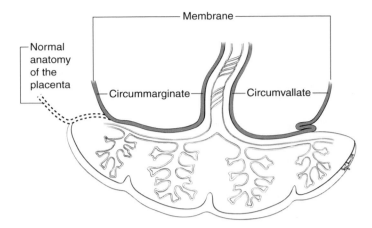

Figure 13.4. Diagram of circummarginate and circumvallate membrane insertion. In both, the fetal membranes do not insert at the edge of the placenta but rather at some point inwards. In circumvallation there is a plication of the membranes evident as a fibrin ridge on gross examination. In circummargination, the membrane insertion is flat and a ridge is not present.

old blood. In **complete circumvallates**, there is a complete circumferential ring that restricts the total surface of the chorion frondosum (Figures 13.5, 13.6). At the periphery, "naked" placental tissue protrudes. The fibrin that is present at the insertion of the membranes causes plication of the membranes, which is characteristic of circumvallates (Figure 13.7). The amnion may follow the chorion into this plica, or most commonly, it flatly covers the plica without infolding. When no plication of the membranes occurs, it is called a

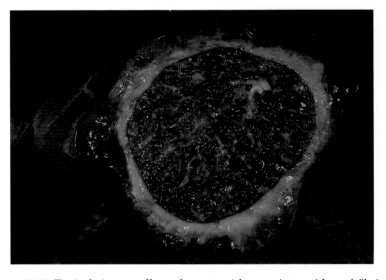

Figure 13.5. Typical circumvallate placenta with prominent ridge of fibrin at the periphery.

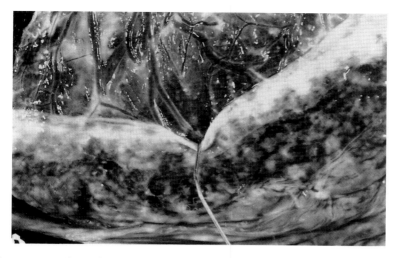

Figure 13.6. Plica of circumvallate margin with a wire holding up the over-hanging margin of the membrane insertion.

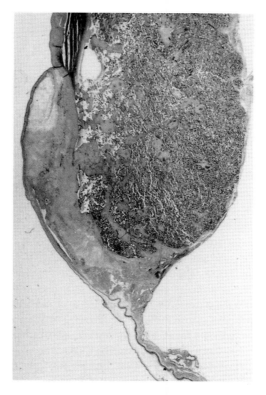

Figure 13.7. Margin of circumvallate placenta. The gray homogeneous material under the plica represents fibrin and degenerated blood.

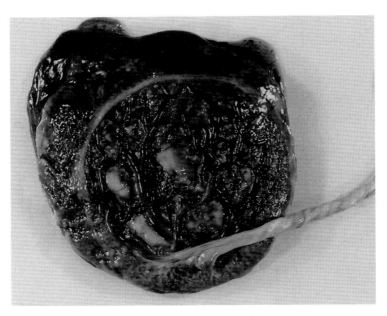

Figure 13.8. Sickle-shaped circummarginate placenta.

circummarginate placenta (Figures 13.4, 13.8). These two forms blend into each other, and partial forms are common.

Gross examination of the placenta *shows yellow-brown marginal fibrin* peripheral to the fibrin present at the membrane insertion. In cases where there is midtrimester hemorrhage and premature delivery, there may be substantial blood at the margin. Hemorrhage may undermine the margin of the placenta, thus imitating abruptio placentae. On microscopic examination, sections taken from the margin of the placenta will show *absence of membranous covering peripherally with hemosiderin deposition and fibrin* (Figure 13.7).

Clinical Features and Implications
The incidence of circumvallation is from 1.0% to 6.5%, and the incidence of circummargination is up to 25% of placentas. They are rarely found in the first trimester. The most common complications of circumvallation are *antenatal bleeding and premature delivery*. Additional, uncommon associations include *premature membrane rupture, perinatal death, congenital anomalies, single umbilical artery, and intrauterine growth restriction*. Cases with extensive hemorrhage and **marginal hematomas** may lead to significant clinical bleeding. Large hematomas may elevate the chorion laeve from its insertion site and cause disruption of the fetal vessels. Thus, the vaginal bleeding in these cases is frequently a mixture of maternal and fetal blood. Significant *neonatal anemia* may result. It has been suggested that circummargination has little clinical impact while circumvallation has some important clinical associations. However, we prefer to view these two entities as aspects of the same process.

Pathogenesis

Several opposing theories have been presented as to the origin of circumvallation. One theory is that circumvallation occurs due to marginal hemorrhage, which undermines the membranes and pushes them over the chorionic plate. Another theory is that circumvallates develop because the embryo implants too superficially and grows outward in a "polypoid" fashion or that it implants too deep. It is possible that there may be different types and origins of circumvallation, and this issue is yet to be resolved.

Extramembranous Pregnancy

Pathogenesis

In **extramembranous** or **extrachorial pregnancy**, there is *early rupture of both the amnion and chorion, leading to escape of the fetus into the uterine cavity* (Figure 13.9). Evidence that the fetus must have escaped out of

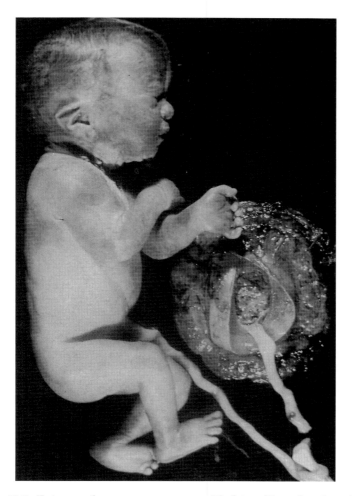

Figure 13.9. Extramembranous pregnancy with fetus. Note the size of fetus and the membrane opening. The placenta shows marked circumvallation.

the membranes much earlier is manifested by the *diminutive hole* through the membranes, which may barely admit the umbilical cord, let alone the fetus (Figure 13.9). It is a rare condition, and as with other conditions associated with early membrane rupture, such as amnionic bands (see Chapter 14), the etiology remains obscure.

Pathologic Features

The placenta shows *marked circumvallation* (Figure 13.10), *the cord may be short, and the fetal surface shows lack of membranous covering*, being covered instead with fibrin and a brownish discoloration consistent with hemosiderin (Figure 13.11). The remaining membranes are relatively normal. Microscopically, one finds substantial quantities of posthemorrhagic *hemosiderin in the membranes*. There also may be sparse amnion nodosum (see Chapter 14) over the placental tissue, but this is usually not striking.

Clinical Features and Implications

Because of membrane rupture and loss of amniotic fluid, extramembranous pregnancies are usually associated with prolonged *amniorrhea* as a result of periodic fetal urination. In addition, there are *severe positional deformities of the fetus and pulmonary hypoplasia* due to the *oligohydramnios*. Ascending infection is occasionally associated with extramembranous pregnancy, but this is not a constant finding. The majority of these pregnancies abort or terminate prematurely, and such fetuses only occasionally survive.

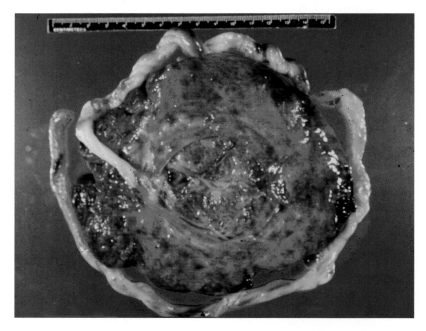

Figure 13.10. Extramembranous pregnancy with circumvallation and diminutive opening.

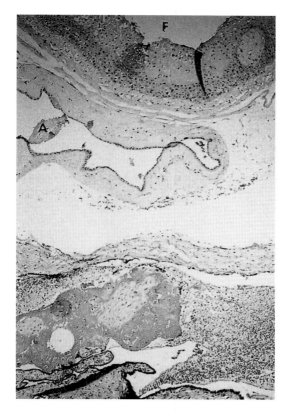

Figure 13.11. Membrane insertion in the extramembranous pregnancy shown in Figure 13.9. Below is the villous tissue, membranes folded at top right, and the fetus lay in space F. A = amnion nodosum.

Suggestions for Examination and Report:
Circumvallate Placenta, Circummarginate Placentas,
and Extramembranous Pregnancy

Gross Examination: Extent of the circumvallation should be noted as well as a lack of amnion over the fetal surface and the presence of hemosiderin (brown discoloration) and fibrin. It should also be noted whether there is plication or the membranes (circumvallate) or not (circummarginate). The presence of extensive marginal hemorrhage (marginal hematoma) and disruption of fetal vessels should also be noted.

Comment: A comment is not necessary except when disrupted fetal vessels are present. In this case, the possible role of circumvallation in the etiology may be suggested. If extreme circumvallation and an extramembranous pregnancy are present, a comment may be made on the association with a history of chronic leakage of amniotic fluid prior to delivery, oligohydramnios, fetal positional deformities, and pulmonary hypoplasia.

Placenta Membranacea (Placenta Diffusa)

Placenta membranacea is a rare abnormality of placental form in which *all, or nearly all, of the circumference of the fetal sac is covered by villous tissue.* The placental tissue is generally quite thin (approximately 1 cm) and is often disrupted (Figures 13.1, 13.12). Partial placenta membranacea can also occur. The etiology is not fully understood, but it seems obvious that those villi destined to atrophy and become the chorion laeve are retained while there is lack of growth of the villi destined to become the chorion frondosum. Underlying reasons postulated for lack of villous growth relate mostly to abnormalities of the endometrium such as *endometrial hypoplasia, poor vascular supply of the decidua basalis, endometritis, multiple curettages, adenomyosis, or atrophy of the endometrium.* Placenta membranacea may manifest clinically as *early bleeding* and *placenta previa.* Affected pregnancies often terminate in *premature delivery,* and *placenta accreta* is relatively common (see Chapter 12). *Spontaneous abortion* and *second trimester fetal demise* have also been reported.

> *Suggestions for Examination and Report:*
> *Placenta Membranacea*
>
> **Gross Examination:** Examination should include documentation of the increased diameter and excessive thinness of the placenta.
>
> **Comment:** Placenta membranacea is of unknown etiology, and the clinical associations are vaginal bleeding, placenta previa, premature delivery, and placenta accreta.

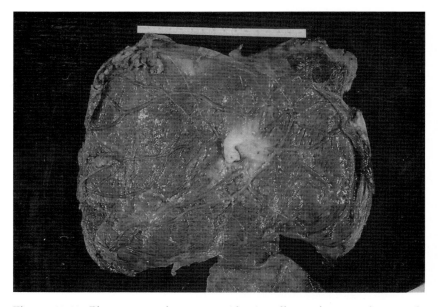

Figure 13.12. Placenta membranacea with virtually no free membranes: the placenta is very thin.

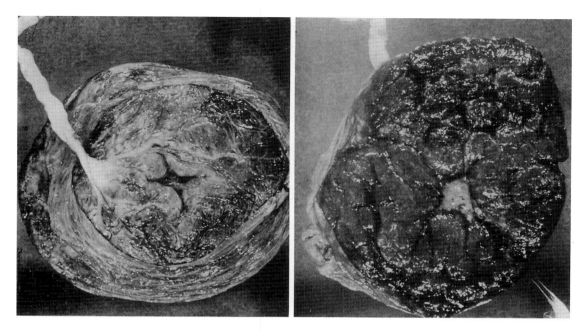

Figure 13.3. Placenta fenestrata. The central area of the placenta has a distinct defect, only chorionic membranes being present. (Courtesy of Dr. L.F. Moreno, Caracas, Venezuela.)

Miscellaneous Shape Abnormalities

In **placenta fenestrata,** a central area of the placenta is atrophied sufficiently to leave only membranes (Figures 13.1, 13.13). One must be careful to rule out the possibility of a missing cotyledon. The etiology is unknown but may be secondary to implantation over a leiomyoma or cornual tube orifice. **Zonary (annular) placentas** have a ring shape (Figure 13.1, 13.14). They are likely derived from a placenta previa with focal atrophy of the low-lying villous tissue covering the internal os.

Placenta Previa

Pathogenesis

The term **placenta previa** refers to the *location of the placenta over the internal os.* The placenta is thus "previous" to the delivering part of the baby. The overall incidence is somewhere between 0.3% and 1%. When, during early pregnancy, a placenta previa is unmistakably diagnosed there is often conversion to a "marginal" or higher-lying placenta. The incidence at midtrimester is 5%, but more than 90% of these "convert" to a non-previa by term. Serial ultrasound examinations throughout pregnancy have shown that the placenta actually "wanders," a phenomenon referred to as "**dynamic placentation.**" This placental movement is not accomplished, of course, by the placenta unseating and

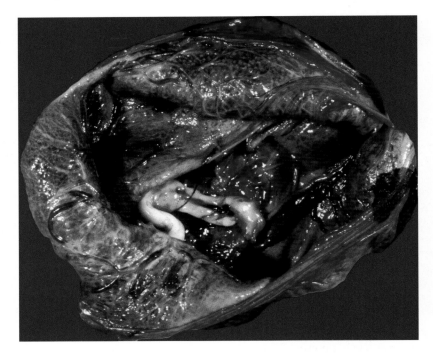

Figure 13.14. Zonary placenta showing a ringlike configuration. The placenta has been placed on its edge to demonstrate the unusual shape. The membranes ruptured and the infant delivered through the opening. The cord inserted to the side (not seen in this figure).

relocating itself, but rather through *marginal atrophy on one side and growth and expansion on the other*, a process called **trophotropism**.

Pathologic Features

It has become customary to subdivide placenta previa into several categories, such as "**central**" (total) and "**partial**" (lateral or marginal) placenta previa. The former generally poses the greater threat and requires early diagnosis. Vaginal delivery is usually permitted only in a marginal previa. In the vaginally delivered marginal placenta previa, the membranes have no free margin and the edge of the placenta frequently is disrupted and hemorrhagic. There are often *old clots at this site, varying from firm, laminated, and brown to friable loose clots or partly necrotic material that is sometimes green or brown.* The fetal vessels of the chorionic surface, when at the edge, may be also disrupted. Portions of placenta are occasionally either *atrophied or infarcted.*

Clinical Features and Implications

Placenta previa is more common in older women, and it is also associated with *multiparity, previous abortion, previous cesarean section, and male infants.* Placenta previa is associated with a higher risk for *abruptio, fetal malpresentation, postpartum hemorrhage, fetal and perinatal mortality, fetal growth restriction, fetal anomalies, prolapsed umbilical cord, and, of course, cesarean section.* It is one of the principal causes of third trimester bleeding and often necessitates an emergency cesarean section as both mother and fetus may experience life-threatening hemorrhage. Maternal hemorrhage may originate from the placental margin or from the disrupted intervillous space. Significant neonatal anemia may result from bleeding that occurs from disrupted placental villous vessels or fetomaternal hemorrhage (see Chapter 20).

Placenta previa is often associated with **placenta accreta** and then is called **placenta previa accreta** (see Chapter 12). In placenta previa, there is implantation in the lower uterine segment and cervix where there is a lack of normal endometrium, and the mucosa does not respond well to the normal hormonal signals for decidualization. Thus, decidualization is deficient, which is the underlying mechanism in placenta accreta. Although placenta previa accreta and cervical pregnancy are relatively rare, the clinical consequences may be dire due to massive hemorrhage and other complications of blood loss.

Suggestions for Examination and Report: Placenta Previa

Gross Examination: In a vaginal delivery, membrane rupture site at the placental margin is consistent with a marginal placental previa and should be recorded.

Comment: None.

Selected References

PHP4, Chapter 13, pages 399–418 (Placental Shape Aberrations), and Chapter 11, pages 320–322 (Extramembranous Pregnancy).

Ahmed A, Gilbert-Barnass E. Placenta membranacea. A developmental anomaly with diverse clinical presentation. Pediatr Dev Pathol 2003;6: 201–202.

Benirschke K. Effects of placental pathology on the embryo and the fetus. In: Wilson JG, Fraser FC (eds) Handbook of teratology, vol 3. New York: Plenum Press, 1977:79–115.

Finn JL. Placenta membranacea. Obstet Gynecol 1954;3:438–440.

Fox H, Sen DK. Placenta extrachorialis. A clinico-pathologic study. J Obstet Gynaecol Br Commonw 1972;79:32–35.

Fujikura T, Benson RC, Driscoll SG. The bipartite placenta and its clinical features. Am J Obstet Gynecol 1970;107:1013–1017.

Lademacher DS, Vermeulen RCW, Harten JJ, et al. Circumvallate placenta and congenital anomalies. Lancet 1981;1:732.

Mathews J. Placenta membranacea. Aust NZ J Obstet Gynaecol 1974;14:45–47.

Naeye RL. Placenta previa: predisposing factors and effects on the fetus and surviving infants. Obstet Gynecol 1978;52:521–525.

Naftolin F, Khudr G, Benirschke K, et al. The syndrome of chronic abruptio placentae, hydrorrhea, and circumvallate placenta. Am J Obstet Gynecol 1973;116:347–350.

Perlman M, Tennenbaum A, Menash M, et al. Extramembranous pregnancy: maternal, placental and perinatal implications. Obstet Gynecol 1980;55: 34S–37S.

Steemers NY, De Rop C, Van Assche A. Zonary placenta. Int J Gynecol Obstet 1995;51:251–253.

Torpin R. Placenta circumvallata and placenta marginata. Obstet Gynecol 1955; 6:277–284.

Torpin R. Human placental anomalies: etiology, evolution and historical background. Mo Med 1958;55:353–357.

Chapter 14

Pathology of the Fetal Membranes

Cysts

Pathologic Features

Localized edema with resultant cyst formation is occasionally seen on the fetal surface. Infrequently, such cysts represent **amnionic epithelial inclusion cysts**. These are simple cysts lined by a *single layer of amnionic epithelium* and usually contain clear fluid (Figure 14.1). Uncommonly, an **epidermal inclusion cyst** or **epidermoid cyst** may be seen within the amnion lined by *keratinizing stratified squamous epithelium* (Figure 14.2). Much more common are **subchorionic cysts** (Figures 14.3, 14.4), which are found in 5% to 7% of mature placentas. They are often multiple and may be quite large; cysts as large as a fetal head have been described. The cyst content is *viscid and mucus like* but does not contain true mucin. It is a rich source of major basic protein and other proteins. This can be appreciated by the presence of the precipitate found in histologic sections (Figure 14.5). The fluid is sometimes intermixed with sanguineous material. These cysts originate from *collections of extravillous trophoblastic cells in which degeneration and central liquefaction have occurred*. Bleeding into such cysts may also occur. Sub-

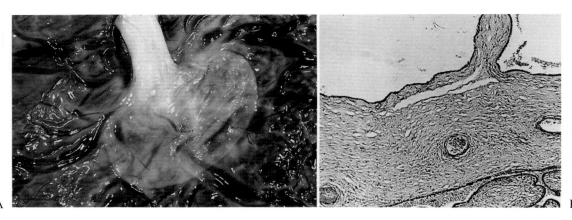

A   B

Figure 14.1. Amnionic cyst surrounding the umbilical cord. The cyst (A) contained 5 ml clear fluid. Microscopic examination (B) revealed a single layer of amnionic epithelium. H&E. ×160.

chorionic cysts are rarely encountered at the margin of the placenta and are not present on the extraplacental membranes. They are similar to those present in the septa and cell islands, which are present in approximately 14% to 17% of mature placentas, and can be found in the chorionic plate, the septa, and cell islands but not in the basal plate.

Pathogenesis

Amnionic and epidermal cysts have an etiology similar to other types of epithelial inclusion cysts. **Subchorionic**, **septal**, and **cell island cysts** are often found in placentas that show increased perivillous fibrin, maternal floor infarction (see Chapter 19), or changes of placental malperfusion (see Chapter 18). They are also more numerous in placentas from high altitudes. These findings support the view that cyst

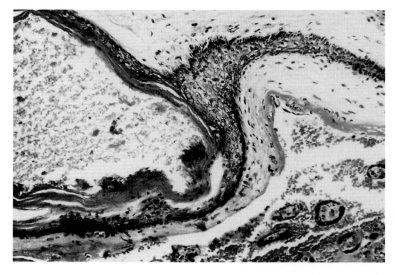

Figure 14.2. Subamnionic squamous epithelium lined cyst with keratinization. H&E. ×160.

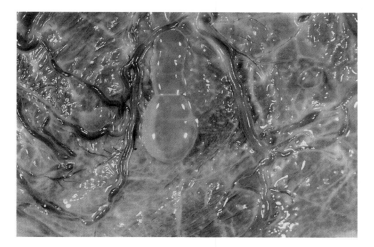

Figure 14.3. Subchorionic cysts on the fetal surface of a mature placenta.

formation is the result of *degenerative processes due to malnutrition and hypoxia in the center of large accumulations of extravillous trophoblast.*

Clinical Features and Implications

Amnionic and epidermal cysts are not usually associated with clinical problems. Large or multiple subchorionic cysts may compress chori-

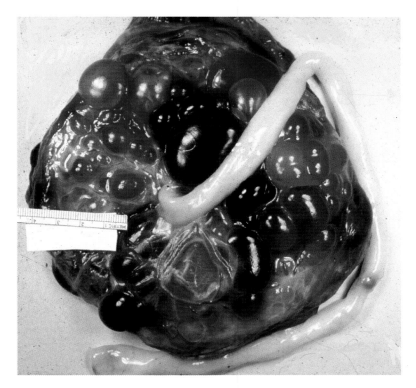

Figure 14.4. Multiple subchorionic cysts, many discolored by previous hemorrhage.

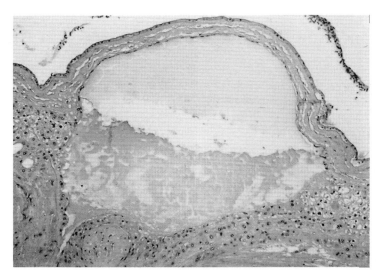

Figure 14.5. Subchorionic cyst of the placenta. Note that the cyst contains precipitated protein. H&E. ×40.

onic or umbilical vessels (see Figure 14.4), but there is no evidence that this actually compromises the fetal circulation. Therefore, subchorionic cysts are thought to have no clinical significance.

> *Suggestions for Examination and Report: Cysts*
>
> **Gross Examination:** Size, location, character of cysts should be noted. Sections need only be taken if the true nature of the cyst is in question and to document large or multiple cysts.
>
> **Comment:** Not generally necessary.

Tumors

Teratomas have been reported to arise in the fetal membranes. The typical description is of *a mass in the placenta, covered with skin, broadly attached to the chorion, which contains a relatively disorganized mass of glia, intestine, cartilage, fat, and/or other tissues.* These descriptions are reminiscent of **acardiac twins** (see Chapter 10) despite the lack of umbilical cord, a feature that is usually held to be a sine qua non for acardiac twins. We are of the opinion that these likely represent a variant of acardiac twinning and that to invoke their origin from aberrant germ cells seems unwarranted without supportive evidence. Other teratomas of the placenta fall into the same category.

Embryonic Remnants

Rarely, embryonic **rests** *of cartilage, skin, or bone may be found underneath the amnionic epithelium* (Figure 14.6); these are of no clinical significance. Some of these structures may represent the remains of aborted or "vanished" twins (see Chapter 10). After regression of the omphalomesenteric duct, remnants of the detached **yolk sac** persist in many placentas. They appear as *3- to 5-mm, white-yellow, chalky disks in the chorionic plate* (Figure 14.7 A). The yolk sac remnant is almost invariably located near the margin of the placenta, underneath the amnion. Histologically, it has a lacy appearance, staining deeply purple with hematoxylin, and *appears calcified* (Figure 14.7 B). Minute omphalomesenteric vessels may occasionally accompany these yolk sac remnants and then can be seen coursing toward the umbilical cord and run along the surface of the cord. These remnants have no associated clinical sequelae.

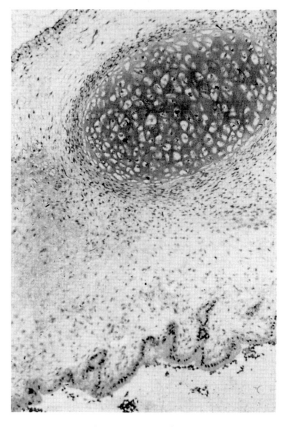

Figure 14.6. Subamnionic embryonic rest of mature cartilage in a normal placenta. H&E. ×100.

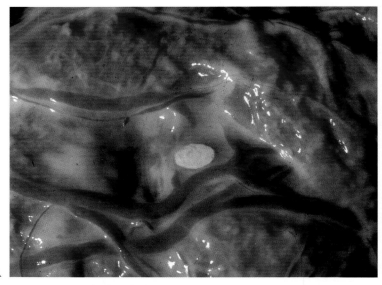

A

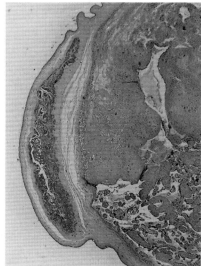

B

Figure 14.7. (A) Yolk sac remnant on the fetal surface of the placenta. (B) Microscopic appearance of a yolk sac remnant consisting of irregular fragments of calcium phosphate deposits between the amnion and chorion. H&E. ×50.

Vernix Caseosa

Vernix caseosa is *sebum, hair, and other skin secretions from the fetus present in the amniotic fluid*. It is a thick, white, and hydrophobic material that may appear as *white flakelike particles*. It is sometimes found submitted with the placenta or attached to the membranes (Figure 14.8). Such accumulations of vernix also occur occasionally in large patches of greasy material that may be mistaken for a fetus papyraceous. After spontaneous rupture of the membranes, it may *dissect underneath the amnion or chorion*. Generally, no cellular reaction to this material takes place. When dissection occurs, fragments *of anucleate squames, fat, hair, and other debris* can be seen under the amnionic epithelium, at times in impressive amounts (Figure 14.9). It has no clinical significance. Vernix has also been identified in the decidua and myometrium of placental bed biopsies and within uterine veins.

Hematomas and Breus' Mole

Subamnionic Hematoma

Subamnionic hematomas are seen quite commonly. They usually originate from chorionic vessels that have been sampled for tests (pH, blood banking, etc.) or are caused by excess traction on the umbilical cord during delivery. Gross examination reveals a thin layer of *recent blood clot between the amnion and chorion* (Figure 14.10). Subamnionic hematomas are particularly common in specimens from cesarean section when the placenta is delivered manually. *Rarely is such subamnionic blood of prenatal origin.* However, trauma to fetal vessels may occur from invasive antenatal procedures. In this case, evaluation of the extent of the bleeding and correlation with clinical history is essential.

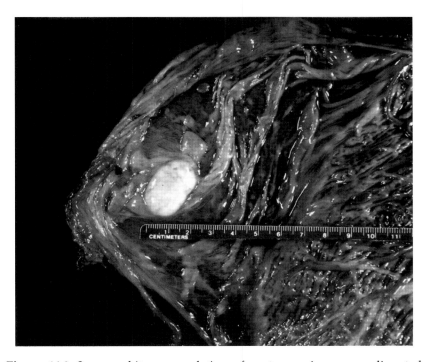

Figure 14.8. Large, white accumulation of pasty vernix caseosa dissected beneath the amnion. It is grossly similar to a yolk sac remnant but is much larger. It may be confused with a fetus papyraceous.

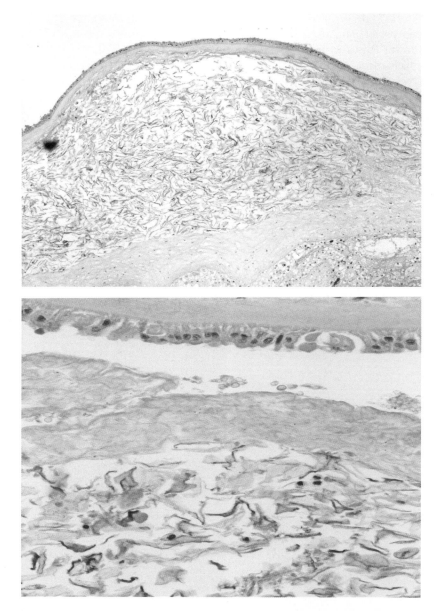

Figure 14.9. Microscopic view of vernix below amnion with readily identifiable squames and occasional hairs and other debris. H&E. Top ×20; bottom ×400.

Retromembranous Hematoma

In the delivered placenta, one often finds small plaques beneath the extraplacental membranes, which consist of *recent or old clot* (Figure 14.11). Older clots may look as though they are composed of fibrotic or necrotic tissue. Microscopically, there may be associated decidual necrosis. **Retromembranous hematomas** are most commonly sequelae of amniocentesis and usually of no clinical importance.

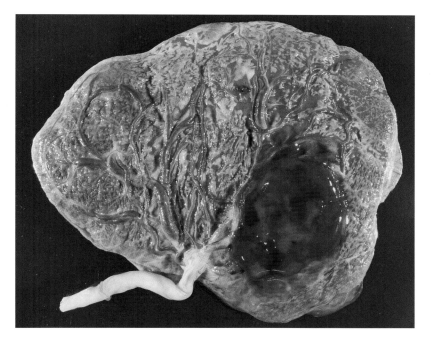

Figure 14.10. Recent subamnionic hemorrhage due to excess traction during delivery. In this case the hematoma forms a plaque. Often the blood dissects underneath the amnion in a thin layer.

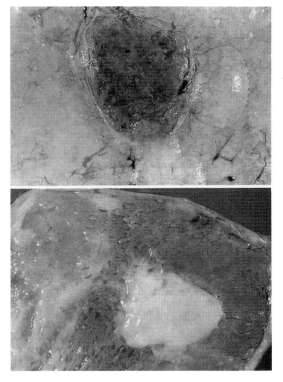

Figure 14.11. Localized retromembranous hematoma. At the top there is a dark ovoid blood clot. The bottom shows an old, white hematoma. Both are from uncomplicated pregnancies.

Subchorionic Hematoma and Breus' Mole

Pathologic Features

Laminated **subchorionic thrombi** form in small quantities almost regularly in the *subchorionic space*. It is at this site where the intervillous (maternal) blood is deflected backward and eddying of intervillous blood accounts for the small amounts of fibrin that normally accumulate here. Macroscopically, they appear as *white patches or plaques* of **fibrin** and **laminated clot** under the chorion (see Figure 3.4, page 29). They often cause *bosselation of the fetal surface of the placenta*. The fibrin accumulations normally increase with maturation, but material that is much more thrombotic accumulates underneath the chorion in some abnormal placentas, forming distinct **subchorionic hematomas**, which may measure up to 15 cm in diameter (Figure 14.12).

Clinical Features and Implications

Subchorionic hematomas have been reported in up to 60% of pregnancies evaluated by ultrasonography. They have been associated with *preterm delivery, spontaneous abortion, vaginal bleeding, midtrimester losses, elevated alpha fetoprotein levels, intrauterine growth restriction, and fetal demise.* However, it is estimated that 80% of the subchorionic hematomas recognized before 20 weeks result in a normal term delivery. They are more often found when maternal circulatory disorders exist such as *complex heart disease, and with maternal antinuclear antibodies and thrombophilias.*

Also present and somewhat overlapping with subchorionic hematoma is the **subchorionic tuberous hematoma, or "Breus' mole"** (Figure 14.13). Breus' mole *differs from subchorionic hematomas in that it*

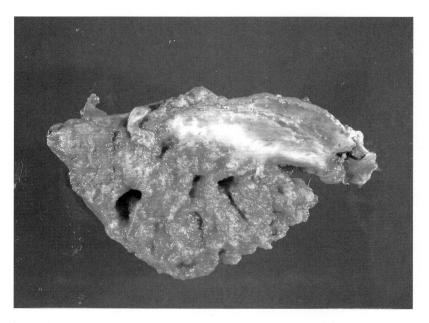

Figure 14.12. Laminated subchorionic hematoma in an uncomplicated term pregnancy.

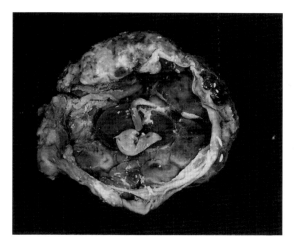

Figure 14.13. Breus' mole in an immature placenta from a missed abortion. Note the numerous blood-filled protrusions on the surface.

is diffusely nodular and forms "pockets." Breus' mole was originally described in association with missed abortions and was interpreted as sacculations or diverticula produced by the continued intervillous blood pressure against a decreased amnionic sac pressure. They have also been associated with *circumvallation, neonatal demise, monosomy X (Turner's syndrome),* and various maternal diseases such as *diabetes and hypertension.* The incidence is estimated to be 1 in 1200 placentas. At present, there is no consensus as to their etiology.

> *Suggestions for Examination and Report: Subamnionic, Retromembranous, and Subchorionic Hematomas*
>
> **Gross Examination:** Documentation of the size, extent, and percentage of the fetal surface involved in a subchorionic hematoma is important, as is estimation of the age of the clot. Subamnionic and retromembranous hematomas should also be measured and described.
>
> **Comment:** Subchorionic hematomas have been associated with an increased risk of preterm delivery, fetal loss, vaginal bleeding, growth restriction, and fetal demise. Correlation with clinical history is suggested. Subamnionic hematomas are usually iatrogenic. Retromembranous hematomas are generally of no clinical significance.

Meconium and Other Pigments

Meconium is the *bile-stained intestinal content of the fetus.* It is present in the fetal intestines long before midgestation but is generally not eliminated until after birth. Its chemical composition is variable and has only been partially determined, but it is known to often contain *mucus, mucopolysaccharides, blood group antigens, enzymes, and a small amount of protein*. Meconium discharge in utero is a common event, occurring in approximately 17% to 19% of placentas.

Pathologic Features

When meconium is discharged before parturition, the *baby and placenta may be meconium stained and deeply green* (Figure 14.14 A). An additional feature of meconium is that it causes edema of the membranes, giving them a slimy quality. Microscopically, meconium pigment may be

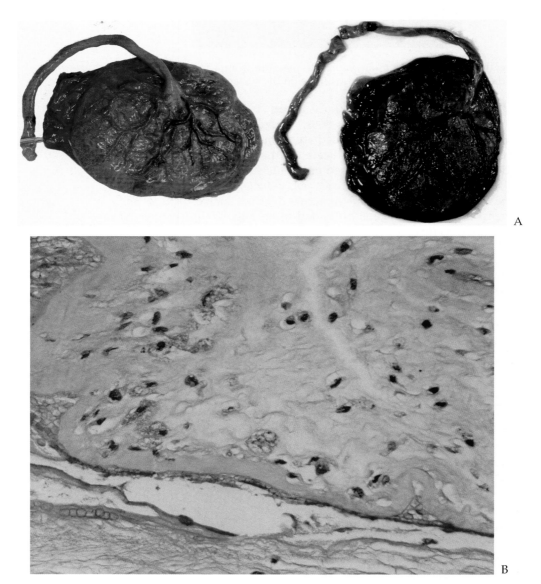

Figure 14.14. (A) Meconium staining of fetal membranes and umbilical cord of two term placentas. (B) Many meconium-filled macrophages are present in the amnion of the placenta in (A). H&E. ×400.

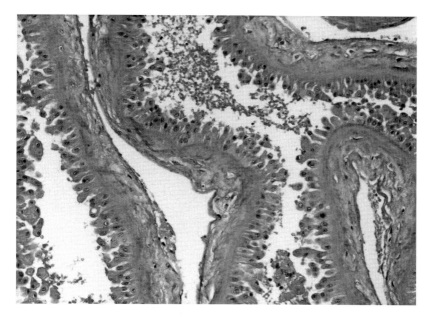

Figure 14.15. Meconium-induced degenerative change of the amnion. Note the piling up of the epithelium. H&E. ×200.

present within macrophages in the fetal membranes, fetal surface, and even the umbilical cord. These **meconium-laden macrophages** are *large, ovoid, or round cells with a slightly translucent, yellow-brown content. They tend to be vacuolated* (Figure 14.14 B). On electron microscopy, phagolysosomes full of debris are present. The macrophages are normally inactive and thus "lie in waiting" in the membranes until meconium or other substances come by and they spring into functional activity.

When meconium has been present in the amniotic cavity for many hours, the amnionic epithelium begins to show degenerative changes. There is *vacuolization of the cytoplasm, heaping up of cells, dissociation, loss of cells, and necrosis* (Figures 14.15 and 4.4, page 52). The heaping up of the cells has been called "villous change" or "hyperplasia," but these terms are misnomers because these changes are degenerative in nature. With meconium staining of greater duration, *the smooth muscle cells of the umbilical vessels and their ramifications on the fetal surface may degenerate and show necrosis of individual muscle fibers* (Figure 14.16). The muscle cells round up, the cytoplasm becomes more eosinophilic, and the nucleus undergoes pyknosis. Eventually, they die with complete loss of the nucleus, leaving a degenerated fragment of cytoplasm. How long the vessel must be exposed to meconium to lead to these vascular alterations on histologic examination is not known precisely, but it is likely to be many hours.

The time from meconium discharge to delivery of the infant and placenta may be estimated as follows:

- **Less than 1 hour**—meconium may be washed off the placental surface without leaving a stain or microscopic evidence;
- **1 to 3 hours**—the amnion, but not the chorion, will be grossly stained and will contain pigment-laden macrophages;

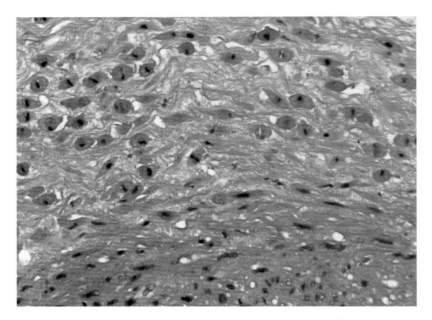

Figure 14.16. Meconium-induced muscle damage to the umbilical artery. Note the rounding up of the myofibers and pkynotic nuclei. H&E. ×200.

- **>3 hours**—the amnion and the chorion will be stained and will contain pigment-laden macrophages;
- **4 to 6 hours**—the fingernails and toenails of the infant will be stained;
- **12 to 14 hours**—the vernix will be stained.

After initial staining of the membranes, meconium will stain the decidua capsularis and, after many hours, the umbilical cord. Staining of the umbilical cord may be seen grossly but is difficult to identify histologically as there are few macrophages in Wharton's jelly. With very long standing meconium exposure, meconium-stained macrophages may be identified within the myometrium. When attempting to time meconium discharge before birth, one must keep in mind that meconium is being removed by the macrophages and by fetal swallowing and inhalation, and that in some instances, fetuses discharge meconium repeatedly.

Other pigments such as **hemosiderin** and **bilirubin** are very similar to meconium. Bilirubin may cause a yellow discoloration of the fetal surface and fetal membranes and is usually associated with maternal hyperbilirubinemia (see Figure 17.1, page 321). Microscopically, pigment-laden macrophages are rare. Hemosiderin derives from hemolyzed red blood cells and is commonly found associated with *circumvallate placentas, erythroblastotic infants, abruptio placentae, thromboses, and other circumstances wherein bleeding has occurred*. Hemosiderin-stained placentas have a more **brownish** tint, as opposed to the green of meconium-stained placentas (Figure 14.17 A). Microscopically, hemosiderin is composed of *brown, granular particles, and it has a characteristic sheen (refringence) when the focus of the light microscope, or its substage, is* *changed* (Figure 14.17 B). In comparison to meconium pigment, hemosiderin is much easier to identify in histologic sections. A **Prussian blue stain** for iron is very helpful for differentiating between these two pigments. Although iron stains readily differentiate hemosiderin, the bile in meconium is not readily confirmed. A **Luna-Ishak stain** will stain bile a greenish color. Unfortunately, this stain is technically difficult to perform and difficult to reliably interpret as well. In addition, hemosiderin becomes metabolized to hematoidin in about 7 days and, regrettably, hematoidin and bilirubin cannot be reliably distinguished from each other by either light microscopy or special histochemical stains.

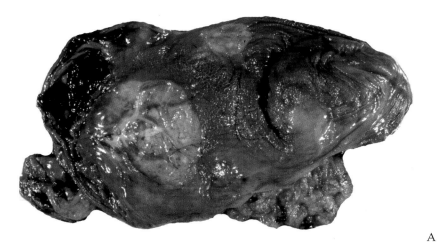

A

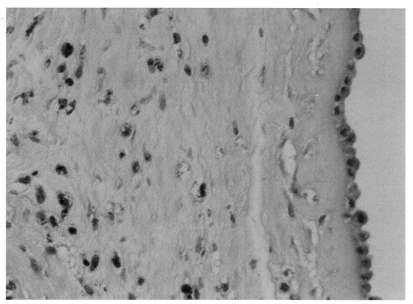

B

Figure 14.17. (A) Placenta with yellow-brown discoloration of the fetal surface consistent with old bleeding. Some recent hemorrhage is also present on the left. (B) Hemosiderin-laden macrophages in the fetal membranes showing yellow-brown particulate material. H&E. ×160.

One should also be aware that the meconium pigment within macrophages bleaches when it is exposed to ambient light.

Pathogenesis

Meconium discharge occurs in approximately 15% of placentas at 39 weeks gestation, in 27% at 41 to 42 weeks, and in 32% over 42 weeks. The reason for the discharge of meconium is complex. It is moved in the intestinal lumen by contractions of the intestinal wall, which is regulated by hormones. One of these is **motilin**. There are lower levels of motilin and other gastrointestinal hormones in immature fetuses than in mature fetuses and higher levels in infants with fetal distress. This is part of the reason why mature fetuses and distressed fetuses often discharge meconium.

Clinical Features and Implications

Meconium discharge is positively correlated with fetal distress but also occurs without fetal distress. Many term stillbirths have never discharged meconium despite prolonged periods of distress that eventually lead to their demise. It is equally true that many infants that discharge meconium have **not** experienced fetal distress. Despite this fact, meconium has assumed great importance in medicolegal pursuits (see Chapter 26). Suffice it to say that *meconium discharge may occur in the setting of fetal distress or be simply due to fetal maturity.*

Despite issues relating to meconium being a result or and indication of in utero hypoxia, meconium itself has deleterious effects. These include sequelae due to *aspiration into the lungs* as well as *direct effects on the amnion and umbilical cord*. One of the major impacts of meconium on fetal morbidity and mortality is related to the meconium aspiration syndrome. Much of the pulmonary damage has been shown to be prenatal in onset, and it is thought that aspirated meconium causes degenerative changes in the alveolar epithelium similar to those seen in the amnionic epithelium and vascular smooth muscle (see above). There is also evidence that damage to the fetal vascular tissue may also have adverse effects. When segments of umbilical veins are exposed in vitro to meconium, the muscular wall contracts markedly and rapidly. Thus, meconium may be a *cause* of hypoperfusion and hypoxia rather than the result.

Suggestions for Examination and Report: Meconium, Hemosiderin, or Other Pigmentation of the Membranes

Gross Examination: Identification of discoloration of the fetal membranes, fetal surface, and umbilical cord should each be noted. Meconium staining is most commonly green, hemosiderin is usually brownish, and bilirubin is more yellow. However, there is much overlap in appearances. If meconium staining is present on the surface of the cord, this should be particularly noted as the presence of meconium macrophages in the cord is difficult to appreciate. Therefore, discolored areas of the cord should be preferentially sectioned.

Comment: Diagnosis of the presence of meconium in the membranes and/or umbilical cord is usually sufficient (meconium-laden macrophages or meconium histiocytosis) and no comment need be made. Associated myonecrosis should always be mentioned if present. If hemosiderin is identified, a comment on possible sources of bleeding may include retromembranous or retroplacental hematoma, deciduitis, marginal hemorrhage, abruptio, placenta previa, and fetal hemorrhage. Yellow discoloration consistent with bilirubin staining should be noted and correlated with the clinical history if possible.

Gastroschisis

Gastroschisis, a fetal anomaly characterized by a defect in the abdominal wall, is associated with a specific abnormality of the amnionic epithelium. The amnionic epithelial cells have a characteristic *fine, uniform, extensive vacuolation* (Figures 14.18 and 4.4, page 52). Although this association was startling when it was first found, it is now known to be regularly present and is virtually diagnostic of gastroschisis. It is not found in fetuses with omphalocele, a similar condition. It appears to have no influence on placental function. The vacuoles contain lipid when examined by electron microscopy, but the origin of the lipid is still obscure. When pregnancies of less than 20 weeks are studied, the vacuolization of the epithelium is not yet present and so it accumulates only later in gestation.

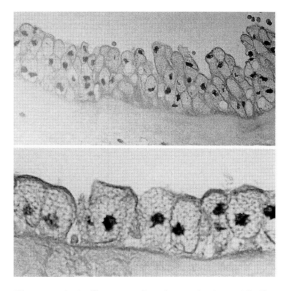

Figure 14.18. Characteristically vacuolated amnionic epithelium in a case of gastroschisis. H&E. ×640.

Squamous Metaplasia

Squamous metaplasia is a change of the amnionic epithelium present in up to 60% of term placentas. The term is a misnomer, because the amnion is a type of immature squamous epithelium, being continuous with the fetal surface and the fetal skin. These areas of "metaplasia" do not form in response to some chronic irritation or inflammation but merely betray maturity. The epithelium becomes *stratified with focal keratinization of the epithelium* (Figures 14.19 and 4.4, page 52), resembling normal epidermis with keratohyaline granules and melanin. Areas of squamous metaplasia are grossly visible as *whitish, hydrophobic foci of small elevations or irregular plaques* (Figure 14.20) and are most commonly found near the cord insertion. They are of no clinical consequence.

Amnion Nodosum

Pathogenesis
Amnion nodosum is associated with conditions that lead to *significant, prolonged oligohydramnios*. It is found in the placentas of fetuses with *renal agenesis, following premature rupture of membranes, in the donor twin of the twin transfusion syndrome, in diamnionic acardiac twins, in sirenomelia,* and in various other disturbances that lead to oligohydramnios. Because the amnion lacks blood vessels, it must subsist almost entirely on the amniotic fluid. Lack of fluid leads to degeneration and death of the epithelium. Once a defect is present in the epithe-

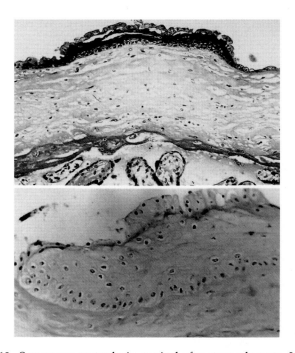

Figure 14.19. Squamous metaplasia, typical of mature placenta. H&E. ×160.

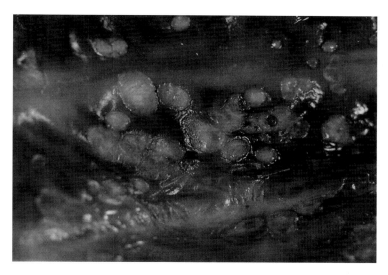

Figure 14.20. Plaques of whitish discoloration on the fetal surface near the umbilical cord characteristic of squamous metaplasia.

lium, vernix becomes deposited on the denuded basement membrane in a nodular fashion. Amnion nodosum develops only late in fetal life because earlier in gestation there is insufficient vernix. When oligo-hydramnios occurs in the second trimester, amnion nodosum does not develop. Instead, the amnion is either completely normal or shows minute foci of cellular degeneration.

Pathologic Features
Most cases of amnion nodosum show *fine granules on the fetal surface* that are best seen in oblique light (Figure 14.21). The nodules may be shiny and relatively translucent but also may be more opaque and brown to yellow. The nodules occasionally extend onto the membranes, but are only very rarely found on the surface of the umbilical cord. They are quite different from the lesions seen in squamous metaplasia, which are typically more plaque like; patchy, and hydrophobic (see above). In addition, amnion nodosum may be scraped off the surface whereas plaques of squamous metaplasia may not. Microscopically, nodules of *vernix composed of squames and hair intermixed with sebum are attached to the surface defect* (Figures 14.22, 14.23; and 4.4, page 52). There is no associated inflammatory or other tissue reaction.

Clinical Features and Implications
Fetal sequelae of prolonged oligohydramnios primarily consist of **pul-monary hypoplasia** and **various malformations** due to fetal compres-sion from lack of fluid, specifically **Potter's sequence** with flattened facies and extremities. Amnion nodosum is another complication of oligohydramnios. *Pulmonary hypoplasia develops due to the inability of the lung to inhale normal amounts of fluid and from compression.* Both breath-ing motions and the availability of amniotic fluid appear to be neces-sary for expansion and development of the lung.

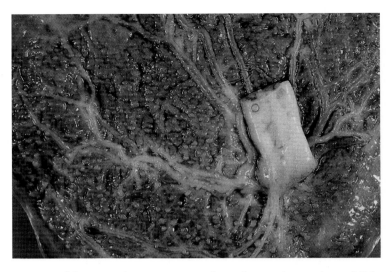

Figure 14.21. Macroscopic appearance of amnion nodosum in a child with renal agenesis. Note the uniform presence of fine granules, mostly sparing the vessel surfaces and not present on the cord.

Suggestions for Examination and Report: Amnion Nodosum

Gross Examination: Lesions should be differentiated from lesions of squamous metaplasia, which are irregular, patchy, and hydrophobic and cannot be rubbed off. Amnion nodosum consists of smaller, more uniform nodules that can easily be removed. Adequate sampling is important, and in some cases gross photographs may be useful.

Comment: Amnion nodosum is generally associated with oligohydramnios and often with congenital malformations, particularly renal malformations. It occurs when there is a significant reduction in amniotic fluid for a period of time.

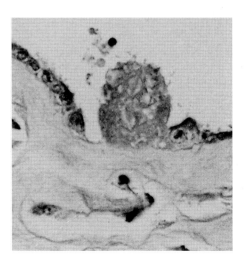

Figure 14.22. Early stages in the development of amnion nodosum. H&E. ×400.

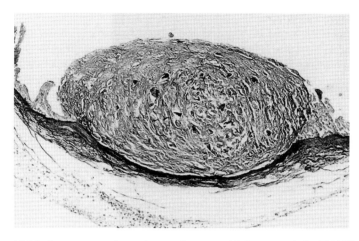

Figure 14.23. Late stage of amnion nodosum with large nodule. PTAH ×1160.

Amnionic Bands

Pathogenesis

The amnion does not become applied to the chorion until the 12th week. If rupture of the amnion occurs before this time, the fetus may escape into the chorionic sac. As growth of the amnion is mediated by stretching of the enlarging sac, rupture will cause the amnion to shrivel and contract, producing **amnionic bands** or **sheets**. Parts of the fetus or umbilical cord may become entangled with the bands, leading to fetal amputations, anomalies, or even demise. Many dysmorphologists refer to these bands and their associated anomalies as the **ADAM complex** (amnionic deformities, adhesions, mutilation) or **TEARS** (the early amnion rupture sequence) **sequence**.

The etiology of the early amnion rupture is unknown. There is no apparent hereditary component, increased risk of recurrence, association with amniocentesis or early chorionic villous sampling, or relation to trauma. Suggested etiologies include excessive fetal activity, defective development of the amnion, and vascular disruption. Although the existence of amnionic bands as a cause of amputations and other fetal debilities can hardly be disputed, such doubts are expressed in the literature with regularity. Current thinking is that there may be two or even three distinct entities rather than one. These can be generally categorized as follows:

- **Amnionic sheets**—attached broadly to the skull or face with associated anomalies
- **Limb–body wall complex**—with gross disruptions and major body wall anomalies
- **Amnionic bands**—constriction of extremities, umbilical cord, etc. with a generally normal fetus

There may be some overlap between categories, and the first two categories seem to be associated not only with amnionic bands but also with *disturbances of early embryogenesis*.

Pathologic Features

Placentas with **amnionic sheets** have broad sheets of amnion tethered to the umbilical cord (Figure 14.24) that tend to be contiguous with the ectoderm of the fetal face or skull. These sheets can often be identified by ultrasonography. Isolated amputations generally are not associated with these sheets but rather certain anomalies are present such as *exencephaly, ectopia cordis, spinal disruptions, meningocele, clubbed feet, and bony defects*. Amnionic sheets are probably associated with early amnionic rupture as well as disturbances in embryogenesis.

The **limb–body wall complex** does not have distinct bands and lacks amputations. They are associated with *single umbilical artery, short umbilical cords, and defects in the abdominal wall*. Characteristic for the limb–body wall complex is an **amnion contiguous with some portion of the body wall, often with the abdomen** (Figure 14.25). The etiology is still disputed but incomplete *embryonic folding and neural tube closure* are likely mechanisms. This idea is supported by the fact that occasionally unrelated anomalies (e.g., truncus arteriosus) are encountered in such fetuses. They are often associated with fetal growth restriction and hydramnios.

With **amnionic bands**, the *fetal surface of the placenta is usually completely devoid of amnion*, as this has previously ruptured in the formation of bands. As such, the fetal surface is covered only with chorion and is grossly opaque due to increased infiltration of macrophages and fibrin deposition. *Remnants of the amnion can be found attached to the base of the umbilical cord;* this is the only portion that does not detach with rupture. Often a small sac is present at the placental end of the cord where the bands originate (Figure 14.26). Occasionally, amnionic bands are identified but the placenta shows a somewhat necrotic, but relatively intact, amnionic surface. In this case, a **focal rupture of the amnion** has occurred with subsequent healing of the amnion over the

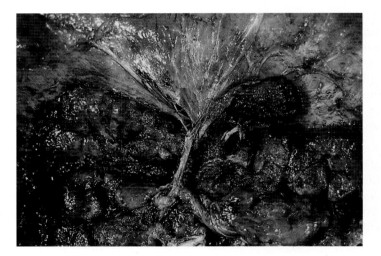

Figure 14.24. Amnionic sheet attached to the fetal surface of the placenta.

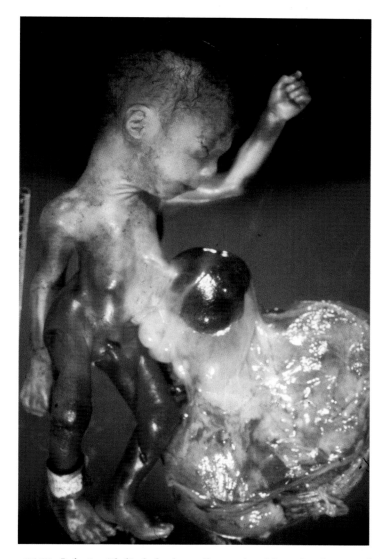

Figure 14.25. Infant with limb–body wall complex. Note the short cord tethering the infant to the placenta and the abdominal wall defect.

defect. When histologic sections are made of the bands, they are found to consist of *normal-appearing amnionic epithelium and underlying connective tissue*. There are usually few signs of degeneration, and inflammation is absent.

Clinical Features and Implications

The *incidence* of amnionic bands is difficult to assess. In previable fetuses, they occur as often as 1 in 53 fetuses. In liveborns, they have been reported to occur in anywhere from 1 per 2,500 to 1 per 10,000 liveborns. The incidence has been reported to be *higher in African-Americans and in younger women*.

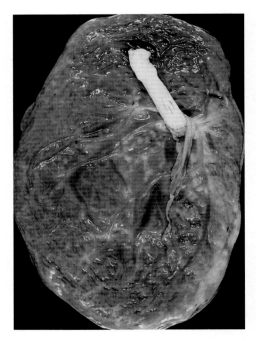

Figure 14.26. Amnionic band attached to the umbilical cord. Note opacity of the membranes.

The most common and best known fetal consequence of amnionic bands is *amputation of a portion of an extremity*. One can usually identify the typical constriction of a limb or other body part surrounded by a membranous fragment of amnion (Figure 14.27). Doubtless the fetus moves and becomes entangled in these remnants of amnion, and because his fingers move most actively, it is this part that is most com-

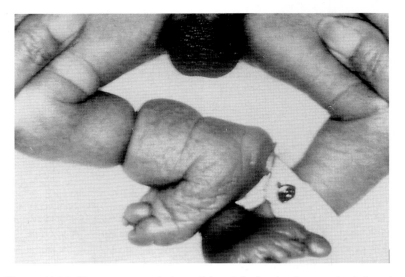

Figure 14.27. Extreme constriction of the right foreleg by amnionic bands.

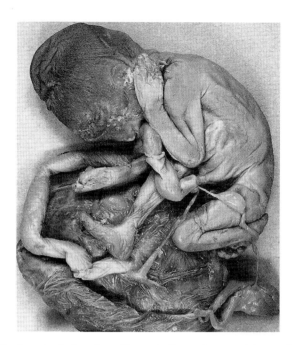

Figure 14.28. Amnionic bands with encircling of extremities and the cord in an aborted fetus. (Courtesy of Dr. G. Altshuler, with permission from Altshuler G, McAdams AJ. The role of the placenta in fetal and perinatal pathology. Am J Obstet Gynecol 1972; 113:616–626, with permission.)

monly involved. Rarely, amnionic bands result in amputations with separate delivery of the amputated part. In this case, the amputated foot or other body part is smaller than the infant, consistent with the gestational age at which the amputation took place. There are also bands that completely encircle the abdomen or an extremity, causing deep furrows and producing sloughing of the skin. Most fetuses with amputations due to amnionic bands are otherwise normal. *Entanglement with the umbilical cord can interrupt its circulation and lead to fetal death* (Figure 14.28), and mortality is estimated at approximately 30%. At the other extreme, one should consider that *not every case of amnionic rupture necessarily leads to entangling and constrictions.* The phenotypic variations are extremely wide, and it is merely a matter of chance which fetal or placental parts become entangled.

Suggestions for Examination and Report: Amnionic Bands

Gross Examination: Careful examination of the fetal surface and extraplacental membranes is essential in identification of amnionic bands and is facilitated by a clinical history that is suggestive of that diagnosis, for example, an isolated amputation. Usually the band or sheet is tethered to the umbilical cord and the remaining fetal surface is devoid of amnion, being covered only by chorion. Photographs are very useful. Histologic sections of the bands are unremarkable, revealing only the presence of amnion.

Comment: The sequelae of amnionic bands have an extremely varied phenotype, and correlation with clinical history is essential.

Selected References

PHP4, Chapter 9, pages 240–242 (Subchorionic Hematoma), Chapter 11, pages 281–334 (Fetal Membranes).

Altshuler G, Arizawa M, Molnar-Nadasdy G. Meconium-induced umbilical cord vascular necrosis and ulceration: a potential link between the placenta and poor pregnancy outcome. Obstet Gynecol 1992;79:760–766.

Ariel IB, Landing BH. A possible distinctive vacuolar change of the amniotic epithelium associated with gastroschisis. Pediatr Pathol 1985;2:283–289.

Heller DS, Rush DS, Baergen RN. Subchorionic hematoma associated with thrombophilia. Pediatr Dev Pathol 2003;6:261–264.

Higginbottom MC, Jones KL, Hall BD, et al. The amniotic band disruption complex: timing of amnion rupture and variable spectra of consequent defects. J Pediatr 1979;95:544–549.

Jacques SM, Qureshi F. Subamnionic vernix caseosa. Pediatr Pathol 1994;14: 585–593.

Joseph TJ, Vogt PJ. Placental teratomas. Obstet Gynecol 1973;41:574–578.

Kalousek D, Banforth S. Amniotic rupture sequence in previable fetuses. Am J Med Genet 1988;31:63–73.

Martinez-Frias ML. Epidemiological characteristics of amnionic band sequence (ABS) and body wall complex (BWC): are they two different entities? Am J Med Genet 1997;73:176–179.

Miller PW, Coen RW, Benirschke K. Dating the time interval from meconium passage to birth. Obstet Gynecol 1985;66:459–462.

Morhaime JL, Park K, Benirschke K, Baergen RN. Disappearance of meconium pigment in placental specimens on exposure to light. Arch Pathol Lab Med 2003;127:711–714.

Nickell KA, Stocker JT. Placental teratoma: a case report. Pediatr Pathol 1987;7:645–650.

Pearlstone M, Bax L. Subchorionic hematoma: a review. Obstet Gynecol Surv 1993;48:65–68.

Perlman M, Tennenbaum A, Menash M, et al. Extramembranous pregnancy: maternal, placental, and perinatal implications. Obstet Gynecol 1980;55: 34S–37S.

Salazar H, Kanbour AI, Pardo M. Amnion nodosum. Ultrastructure and histopathogenesis. Arch Pathol 1974;98:39–46.

Shanklin DR, Scott JS. Massive subchorial thrombohaematoma (Breus' mole). Br J Obstet Gynaecol 1975;82:476–487.

Chapter 15

Pathology of the Umbilical Cord

Embryonic Remnants

Allantoic Duct Remnants

Pathogenesis

The **allantoic duct** arises at about the 16th day postconception, as a *rudimentary outpouching of the caudal portion of the yolk sac* (see Figure 5.4, page 78). Normally, there is complete obliteration of the allantoic duct at 15 weeks gestation. A remnant, which connects the umbilicus to the bladder, persists as the **median umbilical ligament**. Occasionally, the duct persists as a minute connection to the fetal bladder. Allantoic duct remnants may be found in 15% of umbilical cords, and for unknown reasons they are more common in males.

Pathologic Features

Allantoic remnants are most frequently found in the *proximal portions of the umbilical cord* but may exist discontinuously throughout the cord. They are always located centrally *between the two umbilical arteries* and consist of *a collection of cuboidal or flattened epithelial cells, usually without a lumen* (Figure 15.1). The epithelium is generally of the *transitional type although mucin-producing epithelium is occasionally found.* Rarely, it is accompanied by muscle. Small vessels or vasa aberrantia may be distributed around vessels, and rarely extramedullary hematopoiesis is seen.

Clinical Features and Implications

In most cases, allantoic remnants have no clinical significance. In 1 in 200,000 births, however, the duct is patent. In this situation there may be *urination from the clamped umbilical stump or the presence of cysts* that may persist into adult life. Pyelonephritis and abscess formation are common complications of this rare condition. The cysts may become quite large and give the appearance of a "giant" umbilical cord (Figure 15.2).

Omphalomesenteric Duct Remnants

Pathogenesis

Early in development, the midgut communicates with the yolk sac via the umbilical stalk. As the embryo grows the umbilical stalk lengthens and the embryo "prolapses" into the amniotic cavity (see Figure 5.4, page 78). The *connection between the gut and the yolk sac becomes attenuated and forms the* **omphalomesenteric (vitelline) duct**, which is of endodermal origin. When the gut rotates and withdraws to its original cavity between the 7th and 16th weeks, the duct normally atrophies. Persistence of this duct may then be found in 1.5% of umbilical cords. Remnants of vitelline vessels are found in approximately 7% of cords at term.

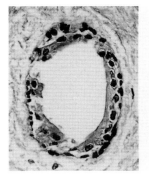 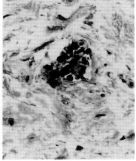

Figure 15.1. Two remnants of allantoic duct: left patent, right obliterated. Note the absence of the muscular coat. H&E. ×525. (Courtesy of G.L. Bourne.)

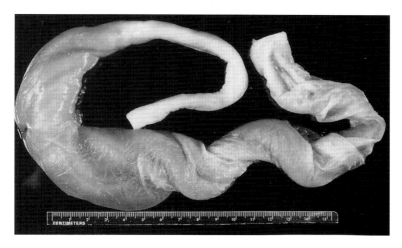

Figure 15.2. Edematous umbilical cord of a 32-week fetus with a large urachal extension into the cord. The cord weighed 180 g (normal weight is 40 g). (Courtesy of Dr. S. Kassel, Fresno, California.)

Pathologic Features

Like allantoic ducts, remnants of **omphalomesenteric ducts** are more common at the fetal end of the cord. Males also outnumber females 4:1. Remnants are usually present *near the periphery of the cord and consist of ducts lined by columnar cells similar to intestinal epithelium* (Figures 15.3, 15.4). They often have muscular coats and may occur in pairs. Having an endodermal origin, it is not surprising that remnants of this duct may contain remnants of *liver, small bowel, pancreatic tissue, gastric mucosa, ganglion cells, or other intestinal structures*. Calcific masses have also been reported. The duct remnants are commonly associated with persistent vitelline vessels (Figure 15.5). These vessels are usually

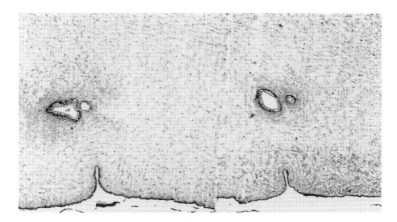

Figure 15.3. Microscopic section of a cord with four remnants of omphalomesenteric duct. The marginal position is typical. H&E. ×50.

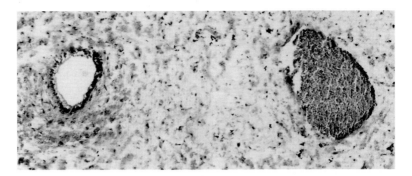

Figure 15.4. The omphalomesenteric duct on the left has mucinous epithelium and a small amount of musculature; on the right are the remains of the vitelline vein. H&E. ×100.

tiny but may contain red blood cells. They always lack a muscular coat and are usually *composed only of endothelium.* Cysts have been described up to 6.0 cm in diameter and are frequently surrounded by a plexus of small vessels.

Clinical Features and Implications

Clinically, these vestiges are unimportant unless there is direct communication with fetal bowel, an uncommon occurrence. Remnants of omphalomesenteric ducts can be associated with *atresia of the small intestine and Meckel's diverticulum* and are a rare cause of abdominal distension.

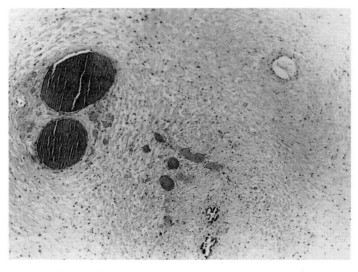

Figure 15.5. A plexus of small vitelline vessels accompanies the duct remnants (bottom center). At top right is the dilated allantoic duct. H&E. ×64.

Umbilical Cord Coiling, Torsion, and Stricture

Pathogenesis

The umbilical cord is usually **coiled, twisted, or spiraled**, more commonly in a counterclockwise direction (a "left" twist) in a ratio of about 4:1 (Figure 15.6). The helices may be seen by ultrasonographic examination as early as the first trimester of pregnancy but they increase significantly during the third trimester. The coils number up to 40, but as many as 380 total turns have been described. The **coiling index** has been used to evaluate the degree of twisting, defined as *the number of coils divided by length of cord*. The average coiling index is 0.21/cm. **Hypocoiled cords** represent about 7.5% of cords, **noncoiled cords** are present in 4% to 5%, and **hypercoiled cords** occur in about 20% (Figure 15.7). Hypocoiling and hypercoiling are both associated with adverse perinatal outcome, including an increase in *perinatal mortality, intrauterine growth restriction, and fetal distress*. Twisting of the cord is thought to be the result of fetal activity. Lack of coiling may then reflect fetal inactivity as coiling is reduced in cases of uterine constraint, anomalies that restrict fetal movement, and possibly central nervous system (CNS) disturbances.

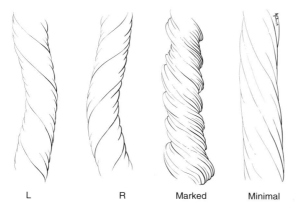

L   R   Marked   Minimal

Figure 15.6. Drawing depicting different types of umbilical cord twist including left (L), right (R), minimal and marked twisting.

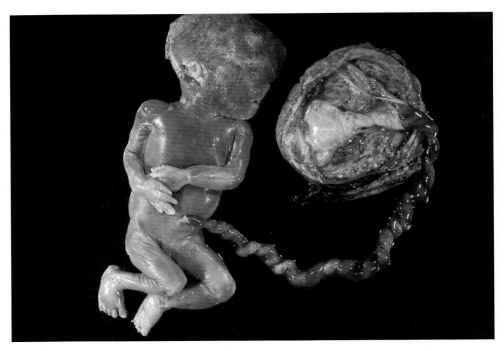

Figure 15.7. Preterm stillborn infant and placenta with a markedly coiled (twisted) umbilical cord. This was the presumed cause of death.

Pathologic Features
The degree of coiling tends to be rather uniform throughout the length of the umbilical cord. However, focal areas may show excessive or decreased coiling or excessive coiling may be localized and form a **stricture** (Figure 15.8). Other terms used for these significant reductions in

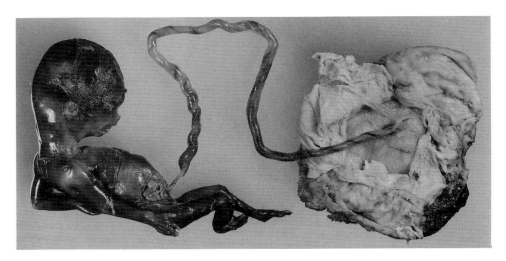

Figure 15.8. Spontaneous abortus at about 14 weeks gestation with markedly spiraled cord and severe constriction of the cord (torsion) near the fetal surface that led to the death.

the diameter of the umbilical cord are **constriction, torsion,** or **coarctation**. They are often seen in fetal demise and most commonly found at the *fetal end of the cord*. This may occur because there is a gradually diminishing amount of Wharton's jelly near the abdominal surface. We are convinced that these are **not** artifacts, as some have suggested, and the pathologic changes associated with strictures support this. In addition, cord strictures are rarely seen in hypocoiled or normally coiled cords. Pathologic findings associated with stricture and/or hypercoiling include *congestion of the cord and vessels on one side of the torsion, compression, and/or distension of the umbilical vein, long-standing degeneration of the umbilical vessels, and thrombi in the umbilical or placental surface vessels*. Because these fetuses are often macerated and coagulation is inadequately developed in embryos, the demonstration of thrombi is often difficult in early gestation.

Suggestions for Examination and Report:
Abnormal Coiling or Stricture

Gross Examination: Ideally, the direction of the coil or twist and the degree of coiling should be noted (see Figure 15.6). The coiling index described above may be used for this purpose, but may not be necessary if the examiner is experienced. Focal areas with increased or decreased twisting should also be noted. Constrictions should be sectioned, and attention should be given to the chorionic vessels as these may contain thrombi.

Comment: Abnormal coiling or strictures may be associated with adverse perinatal outcome. If a stricture is present in the setting of a fetal demise and there is evidence of venous obstruction, such as thrombosis, the constriction can be considered the cause of death. If supporting histologic findings are not present, the constriction may be suggested as a cause of demise.

Umbilical Cord Length

Pathologic Features

The normal length of the umbilical cord at term is approximately **55 to 65 cm**. Excessively long cords occur in 4% to 6% of placentas whereas abnormally short cords have an incidence of approximately 1% to 2%. Short cords are those **less than 35 cm** and long cords are those **greater than 70 to 80 cm**. When evaluating cord length, there are several points that should be remembered. First, it is important to distinguish between "absolute" and "relative" lengths. A cord that is long but wound about the neck multiple times will be functionally short, and this is particularly evident during fetal descent at delivery. Furthermore, the entire cord is almost never submitted to Pathology and so the diagnosis of a short cord must be made with caution. Usually 4 to 7 cm is always left attached to the infant at delivery and other fragments are discarded, used for blood gas determinations or other testing. Last, the length of the cord shrinks as much as several centimeters in the first few hours following delivery. For these reasons, accurate recording at the time of delivery, although difficult to accomplish, is preferable. Abnormally long cords are associated with *cord edema, congestion and hemorrhage, and thrombosis of umbilical or chorionic vessels*. Long cords are also associated with other pathologic changes in the placenta including *meconium, nucleated red blood cells, and chorangiosis*. The latter two findings are seen in the placenta in the setting of intrauterine hypoxia, and meconium may be present in fetal distress.

Pathogenesis

Cord length seems to be determined by several factors—*gestational age, genetics, and fetal movement*. On the 41st day after conception the developing cord has a mean length of about 0.5 cm. By the 4th month it has grown to between 16 to 18 cm and, by the 6th month, to approximately 33 to 35 cm. Most of the cord's length is achieved by the 28th week of pregnancy. Although growth slows progressively after this time, it never ceases until delivery. A genetic predisposition for longer or shorter cords seems to exist and excessively long cords have been shown to have a tendency to recur in subsequent pregnancies. Males also have longer cords than females. Fetal movement has been shown to have an effect on the length of cord as well. Short cords are more common in situations in which there is decreased fetal movement due to congenital anomalies such as skeletal dysplasias or trisomy 21, and where there is intrauterine constraint such as uterine anomalies, ectopic pregnancies, amnionic bands, and twins. In addition, when pregnant animals are administered drugs that decrease fetal movements, such as curare, alcohol, or beta-blockers, short cords result. The possible relation between long cords and excessive fetal movements is more difficult to assess because of the lack of quantitative data on prenatal movements. However, neonates with long cords have been noted to be relatively hyperkinetic when compared with those that had shorter cords.

Clinical Features and Implications

Excessively short cords are clearly correlated with neonatal problems; the essential question, however, is whether the length of the cord is determined by prenatal CNS problems or whether the CNS problems result from perinatal problems attending the delivery of a short cord. Many problems associated with short cords are related to excess traction during delivery. These include *premature separation of the placenta (abruptio), cord hemorrhage or hematoma, cord rupture, uterine inversion, failure of descent, and prolongation of the second stage of labor*. Short cords have also been associated with *fetal distress, low Apgar scores, and depressed intelligence quotient (IQ)*. Short cords are associated with some developmental anomalies such as abdominal wall defects. **Excessively long cords**, on the other hand, are associated with *fetal distress, cord entanglement, cord prolapse, true knots, excessive coiling, constriction, and thrombosis* (Figure 15.9). Clinical sequelae of long cords include *long-*

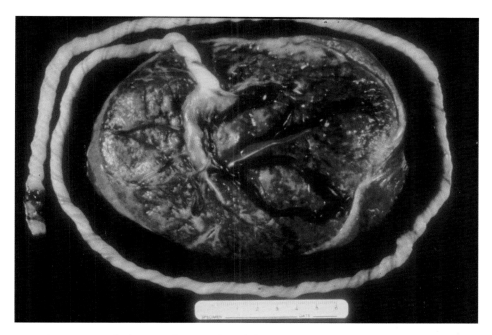

Figure 15.9. An excessively long and twisted umbilical cord. Note the visible thrombus in the fetal surface vasculature seen as a white streak in the vessel.

term neurologic impairment, intrauterine growth restriction, fetal demise, and fetal distress. Cord entanglement, prolapse, and true knots are discussed below.

Cord Diameter

The diameter of the cord is predominantly due to the water content of Wharton's jelly. The diameter increases slowly throughout gestation and then declines slightly in the last few weeks before full maturity. An increased cord diameter is usually due to **edema** (Figure 15.10). Cord edema is found in 10% of infants and is more common in premature infants. The edema may be *diffusely distributed or occur focally and appear as cysts.* Usually, infants with cord edema have a normal outcome but cord edema is occasionally associated with *polyhydramnios, maternal diabetes, and fetal hydrops.*

Excessively thin umbilical cords are a potential cause of fetal problems. The cord may be thin throughout or only portions may be thinned. In the thin areas there is a decreased amount of Wharton's jelly and thus *compression of vessels is a greater possibility than when they are protected.* Thin cords occur more often with *growth-restricted fetuses and in preeclampsia.* Occasionally, the cord has an almost complete lack of Wharton's jelly, which is usually associated with fetal growth restriction.

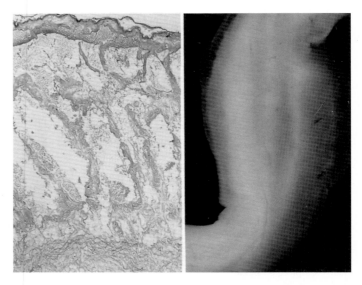

Figure 15.10. Marked edema in the umbilical cord of a normal newborn infant. Note the dissociation of fibrous tissue underneath the surface of the cord. H&E. ×160.

Suggestions for Examination and Report: Excessively Long or Short Cords, Cord Edema, and Thin Cords

Gross Examination: Measurement of the total length of all cord fragments submitted is suggested, although the true length cannot be determined without measurement at delivery. Measurement of the cord diameter should be performed as well with particular attention to focal areas of edema. The chorionic vessels should be evaluated for the presence of thrombi.

Comment: Abnormalities in cord length and thin cords are associated with adverse perinatal outcome. Cord edema is usually not associated with adverse outcome.

Cord Entanglement and Cord Prolapse

Clinical Features and Implications

The incidence of a single **nuchal cord** at term is approximately 20%, while two nuchal cords occur in 2.5% and three nuchal cords in 0.5% of births. Nuchal cords have been identified as early as 20 weeks gestation, and some of these may resolve before delivery. It appears that having a nuchal cord that encircles the neck in a locked pattern is of greater significance to outcome than those with an unlocked pattern. The presence of **nuchal cords** or **cord entanglement** is associated with *more admissions to the intensive care unit, a higher incidence of cesarean section delivery, fetal growth restriction, neonatal anemia, poor long-term* *neurologic outcome, spastic cerebral palsy, and fetal demise.* **Cord prolapse** is estimated to occur in 0.41% of deliveries. It is associated with *multiparity, premature labor, multiple gestation, fetal malpresentation, artificial rupture of membranes with high presenting fetal parts, and with long cords.* The presence of a prolapsed cord may have grave prognostic significance and is associated with a perinatal mortality of approximately 13%. The manner in which nuchal cords, cord entanglements, or prolapse lead to adverse outcome is by vascular occlusion and decreased venous return from the placenta leading to asphyxia (Figure 15.11). Cord compression may have serious fetal neurologic consequences and this is why the "cord compression pattern" of fetal heart monitoring is taken so seriously.

Pathologic Features
The compressed umbilical cord may show profound pathological changes such as *hemorrhage or even rupture* at the site of compression. It leads occasionally to *thrombosis* of umbilical vessels, or more commonly of the chorionic vessels. Therefore, additional sections of chorionic vessels are suggested. However, these findings are not pathognomonic for cord compression and the diagnosis cannot be made on pathology alone.

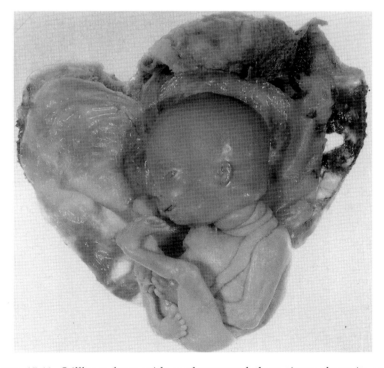

Figure 15.11. Stillborn fetus with cord wrapped three times about its neck. Death presumably came about by obstruction to venous return from the placenta, **not** by obstruction to vessels of the fetal head.

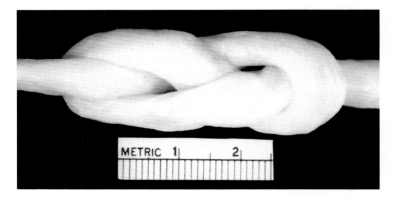

Figure 15.12. Loose true knot in the umbilical cord in infant with no untoward sequelae.

Umbilical Cord Knots

Pathologic Features
True knots of the umbilical cord occur with a *frequency of 0.4% to 0.5%.* They may be loose (Figure 15.12) or tight (Figure 15.13), the latter obviously having greater clinical significance. Tight true knots cause *compression of Wharton's jelly at the site of knotting, congestion of the placental side of the knot (due to decreased venous return to the placenta), and tendency*

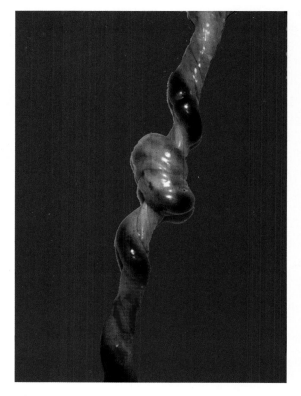

Figure 15.13. Umbilical cord with tight true knot.

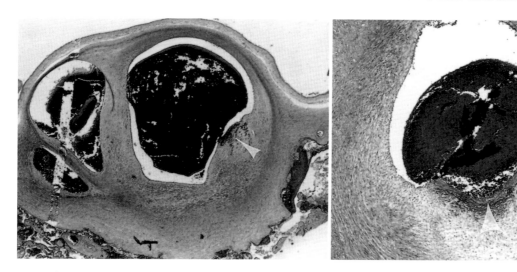

Figure 15.14. Mural thrombi in surface veins. H&E. Left ×16; right, Masson trichome ×64.

of the unknotted cord to curl (if the knot has been present for a period of time). In clinically significant knots, the venous stasis that occurs often results in *thrombosis of placental surface veins or even umbilical vein thrombosis*. Mural thrombosis or complete occlusion may be found, and calcifications may occur in long-standing thrombosis (Figure 15.14). In addition, the veins are frequently thickened and may exhibit "**cushions,**" which are *myxoid-appearing, irregular areas of thickening of blood vessels with the deposition of fibrin within the wall* (see Figure 21.10, page 398).

False knots should not be called knots at all. These are actually local redundancies of the umbilical vessels, mostly the vein (Figure 15.15). So far as can be determined, false knots *have absolutely no clinical importance*. Despite their clinical irrelevancy, questions persist

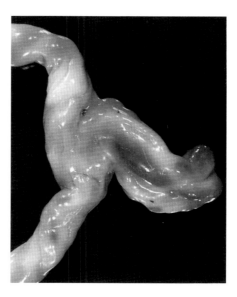

Figure 15.15. "False knots," representing vascular redundancies.

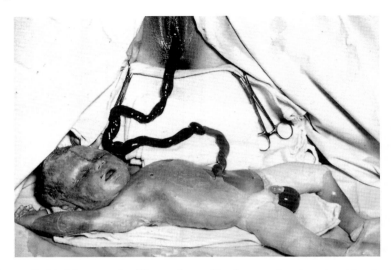

Figure 15.16. Macerated stillborn fetus. Death was due to a true knot with obstruction of venous return from the placenta. Total cord length was 65 cm. Note the marked congestion of the cord distal to the knot.

as to why these redundancies appear at all, but answers are elusive at present.

Clinical Features and Implications

True knots are commonly associated with *long cords*, *multigravidas*, *male fetuses, and monoamnionic twins*. Knots probably develop early in gestation because the marked fetal movement necessary to cause knotting is not possible when the fetus has reached a certain size. The knot may not become tight until the onset of labor when fetal descent into the birth canal increases traction on the cord. Knots may not only cause *intrauterine or intrapartum fetal death* (Figure 15.16), but may lead to significant *hypoxia with lasting neurologic damage in the infant*. True knots have an *overall mortality of about 10%*.

Suggestions for Examination and Report: Umbilical Cord Knots

Gross Examination: Documentation should be made of the presence of the true knot, the tightness of the knot, the presence of congestion, constriction in the area of knot, curling of the unknotted cord, and gross evidence of thrombosis. Additional sections should be taken in the area of the knot. No additional examination is necessary with false knots.

Comment: True knots are more clinically significant when tight and associated with signs of vascular obstruction such as thrombosis, congestion, etc. A comment on the associated findings and an evaluation of the clinical significance of the knot in each case is recommended if possible. No comment is necessary when false knots are present as they have no clinical consequence.

Cord Insertion

The umbilical cord normally inserts on the placental surface, more often near or at the center than elsewhere (Figure 15.17). In nearly 7% of term placentas it has a **marginal insertion**, a "Battledore" placenta.

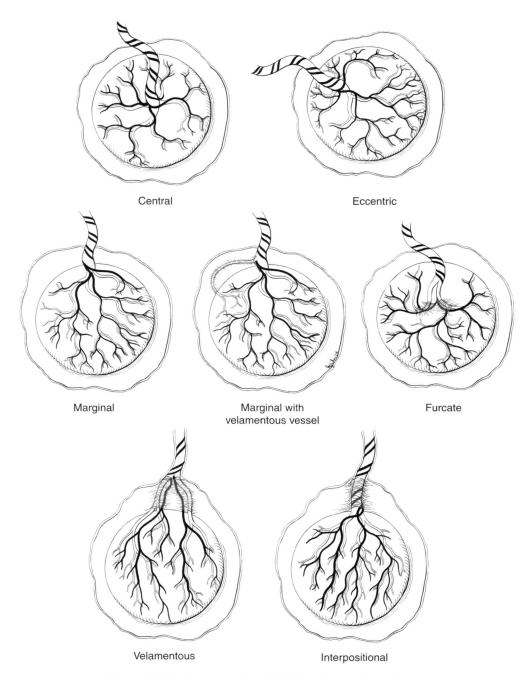

Figure 15.17. Drawing of umbilical cord insertion patterns.

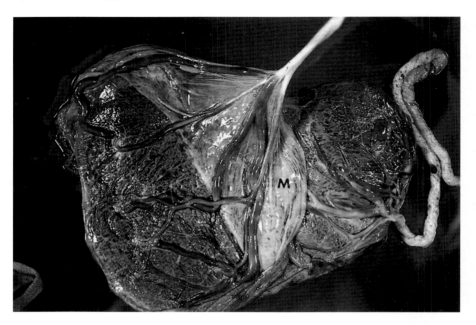

Figure 15.18. Velamentous insertion of umbilical cord on the "dividing membranes" of twin placenta.

In about 1%, the cord inserts into the membranes, a **velamentous** or **membranous insertion** (Figures 15.17, 15.18). Here, the umbilical vessels course over the free membranes and, having lost their protection by Wharton's jelly, are more vulnerable to trauma and disruption. Not only are the sites of insertion variable, the insertion itself may take an abnormal shape. Thus, the branching of vessels before the cord inserts onto the surface of the placenta results in a **furcate cord insertion** (Figures 15.17, 15.19). At times, the cord runs parallel to the placental surface or in the membranes before its vessels branch, called an **interpositional insertion** (Figures 15.17, 15.20).

Velamentous and Marginal Cord Insertion

Pathologic Features
Velamentous insertion of the umbilical cord occurs in around 1% of singleton term deliveries, **marginal insertion** in approximately 7%. They are more common with *twins, higher multiples, and in association with a single umbilical artery.* The cord may insert reasonably close to the edge of the placenta, which is much more common than the extreme situation, where the cord inserts at the apex of the membranous sac. In the latter configuration, the long membranous course of the vessels makes them very *vulnerable to injury.* It should be pointed out, however, that a membranous course of fetal blood vessels is not restricted to a velamentous insertion of the cord. Quite often there are such membranous vessels issuing from marginally inserted cords (Figure 15.17), and they have the same potential consequences. In multiple gestations, the

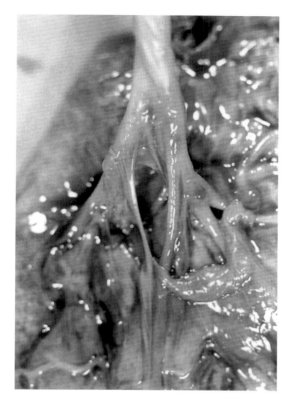

Figure 15.19. Furcate insertion of the umbilical cord. Note that the umbilical vessels leave the protection of Wharton's jelly above the insertion on the placenta. (Courtesy of Dr. W. Tench.)

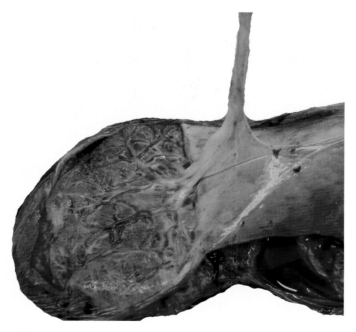

Figure 15.20. Interpositional insertion of umbilical cord. Note that the cord inserts into the membranes, running briefly within the membranes before inserting onto the placental surface. It is clear than the membranous portion of the cord has **not** lost the protection of Wharton's jelly.

velamentous cord insertion often arises on the dividing membranes and the membranous vessels are then similarly prone to disruption.

Thrombosis of the velamentous arteries and veins may be seen in this insertional anomaly (Figure 15.21). *Hemorrhage* arises due to rupture of the velamentous vessels, most commonly from the veins. It is the most frequent complication of membranous vessels (Figure 15.22). Hemorrhage may even commence before labor has begun. In this case there are *numerous hemosiderin-laden macrophages around the necrotic, thrombosed artery, presumably derived from the hemolysis of extravasated blood.* Velamentous vessels over the cervical os are called **vasa previa**. Vasa previa has a particularly serious prognosis in that the vessels may rupture during a vaginal delivery.

Pathogenesis

Two mutually contradictory theories have been put forward to explain marginal and velamentous cord insertions, **abnormal primary implantation** ("polarity theory") and **trophotropism**. The abnormal implantation theory postulates that, at the nidation of the blastocyst, the embryo does not face the endometrium; rather, it is located at the opposite side, or obliquely oriented. Thus, when the early umbilical cord develops, it has to seek its connection with the future area of placentation by extending its vessels from the embryo to the base of implantation. Eventually, the vessels must become membranous in location. However, virtually all early embryos that have been described have

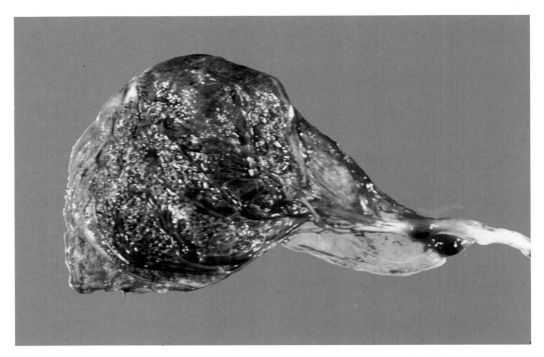

Figure 15.21. Placenta with velamentous cord insertion and thrombosis of velamentous vessels seen at the right.

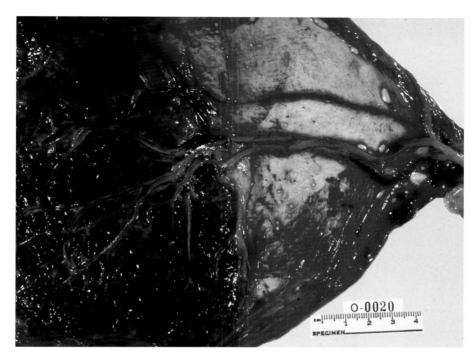

Figure 15.22. Recent hemorrhage in the membranes from rupture of velamentous vessel. Note discoloration of membranes in area of hemorrhage.

had a "normal" endometrial position. The second theory of **trophotropism** is favored for the following reasons. Serial ultrasonograms during early pregnancy show that the placenta changes location. This placental movement is accomplished through *marginal atrophy on one side and growth and expansion on the other*. In abnormal cord insertions, atrophy near the cord insertion with growth and expansion of the opposite site results in the cord insertion *being left behind in the membranes*. Lesser degrees would result in a marginal insertion. Trophotropism also plays a role in the development of abnormal placental shapes as well (see Chapter 13).

Clinical Features and Implications

Velamentous and marginal cord insertions are found relatively frequently in early abortions and are highly correlated with *congenital anomalies*. One of the most serious complications of velamentous vessels is **vasa previa** in which membranous vessels are present over the internal cervical os. In this situation, membranous vessels may be disrupted by the exiting fetal head or by the obstetric attendant who ruptures the membranes (Figure 15.22). *Exsanguination* from ruptured membranous vessels can proceed within minutes. The frequency of hemorrhage is difficult to assess but has been estimated to be 1 in 50 cases of velamentous insertions. The mortality rate from intrapartum rupture and hemorrhage is around 58% overall and 73% when the hemorrhage occurs before delivery. Velamentous vessels are also more susceptible to compression by fetal parts resulting in obstruction of blood flow. Clinical associations of velamentous insertion therefore include *fetal distress, low Apgar scores, neonatal thrombocytopenia, fetal growth restriction, prematurity, growth restriction, cerebral palsy, and death.* Marginal insertions do not have the same sequelae as velamentous insertion, unless membranous vessels are present.

Furcate Cord Insertion

Furcate cord insertion is a rare abnormality in which the *umbilical vessels split and separate from the cord substance before reaching the surface of the placenta* (see Figures 15.17, 15.19). They may lose the protection afforded by Wharton's jelly and are thus *prone to thrombosis and injury.* There is much confusion of furcate insertions with velamentous insertions, which have many features in common. *Stillbirth, fatal hemorrhage, varices, thrombosis of fetal vessels, and intrauterine growth restriction* have all been described in association with furcate cord insertion, but most infants are normal.

Interpositional Cord Insertion

Interpositional insertion is also a type of membranous insertion. Here, the cord inserts in the membranes but, unlike velamentous insertion, *the vessels do not lose the protection of Wharton's jelly* (see Figures 15.17, 15.20). Interpositional insertion therefore does not have the same clinical consequences as velamentous insertion.

Suggestions for Examination and Report:
Abnormal Cord Insertion

Gross Examination: In velamentous insertion, the distance from insertion to the placental margin should be measured and the membranous vessels evaluated for rupture, hemorrhage, or thrombosis. It is recommended that membranous vessels be rolled with the fetal membranes and submitted as a separate section. Photographs of the intact specimen should be considered, particularly in cases of poor outcome.

Comment: If there is rupture or thrombosis of velamentous vessels, the possibility of fetal hemorrhage should be mentioned.

Single Umbilical Artery

Pathologic Features
Single umbilical artery (SUA) is the commonest congenital anomaly of humans (Figure 15.23 A). It has an incidence of 0.5 to 1% in singletons and 8.8% in twins. It can now be detected prenatally by ultrasonography and should **always** be ascertained at birth. A remnant of the second umbilical artery can sometimes be identified on micro-

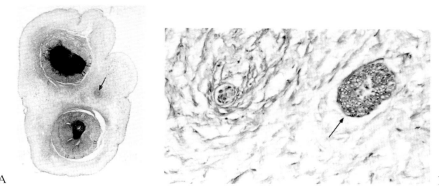

A   B

Figure 15.23. (A) Umbilical cord with single umbilical artery (SUA). A degenerating second artery is seen (arrow). H&E. ×10. (B) Muscular remnant of a "vanished" second umbilical artery (arrow); on the left is a remnant of an allantoic duct. H&E. ×60.

scopic examination (Figure 15.23 B). *It must be cautioned that SUA may be found at one end of the cord and not the other.* At times, the arteries fuse far above the cord insertion on the placenta in a manner that is similar to their normal communication near the placenta. Occasionally, this communication is many centimeters from the cord insertion onto the placenta.

Clinical Features and Implications
SUA has been associated with *growth restriction, maternal diabetes, antepartum hemorrhage, polyhydramnios, and oligohydramnios.* Cord accidents are more common in these cords. Congenital anomalies are present in 30% to 44.7% of infants, and other placental abnormalities are found in 16.4%. Because *renal anomalies* are relatively frequent with an incidence of 18.5%, neonatal renal sonography is often recommended when SUA is found. Hollow organ anomalies, such as *intestinal atresia*, are also relatively frequent in these infants. An isolated SUA (without other sonographic anomalies) overall does not usually affect outcome and is often found in perfectly healthy infants. To be sure, the pediatrician should be notified of its existence to perform a more detailed physical examination to ensure that the infant has no hidden anomalies.

Pathogenesis
In 73%, the defect locates to the left artery. Cytogenetic and complex anomalies are associated nearly exclusively with the left-sided absence. *Absence of one umbilical artery may occur as aplasia or as the consequence of atrophy of one artery.* The latter mechanism is probably more frequent and can be seen to have occurred in many specimens when histologic examination is undertaken (Figure 15.23 B). Atrophy occasionally occurs late in pregnancy, but when it takes place long before birth, the arterial lumen gradually vanishes and only a tiny muscular remnant may remain. In some cases, atrophy of an artery when a portion of the placenta atrophies and one umbilical artery loses its "territory." Thus,

SUA may be associated with trophotropism and therefore with placental shape aberrations or abnormal insertions.

Supernumerary Vessels

More than three umbilical vessels are normal for many species, but are *rare in humans*. **Persistence of the right umbilical vein** has been reported associated with anomalies. However, considering its rarity, one must take care, when assessing an increased number of vessels, not to be misled by the frequent looping that occurs in many cord vessels or by false knots.

Suggestions for Examination and Report: Single Umbilical Artery and Persistence of the Right Umbilical Vein

Gross Examination: Several cross sections of the cord must be examined to ensure that the correct number of vessels is documented. Sections away from the insertion site are recommended as these may show only one artery due to anastomoses or may show more vessels due to false knots.

Comment: Single umbilical artery and persistence of the right umbilical vein are both associated with an increased risk of congenital anomalies. Therefore, evaluation for anomalies may be suggested.

Thrombosis of Umbilical Vessels

Pathologic Features
The incidence of **umbilical vessel thrombosis** is 1 in 1300 deliveries, 1 in 1000 perinatal autopsies, and 1 in 250 high-risk gestations. *Venous thromboses are more common than arterial thromboses, but the latter are more often lethal.* Old thrombi in umbilical vessels, primarily the vein, may calcify and occasionally massive calcification has made it difficult to ligate the cord at delivery (Figure 15.24).

Pathogenesis
Thrombosis of umbilical vessels most frequently occurs near term. It may develop due to *velamentous insertion, inflammation, varices, entanglement, knotting, torsion, abnormal coiling, amnionic bands, maternal diabetes, and funipuncture.* Coagulation problems caused by thrombophilias of mother or infant are sometimes the cause. The formation of thrombi with velamentous insertion of the cord is readily understandable. It is also easy to understand that thrombosis of cord vessels may occur in varices and from knotting as well as the entangling of cords in monoamnionic twins (see Chapter 10).

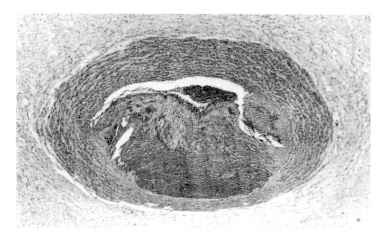

Figure 15.24. Nearly occlusive venous thrombus in a long cord associated with fetal death. H&E. ×40.

Clinical Features and Implications

Thrombosis can compromise the circulation and lead to *growth restriction, fetal death, or neurologic injury*. Thrombi may also break off and potentially embolize to the fetus or to the placenta, where they may cause infarction. More remarkable are the thrombi that occur in the absence of all these more readily understood complications, and they are perhaps the most common. Very frequently thromboses of vessels in the cord are associated with similar events in the villous ramifications (see Chapter 21). Thrombosis due to coagulation defects has been associated with extensive CNS lesions in the infants as well as stroke and neonatal thrombosis.

Suggestions for Examination and Report:
Thrombosis of Umbilical Vessels

Gross Examination: Thrombi that are grossly identified should be submitted for microscopic examination. As the cord is often multiply clamped at delivery, local hemorrhage (which may mimic thrombosis) is common. This should not be misinterpreted as thrombosis. However, the serrations of the clamp usually remain visible.

Comment: Thrombosis of umbilical vessels may be associated with underlying coagulopathies, or other maternal or fetal disorders.

Tumors

Hemangiomas

Angiomas are benign neoplasms. They tend to occur at the placental end of the cord and arise from one or more umbilical vessels. Unlike chorangiomas that occur in the villous tissue (see Chapter 22), they are not usually associated with hydramnios. The neoplasms may attain a large size, up to 18 cm in length and 14 cm in diameter, with weights up to 900 g. They have a fairly uniform histologic appearance (Figure 15.25), consisting of a *proliferation of small capillaries in a loose connective tissue stroma. Some have myxoma-like stroma and are then called angiomyoxomas;* however, some have referred to these as hamartomas. Hemangiomas are associated with *fetal hemorrhage, high-output cardiac failure, elevated maternal alpha fetoprotein (AFP) levels, disseminated intravascular coagulation (DIC), fetal hemangiomas, fetal anomalies, and fetal death.*

Teratomas

Teratomas are much less common than angiomas. There is some controversy about the diagnosis of these lesions and their differentiation from acardiac twins (see Chapter 10). If the lesion does not contain axial skeleton or umbilical cord, it likely represents a true tumor. As with other teratomas *skin, connective tissue, and various other tissues* such as colonic or respiratory epithelium are often present.

Miscellaneous Cord Lesions

Hemorrhages and **hematomas** of the umbilical cord are relatively rare. They have serious consequences as the fetus may *exsanguinate or sustain significant neurologic injury from compression of umbilical vessels.* A 50% fetal mortality has been reported (Figure 15.26). Spontaneous cord hematomas are associated with *short cords, trauma (amniocentesis, cor-*

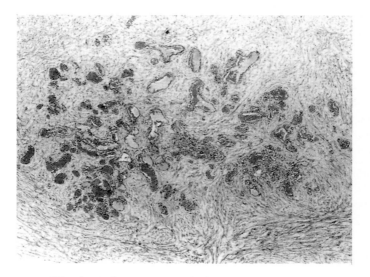

Figure 15.25. Histological appearance of a hemangioma of the umbilical cord. H&E. ×20. (From Benirschke K, Dodds JP. Angiomyxoma of the umbilical cord with atrophy of an umbilical arter. Obstet Gynecol 1967;30:99–102, with permission.)

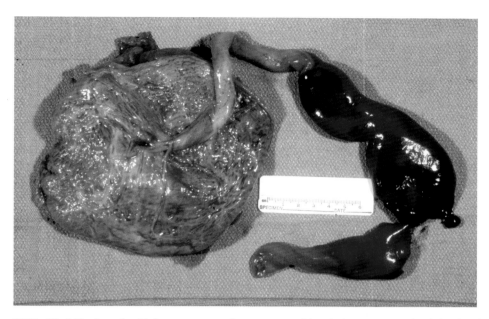

Figure 15.26. Umbilical cord with hematoma and rupture resulting in intrapartum fetal death. The cord shows marked discoloration and hemorrhage with a somewhat fusiform shape due to accumulation of blood.

docentesis), aneurysms, and cord entanglement. At times there are associated thrombi.

False knots, which are actually vascular redundancies, often appear as varicosities in the umbilical cord. However, real **varix** formations are rare (Figure 15.27). When present, they show *marked, focal thinning of the wall of the umbilical vein* that may be associated with *muscle necrosis.* Fetal death may occur from *fetal hemorrhage or compression of the aneurys-*

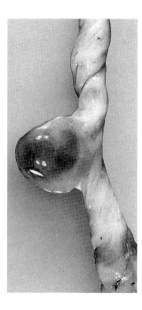

Figure 15.27. Partially thrombosed varix near the fetal end of the cord. The fetus was normal.

mally dilated veins (Figure 15.28). When elastic stains are done on such cords it has been repeatedly found that the elastic fibers of the vein are focally deficient.

The umbilical cord may **rupture**, either completely or partially (see Figure 15.26). This will inevitably lead to bleeding and often results in cord *hematomas*. Excessively *short cords* may rupture during descent, but *velamentous cord insertion* is the most frequent antecedent of this complication. Rupture has also been reported associated with *varices, cord entanglement, trauma from amniocentesis, or therapeutic intrauterine transfusion and severe acute funisitis*. If rupture occurs, it is most often at the site of its placental attachment, but can occur anywhere. Spontaneous complete rupture is an uncommon event; *most ruptures are partial and cause local hematomas or hemorrhage.*

Necrosis of umbilical vessel walls may result from chronic and severe **meconium exposure**. The cord will usually be discolored green or greenish-brown. On histologic section one sees *rounded, degenerating myocytes with loss of nuclei and cell death* (see Figure 14.16, page 236). Such areas of degeneration not only occur in the vein but may affect arteries as well. On occasion, they are the sequelae of thrombosis, but they may occur without it. Necrosis of umbilical arteries and a linear **ulceration** of Wharton's jelly have been described associated with intestinal atresia. Obviously, this leads to hemorrhage into the umbilical cord and amniotic fluid, with resultant fetal anemia and the potential for fetal exsanguination. **Segmental thinning** of umbilical vessels has also been described as a focal thinning of the vessel wall with virtual absence of the vascular media. It is seen predominantly in the umbilical vein (Figure 15.29) and has been associated with congenital malformations and fetal distress.

Squamous metaplasia of the amnionic epithelium covering the umbilical cord may occur as it does in the fetal membranes. These may grossly visible as *irregular, white, hydrophobic patches on the surface of cord.*

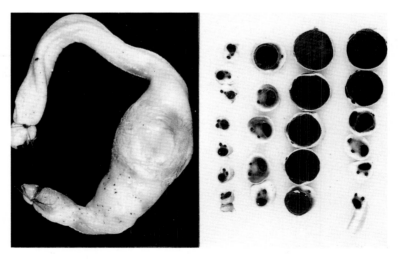

Figure 15.28. Aneurysmal dilatation of the umbilical vein with fatal compression of arteries. No cause was identified for this lesion.

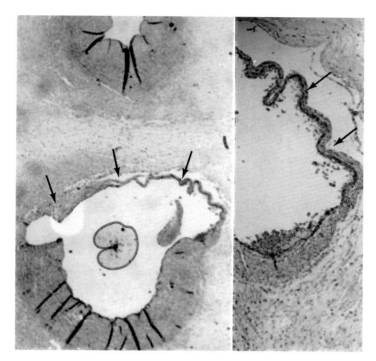

Figure 15.29. Segmental thinning of the umbilical vein (arrows) in a child with cerebral palsy. No cause was apparent. H&E. Left ×60; right ×160.

Microscopically, *keratinizing squamous epithelium* partially replaces the more usual cuboidal epithelium. These plaques may be confused with the surface nodules present in **Candida** infection. In the latter situation, the nodules tend to be *slightly elevated, more circumscribed, round, and may be white to yellow in color* (see Chapter 16). Finally, the cord may show various **discolorations** similar to those seen in the fetal membranes (see Chapter 14). Green discoloration may be present in meconium exposure, brown discoloration is usually due to hemosiderin from old hemorrhage, yellow discoloration from maternal bilirubinemia, and red-brown discoloration is usually secondary to **hemolysis** after fetal death.

Suggestions for Examination and Report: Hemangioma, Hematoma, Hemorrhage, Varices, and Rupture

Gross Examination: Any time a hemorrhagic lesion of the cord is identified, multiple serial sections should be cut to determine the underlying cause. If this is not readily apparent, serial sections of the entire lesion should be submitted.

Comment: If there is extensive hemorrhage in the cord, compression of umbilical vessels may occur, leading to significant embarrassment of blood flow to the fetus with potentially dire consequences.

Selected References

PHP4, Chapter 12, pages 335–398.

Baergen RN, Malicki D, Behling CA, Benirschke K. Morbidity, mortality and placental pathology in excessively long umbilical cords. Pediatr Dev Pathol 2001;4:144–153.

Bendon RW, Tyson RW, Baldwin VJ, et al. Umbilical cord ulceration and intestinal atresia: a new association? Am J Obstet Gynecol 1991;164:582–586.

Benirschke K. Obstetrically important lesions of the umbilical cord. J Reprod Med 1994;39:262–272.

Benirschke K, Bourne GL. The incidence and prognostic implication of congenital absence of one umbilical artery. Am J Obstet Gynecol 1960;79:251–254.

Heifetz SA. Single umbilical artery: a statistical analysis of 237 autopsy cases and review of the literature. Perspect Pediatr Pathol 1984;8:345–378.

Heifetz SA. Thrombosis of the umbilical cord: analysis of 52 cases and literature review. Pediatr Pathol 1988;8:37–54.

Heifetz SA, Rueda-Pedraza ME. Hemangiomas of the umbilical cord. Pediatr Pathol 1983;1:385–398.

Jauniaux E, De Munter C, Vanesse M, et al. Embryonic remnants of the umbilical cord: morphologic and clinical aspects. Hum Pathol 1989;20:458–462.

Lacro RV, Jones KL, Benirschke K. The umbilical cord twist: origin, direction, and relevance. Am J Obstet Gynecol 1987;157:833–838.

Naeye RL. Umbilical cord length: clinical significance. J Pediatr 1985;107:278–281.

Qureshi F, Jacques SM. Marked segmental thinning of the umbilical cord vessels. Arch Pathol Lab Med 1994;118:826–830.

Strong TH, Jarles DL, Vega JS, et al. The umbilical coiling index. Am J Obstet Gynecol 1994;170:29–32.

Sun Y, Arbuckle S, Hocking G, et al. Umbilical cord stricture and intrauterine fetal death. Pediatr Pathol Lab Med 1995;15:723–732.

Section V

Disease Processes and the Placenta

This section is concerned with diseases or disease processes that affect the placenta and includes both maternal and fetal conditions. It begins, in Chapter 16, with a discussion of infection. This chapter covers acute chorioamnionitis, ascending infection, and chronic villitis and includes discussion of causative organisms. Chapter 17 covers maternal diseases and the various drugs and physical agents that may affect the placenta. There are numerous maternal diseases that complicate pregnancy, but only the most important of those that affect placental function are covered here. Because of their particular importance, preeclampsia, systemic lupus erythematosus, and thrombophilia are discussed separately in Chapter 18. Chapter 19 presents a miscellaneous group of placental lesions, some of which are associated with maternal or fetal disease. However, these lesions either do not have one specific etiology or the etiology is unknown and so they do not fit easily in other chapters. Therefore, they are placed in this chapter for convenience. The final two chapters discuss fetal conditions. Placental changes in hydrops, fetomaternal hemorrhage, and metabolic disorders are covered in Chapter 20, while fetal thrombotic lesions are discussed in Chapter 21.

Chapter 16

Infectious Diseases

General Considerations

The pathogenesis of prenatal infections and related circumstances must be understood if the associated pathologic lesions are to be interpreted correctly. Infections may reach the placenta and fetus in several ways:

- By **ascension** from through endocervical canal,
- By **hematogenous transmission** from maternal blood,
- By **direct introduction** via amniocentesis, chorionic villus sampling, amnioscopy, percutaneous umbilical blood sampling or intrauterine fetal transfusion, and

• By **direct extension** from infection in the endometrium.

The majority of infections arise by one of the first two routes, and these are the focus of this chapter.

Ascending Infection and Acute Chorioamnionitis

Acute chorioamnionitis is common, with an incidence of 20% to 24% of live births and up to 67% of preterm deliveries. It is an important cause of *preterm labor* and *preterm deliveries*, which are significant causes of perinatal morbidity and mortality. Acute chorioamnionitis has also recently been implicated in the development of poor *long-term neurologic outcome and cerebral palsy*.

Pathogenesis

Ascending infection, also called "amniotic sac infection syndrome," develops from *an infection that commences in the vagina and endocervix and then ascends to the uterine cavity* (Figure 16.1). Acute chorioamnionitis is *always* due to infection, and the ascending nature of this infection is supported by three pathologic findings:

• It is usually associated with severe acute deciduitis.
• In twin gestations, it is invariably the lower twin that has chorioamnionitis or whose membranes are more severely inflamed.
• The point of spontaneous membrane rupture, which is in proximity to the cervical os, has the most severe inflammation.

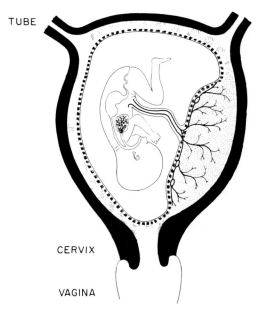

Figure 16.1. Intrauterine position of fetus and placenta. Infectious organisms ascend through the endocervical canal. They first infect the membranes covering the internal os and then penetrate the amniotic cavity.

It is often stated that infection occurs secondary to membrane rupture, but in actuality *it is the loss of membrane integrity resulting from inflammation that makes rupture a probability*. In fact, ascending infection occurs most often in the **presence of intact fetal membranes.** Furthermore, it is now the predominant opinion that *amniotic sac infection is the primary cause of premature labor and delivery*, at least in those pregnancies that terminate spontaneously before 30 weeks gestation, and that antimicrobial therapy usually fails to prolong pregnancy when chorioamnionitis is already extant.

Acute Chorioamnionitis and Preterm Delivery: Causes or associations of preterm labor include *acute chorioamnionitis, chronic endocervicitis, maternal smoking, parity,* and *prior cervical surgery.* It has also been suggested that *intercourse during late pregnancy* may initiate premature delivery, but this is still controversial. There is now a very large body of investigation *incriminating inflammatory mediators in the initiation of labor during the process of ascending infection.* Interleukin-1 (IL-1), IL-6, and IL-8 are elevated in the amniotic fluid and cord blood in the presence of an ascending infection. Tumor necrosis factor (TNF) activates the cytokine machinery and may well be at the starting point of labor initiation by stimulating prostaglandin production from the decidua. Deciduitis, decidual macrophage activation, and neutrophils exudation, in particular, play an important role in the initiation of premature labor. However, the precise chemical cascade that ultimately leads to myometrial contractions is not yet elucidated. Suffice it to say that the cytokine system is intimately involved in premature labor when it is caused by infection.

Incompetent Cervix: It has been suggested that 1% of pregnancies and up to 20% of midtrimester abortions result from an "**incompetent cervix.**" It is clinically defined as painless cervical dilatation occurring preterm. We are of the opinion that a truly incompetent cervix is an *anatomical defect* that develops due to *congenital anomalies or trauma.* Trauma, specifically a history of previous surgery, is the most common antecedent. In a study of cervical laser conization, the frequency of premature births increased from 6% to 38%. However, in the majority of cases of preterm labor, the cervix is anatomically normal and is *affected by severe chronic cervicitis, causing the cervix to be patulous and prone to premature dilatation.* Often, an incompetent cervix is diagnosed, the pregnancy delivers prematurely, and the histology shows a significant acute chorioamnionitis. In these cases, the painless cervical dilatation is most likely *not* due to an "incompetence" of the cervix but rather the result of underlying ascending infection. This underlying inflammation may be associated with, if not caused by, deficient endocervical mucus production.

"Clinical" Acute Chorioamnionitis: Making the diagnosis of **"clinical" chorioamnionitis** is problematic as only some gravidas with amniotic sac infection experience *fever, leukocytosis, uterine tenderness, or maternal or fetal tachycardia.* Indeed, close to 75% of women with histologic acute

chorioamnionitis do not fulfill the criteria for clinical chorioamnionitis, and many have no symptoms at all. On the other hand, only a minority of patients with a diagnosis of clinical chorioamnionitis ultimately show histologic chorioamnionitis. Other tests such as culture and Gram stain of the amniotic fluid, assays of the amniotic fluid for cytokines, esterase, or endotoxin, and fetal fibronectin have provided better correlation with histologic chorioamnionitis than clinical evaluation.

Pathologic Features

The pathologic features of an **ascending infection** are those of **acute chorioamnionitis**. Inflammatory lesions are present **only** when microbacterial contamination exists in the amniotic cavity. Typically, the fetal surface of the placenta lacks the blue sheen of the normal organ, and both *the membranes and fetal surface are white and opaque*, being obscured by the inflammatory exudate of polymorphonuclear leukocytes (PMNs) (Figure 16.2). The surface may become *yellow or green when much leukocytic exudate has accumulated or the process has been of long duration*. The placenta is frequently malodorous, and the very astute observer may sometimes identify the prevailing organism by the odor. The fecal odor of *Fusobacterium* and *Bacteroides* infections and the sweet odor of *Clostridium* and *Listeria* infections are useful identifiers for the adept examiner. *The membranes are typically more friable, and the decidua capsularis is frequently detached and hemorrhagic*. In many cases, the membranes are incomplete and consist of mere fragments of amnion without chorion or decidua capsularis. Particularly in preterm placentas, the inflammation is often accompanied by *acute marginal*

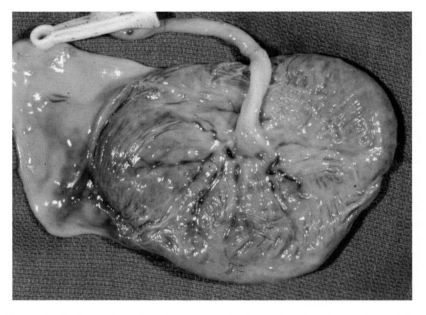

Figure 16.2. Term placenta with severe chorioamnionitis. The surface of the placenta is obscured by a whitish exudate; the vasculature is also indistinct.

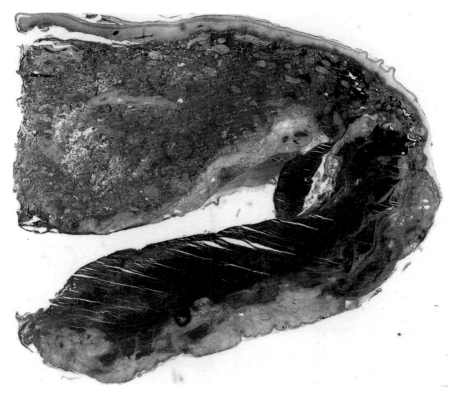

Figure 16.3. Placenta at 23 weeks gestation with massive chorioamnionitis and marked marginal hemorrhage that undermines the placenta and originates from deciduitis and disrupted vessels. H&E. ×3.5.

hemorrhage that undermines the edge of the placenta. Although this mimics abruptio placentae clinically, this process (Figure 16.3) markedly differs from the typical abruptio placentae as it originates from the associated acute deciduitis.

Acute chorioamnionitis, by definition, is *the presence of acute inflammatory cells, PMNs in particular, within the fetal membranes* (Figure 16.4). Eosinophils are found at times but usually only in protracted infections. Macrophages may participate to a variable extent. Chronic inflammatory cells, such as lymphocytes and plasma cells, are generally **not** present in acute chorioamnionitis. When present and admixed with acute inflammatory cells, the diagnosis of **subacute chorioamnionitis** may be made (see below). There is a grading system for acute chorioamnionitis; the idea being that grade correlates with neonatal outcome. However, grading is not reliable for this purpose. We believe that *the most important features of ascending infection are the infectious agent and whether there is a fetal response*. For example, *Trichomonas* can be enormously leukotactic, yet have little effect on neonatal morbidity and mortality. Conversely, *group B Streptococcus* may be associated with minimal leukocyte infiltration but have a devastating effect upon fetal and neonatal life.

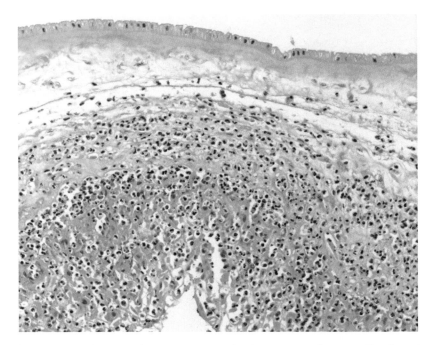

Figure 16.4. Massive chorioamnionitis in immature placenta. Exudate is present in the amnion and chorion. The placenta had a purulent surface and marked funisitis. H&E. ×60.

Maternal Response, Fetal Response, and Fetal Infection: In acute chorioamnionitis, the inflammatory infiltrate may be **maternal** or **fetal** in origin. The **maternal component** of the leukocytic reaction originates in the intervillous space and in the maternal vessels of the decidua in the free membranes. The *emigration of leukocytes is always directional, toward the amniotic cavity*, presumably toward an antigenic source in the amniotic fluid. Initially, when organisms first gain access to the uterine cavity, the fetal membranes covering the internal cervical os may show an inflammatory infiltrate (Figure 16.5). This is often accompanied by acute deciduitis (Figure 16.6). This local phenomenon does not indicate an intraamniotic infection is present. *The first evidence that* **true** *intraamniotic infection has occurred is the presence of leukocytes that marginate from beneath the fibrin under the chorionic plate.* As the infection progresses, the leukocytes then infiltrate the chorion and eventually the amnion of the chorionic plate. Abscess formation underneath the chorionic plate and dissemination of exudate between villous trunks are rare events.

After the organism gains access to the amniotic cavity, a fetal response to the infection may occur. Fetal inflammatory *cells migrate from the umbilical vessels and the superficial fetal vessels in the chorionic plate*, constituting a **fetal inflammatory response**. Fetal response is, however, rare before the 20th week of gestation due to immaturity of the fetal immune system. In general, **acute funisitis** occurs first. The

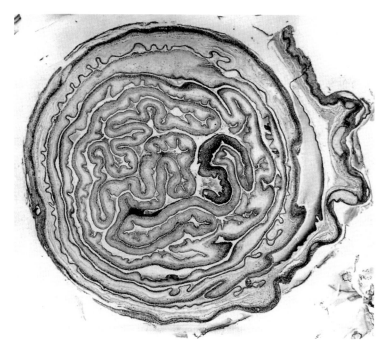

Figure 16.5. Membrane roll of placenta with chorioamnionitis. The edge of the membrane rupture is in the center and shows a dark exudate. H&E. ×12. (From Benirschke and Altshuler, 1971, with permission.)

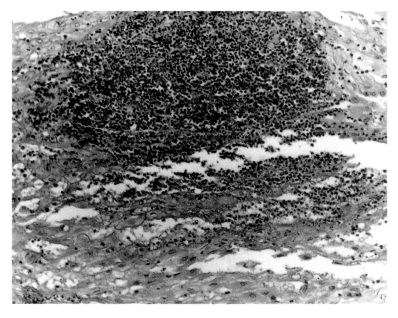

Figure 16.6. Acute deciduitis in an immature placenta with chorioamnionitis. H&E. ×160.

inflammatory cells migrate toward the amnionic surface, marginate first at the vascular intima, *and then begin to dissect among the muscle bundles of the umbilical vein and arteries, finally infiltrating Wharton's jelly* (Figure 16.7). They also reach the cord's surface and may accumulate there in substantial numbers. Funisitis does ***not*** signify the existence of fetal sepsis. Fetal sepsis is a relatively late event in the course of an ascending bacterial infection and often results from invasion of organisms into the fetal lung, intestinal tract, and even the middle ear. *If fetal infection occurs, PMNs can be found in the lung and stomach of the neonate intermixed with squames.* Initially, this pus is likely aspirated from the amniotic fluid and not produced in the fetal lung, as only later in the infectious process can one find an inflammatory accumulation within the alveolar tissue.

In longer-standing infections, **necrotizing funisitis** may occur. Compared to the fetal membranes, the umbilical cord is not able to efficiently remove the chronic accumulation of inflammatory debris. The connective tissue cells of the umbilical cord often then degenerate completely. This results in *exudate being deposited in successive waves, which accumulate in concentric perivascular rings* giving the appearance of Ouchterlony immunodiffusion plates (Figure 16.8). This exudate is more prone to develop mineralization than the exudate of the fetal membranes and thus may become *calcified*. The calcification may reach extraordinary proportions at times, so that the cord cannot be readily clamped at delivery. *Mural thrombosis* may also be present. Necrotizing funisitis is classically associated with congenital syphilis infection (see

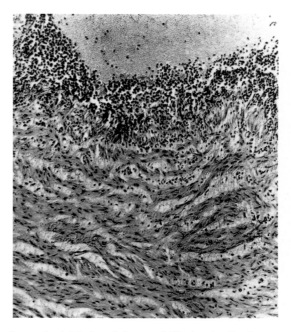

Figure 16.7. Acute funisitis involving umbilical vein. Leukocytes have penetrated between muscle fibers toward the cord surface. H&E. ×260.

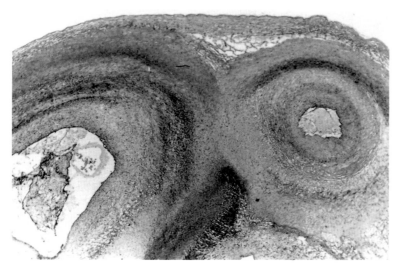

Figure 16.8. Necrotizing funisitis with rings of exudates, some of which are degenerated. H&E. ×40.

below) but is not specific as other organisms, such as *Candida*, streptococci, and other bacteria, have been isolated. **Mural thrombosis in chorionic veins** is also frequently present when the infection has been of longer duration and there is some destruction of the vessel walls through which the neutrophils migrate. The thrombi may be grossly apparent as yellow-white streaks and are usually attached to the intima of the veins, toward the amnionic surface (Figure 16.9).

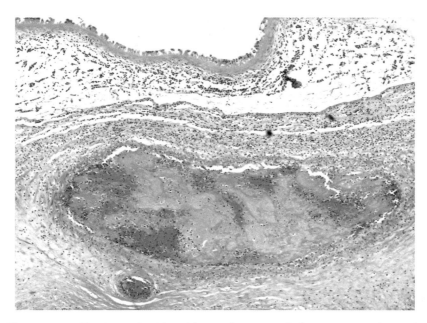

Figure 16.9. Chorioamnionitis with involvement of chorionic vessels. Early mural thrombosis is present at the surface of the vein. H&E. ×20.

Subacute Chorioamnionitis: In the amniotic infection syndrome, the amnionic epithelium may be *degenerated or necrotic*, especially in areas of severe inflammation. If the infection progresses, the PMNs die and the *dead inflammatory cells* may accumulate in large quantities underneath the amnion in the potential space that exists between amnion and chorion. There may be accumulation of *mononuclear cells* as well. This has been referred to as **subacute chorioamnionitis** (Figure 16.10). It occurs in situations where the causative organism is of *low pathogenicity* and does not result in immediate delivery or when there are *repetitive bouts of infection*. Thus, similar to necrotizing funisitis and thrombosis, it is indicative of a longer-standing infection. Like the exudate in the umbilical cord, some of the necrotic exudate underneath the amnion may ultimately calcify, but the fetus usually delivers before this happens. Subacute chorioamnionitis should be distinguished from chronic chorioamnionitis (see below) in which the infiltrate is predominantly mononuclear.

Suggestions for Examination and Report: Acute Chorioamnionitis

Gross Examination: The discoloration and opacity of the fetal surface and membranes should be described. Sections of the membrane roll should include the rupture point of the membranes (furthest from the margin of the placental disc) as this gives the highest yield. If desired, bacterial cultures may be done before examination by lifting the amnion and swabbing between the amnion and chorion. Visible calcifications or thrombi in the umbilical cord should also be noted.

Comment: The diagnosis should include descriptions of the *severity, location, and characterization* of the inflammatory infiltrate. Additional findings of necrosis indicative of *subacute chorioamnionitis*, inflammation-associated *thrombosis of chorionic vessels*, *acute villitis, intervillous abscesses*, and *funisitis* should always be specifically mentioned.

Specific Microorganisms

The organisms most frequently associated with **preterm infants** are *group B Streptococcus, Fusobacterium*, and *Peptostreptococcus*, while the organisms associated with **term infants** are *group B Streptococcus, Fusobacterium, Escherichia coli, Bacteroides*, and *Ureaplasma*. Microorganisms are difficult to identify on histologic sections of infected placentas, and Gram stains are rarely helpful. However, some organisms such as *Listeria, Candida, Fusobacterium*, and some cocci may be visible on careful microscopic examination and with the use of additional special stains (see below). The *pattern of inflammation* is often the most important clue to diagnosis of a specific organism. The most common organ-

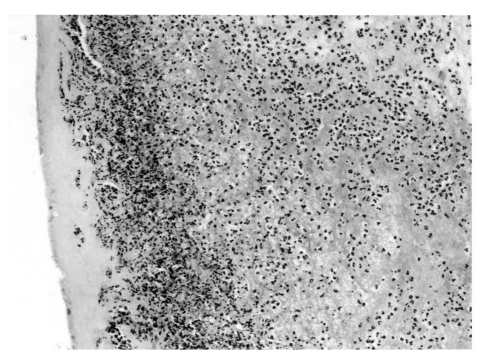

Figure 16.10. Subacute chorioamnionitis with massive infiltration of acute and chronic inflammatory cells and necrosis. H&E. ×60.

isms causing acute chorioamnionitis are discussed in some detail; features of the less common infections are summarized in Table 16.1.

Group B *Streptococcus*

Clinical Features and Implications

Group B streptococci are *gram-positive cocci* that are often, but not always, beta hemolytic. Infections with this organism are frequent, and it is considered one *of the most virulent perinatal infections*. Prematurity and premature rupture of membranes are strongly correlated with group B streptococcal infections. *Sepsis, pneumonia, and meningitis* are common sequelae, and infection is an important cause of *fetal hypoxia, stillbirth, and neonatal death.* A significant number of women will have a positive screen for this organism. Antibiotic treatment does not ensure eradication of the organism throughout pregnancy. Although rapid detection and screening are possible currently using DNA probes, there is no agreement on when to screen for the colonization, or how to respond when positive results are obtained. Recent studies show rapid neonatal and/or intrapartum administration of antibiotics does not prevent neonatal sepsis, nor does it reduce mortality. There is still a great deal of controversy on how and when to treat mothers and infants in this setting.

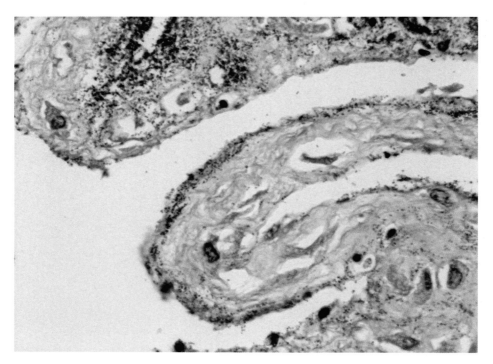

Figure 16.11. Group B streptococcus infection. Note the abundance of bacterial organisms and the minimal associated inflammation. H&E. ×250.

Pathologic Features

Intraamniotic infection with group B *Streptococcus* and even neonatal sepsis may occur *without chorioamnionitis being present*. In fact, there is little to no inflammation in the placentas of 75% of newborns in which the organism has been cultured. This is one of the peculiarities of this organism and is primarily due to host-related factors and the toxins produced by the bacteria that enable its proliferation. This lack of inflammatory response is one of the factors responsible for the virulence of the organism. With careful search, it is often possible to identify the cocci, particularly on the amnion (Figure 16.11). In fact, *the presence of minimal inflammation and readily identifiable cocci in the membranes is almost pathognomonic for group B Streptococcus*. In some cases, focal abscesses may form underneath the amnion, associated with epithelial necrosis and accumulation of bacterial colonies.

Listeriosis

Clinical Features and Implications

Listeriosis is caused by a *gram-positive bacillus*, **Listeria monocytogenes**. The organism is a danger principally to *pregnant women, newborns, and immunocompromised individuals*. In infants, listeriosis is known as **granulomatosis infantiseptica** and is characterized by visible abscesses and a 60% perinatal mortality. *Neonatal meningitis* is another serious complication of fetal infection with this organism. A rash is often present in the neonate, and Gram stains of the skin or gastric aspirates are helpful in identification. The diagnosis is also easily established from cultures. Anti-listeriolysin O titers quickly develop after infection and so may be useful in diagnosis.

Pathogenesis

Listeriosis occurs in a wide variety of mammals and birds, as well as in humans. There is transmission to neonates from mother's milk or as a nosocomial infection in nurseries. Direct contact with infected animals and consumption of certain foods such as *pasteurized milk, certain fresh cheeses, cabbage, poorly cooked sausage and chicken, and pâté.* The organism survives moderate heat and thrives at low temperature so that it grows in refrigerated food. The presence of organisms in the vagina and in stool and the *typically severe chorioamnionitis* suggest that the mode of infection is ascending.

Pathologic Features

Aside from the usual *opacity of the fetal surface and membranes* of the placenta, which is occasionally described as greenish, the typical **intervillous abscesses** may be visible in cross sections of the placenta (Figure 16.12). If smears are done on these lesions, a Gram stain will often reveal the organism. On microscopic examination, one sees *villous*

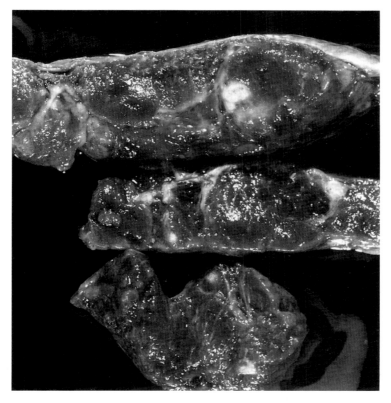

Figure 16.12. Numerous placental abscesses (white nodules) due to *Listeria* infection in a premature infant.

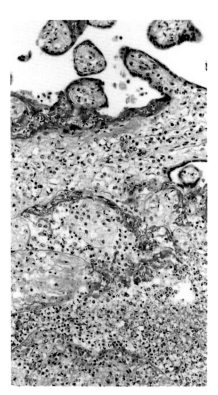

Figure 16.13. *Listeria* abscess in an immature placenta. There is much necrosis of villi, fibrinoid deposition, and infiltration with polymorphonuclear leukocytes (PMNs). Numerous organisms were found on Gram stain. H&E. ×240.

abscesses, villous necrosis, and acute villitis. The abscesses frequently have a central area of necrosis and are usually composed of massive numbers of neutrophils, which surround and infiltrate the villi (Figure 16.13). The villitis may be necrotizing and associated with villous destruction. This pattern may also occur occasionally in maternal septicemias due to *Staphylococcus* and *E. coli,* and uncommonly with other organisms such as *Campylobacter* and *Chlamydia.* Generally, in maternal sepsis the mothers are usually so ill that labor and delivery occur before abscesses develop. The villi are otherwise almost never involved in common cases of chorioamnionitis, however severe that process may be. In the case of *Listeria,* the presence of *placental abscesses* may be due to fetal septicemia, corresponding to similar abscesses in the fetus.

The amnion commonly contains abundant bacterial growth and the *acute chorioamnionitis is usually severe. Acute funisitis* may also be present. Because the *bacteria thrive under low-temperature conditions,* they will often proliferate during cold storage of the placenta before examination. Rapid diagnosis is important because prompt therapy with ampicillin rapidly cures the maternal and fetal infection. When listeriosis is recognized during pregnancy and adequately treated, the *placental abscesses may undergo "scarring."* They are then sometimes still recognizable histologically as a former abscess. The abscesses in the fetus probably have a similar fate.

Escherichia coli

Gram-negative bacilli, in particular ***Escherichia coli***, are a frequent cause of acute chorioamnionitis. They normally colonize the gastrointestinal tract and commonly cause urinary tract infections. There is a strong association with maternal rectal colonization of the organism and subsequent vertical transmission. Infection of the infant may result in *pneumonia, intestinal infection, sepsis, or meningitis.* Neonatal meningitis may occur through the aspiration of amniotic fluid via the middle ear. Uncommonly, acute chorioamnionitis *may be associated with intervillous abscesses and acute villitis.*

Fusobacterium

Fusobacterium necrophorum and ***Fusobacterium nucleatum*** are *pleomorphic, filamentous, gram-negative, anaerobic organisms* that are common causes of acute chorioamnionitis. They normally colonize the mucous membranes or the mouth, intestines, and urogenital tract. It is estimated that as many as 30% of patients with "occult" chorioamnionitis may be infected with *Fusobacterium* species. They are considered an important cause of premature labor. *Acute chorioamnionitis may be severe* but the organisms are often invisible on routine stains and difficult to identify on tissue Gram stains. Bouin's fixative makes their demonstration particularly difficult. *Giemsa* and *Wharthin-Starry stains* may be used for identification of these organisms (Figure 16.14).

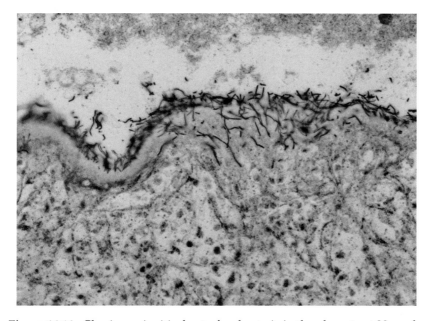

Figure 16.14. Chorioamnionitis due to fusobacteria in the placenta at 23 weeks gestation. The placental surface was opaque. The silver stain shows massive bacterial growth. The dark filaments radiating from the amnionic basement membrane are easily identified as the filamentous organisms. GMS ×240.

Clostridia

Infection with **Clostridium perfringens**, *a gram-positive rod*, occasionally complicates pregnancy. Among anaerobic infections it is particularly feared because it causes postabortal sepsis and uterine gas gangrene, which may be life threatening for the mother. The infection is often quite severe and associated with frequent *abortion and fetal loss*. The placenta may have a *greenish amnionic surface and a putrefactive odor. Purulent exudate* will be present within the membranes and fetal surface, and it may contain *gram-positive rods* (Figure 16.15). Inflammation and necrosis of villous tissue may be found in septic cases. Fetal infection may also occur.

Mycoplasma

Mycoplasma hominis and **Ureaplasma urealyticum** are known urogenital pathogens for humans. *M. hominis* is a known cause of pelvic inflammatory disease and febrile conditions during the postpartum period. *U. urealyticum* is known to cause nongonococcal urethritis in men. The organism attaches itself to spermatozoa and may thus more readily penetrate the endocervical mucous barrier. *U. urealyticum* may be the cause of *repetitive abortions, sterility, and premature birth*. Both organisms are a cause of *neonatal meningitis* and have been associated with *chronic neonatal lung disease*. The organisms may cause *acute chorioamnionitis* similar to that caused by other bacteria. Some villous alterations such as *villous sclerosis, degenerative changes of villous vessels, thrombosis, and villous edema* have been reported. Study of these organ-

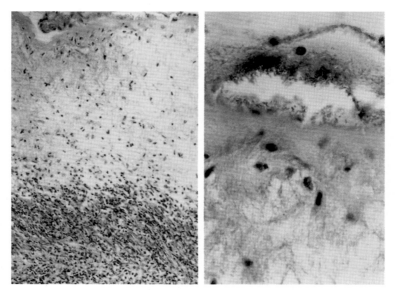

Figure 16.15. Clostridial chorioamnionitis at term. There was intensive deciduitis and chorionitis. Note the pocket of gram-positive rods underneath the amnion. H&E. ×640.

isms is hampered by our current inability to demonstrate the organism in tissue sections and their specific culture requirements.

Chlamydia

Chlamydia trachomatis is responsible for the most common sexually transmitted disease in the United States. C. trachomatis also causes *trachoma, lymphogranuloma venereum*, and *nongonococcal urethritis in men* and *mucopurulent cervicitis, chronic salpingitis*, and *sterility in women*. It is estimated that between 10% and 20% of sexually active men and women are infected with this organism. Approximately one-half of infants born to infected mothers develop *ophthalmia neonatorum ("inclusion body blennorrhoea")* and others develop *pneumonitis*. Approximately 3% to 4% of all neonates have ophthalmia and 1% to 2% have pneumonitis from infection with this organism. This organism has not been isolated from the placenta and thus has not been conclusively demonstrated to be a direct cause of acute chorioamnionitis, but it *has* been found in the amniotic fluid, and in the eye and nasopharynx of neonates. The *bacterium-like intracellular microbe* can be visualized in the cytoplasm of infected cells by *direct immunofluorescence*. The infection can also be diagnosed by culture, by immunoperoxidase, and by polymerase chain reaction (PCR) amplification.

   Chlamydia psittaci infection is rarely recognized as a cause of human abortion although it commonly causes abortions in sheep and other domestic species. Sheep farmers and their wives have a high exposure to this pathogen, and abortion has been described in this population. When abortion ensures, it is then associated with *acute intervillositis, villous necrosis*, and *inclusions in syncytiotrophoblast*. Electron microscopy and immunofluorescence have confirmed the presence of the organism.

Bacterial Vaginosis

Bacterial vaginosis has been defined as the *"replacement of the lactobacilli of the vagina by characteristic groups of bacteria accompanied by changed properties of the vaginal fluid."* The bacterial species include *Bacteroides, Gardnerella vaginalis, Mycoplasma hominis, Ureaplasma urealyticum*, and perhaps others. A relationship to premature rupture of membranes, preterm birth, and amniotic sac infection has been reported to exist.

Candida Species

Clinical Features and Implications
Vaginal infection with **Candida albicans** is common during pregnancy, and it is estimated that 26% of women harbor these organisms. Neonatal candidiasis can be traced to maternal vaginal infection in most cases and may manifest as *skin rash, dark red skin discoloration, pneumonia, meningitis, sepsis, and intestinal contamination*. Although infection may cause neonatal demise, successful treatment has been reported. *Candida* infection has also been associated with abortions. Although C. albicans

is the most common candidal organism, infection with *C. parapsilosis*, a common skin inhabitant, has also been reported, as has infection with *C. tropicalis*.

Pathologic Features

Prenatal infection of the placenta, cord, and fetus may be associated with severe acute chorioamnionitis but *typically involves only the umbilical cord*. Grossly, *the umbilical cord shows numerous tiny, round, white or yellow plaques* (Figure 16.16). Histologically, the nodules consist of *focal infiltrates of acute inflammatory cells underneath areas of epithelial necrosis* in the periphery of the umbilical cord (Figure 16.17 A). *Fungal pseudohyphae and yeast forms* are readily demonstrated with silver stains but are quite difficult to identify in routine preparations (Figure 16.17 B). Villous lesions are rarely identified, but when they occur consist of *focal necrosis, chronic villitis, and intervillous abscesses*.

Suggestions for Examination and Report: Specific Infections Causing Acute Chorioamnionitis

Gross Examination: There are no gross techniques or sections to submit to identify specific organisms except in the case of *Candida*. Extra sections of cord are suggested in this case.

Comment: Use of special stains for microorganisms is not generally helpful, but if the pattern of inflammation is suggestive of a particular organism, such as group B *Streptococcus*, *Candida*, *Fusobacterium*, or *Listeria*, special stains may be useful.

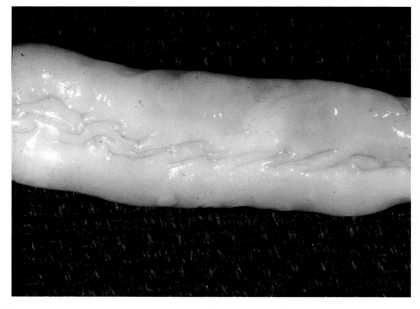

Figure 16.16. Congenital candidiasis showing numerous small white plaques, representing abscesses.

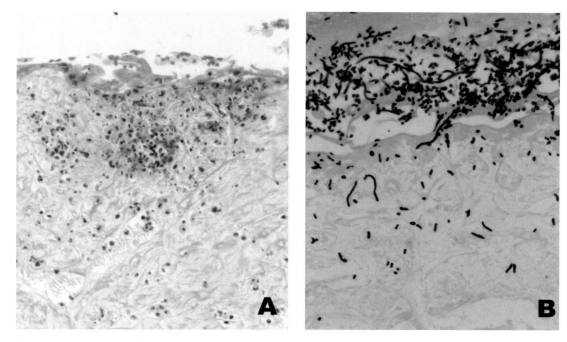

Figure 16.17. (A) Candidiasis of umbilical cord. There are accumulations of inflammatory cells, debris, and organisms associated with epithelial necrosis. H&E. ×200. (B) Gomori methenamine-silver (GMS) stain showing pseudohyphae and yeast forms. GMS ×200.

Chronic Villitis

Chronic villitis is defined by a *chronic inflammatory infiltrate in the chorionic villi*. Chronic villitides are divided into two general groups, those of *infectious* etiology and those of *unknown* etiology (**villitis of unknown etiology or VUE**). In infectious villitides, maternal infections are transmitted *hematogenously* and *transplacentally* from the mother to fetus. Causative organisms include the TORCH infections: *Toxoplasma gondii*, rubella virus, cytomegalovirus, herpes simplex virus, hepatitis, and human immunodeficiency virus (HIV). However, many other organisms such as spirochetes, parasites, and other viruses are implicated. Close to 90% of infectious villitides are due to cytomegalovirus and syphilis. Selected infections are covered in some detail, while features of the remaining organisms are summarized in Table 16.2.

Syphilis

Pathogenesis
Infection with **Treponema pallidum** may occur at any time during pregnancy. The organism may pass to the fetus via the placenta during all stages of maternal syphilis infection. Most frequently, disseminated infection in the neonate arises from *hematogenous spread of the spirochetes between the first and second stages of infection of the mother*. Spirochetes can

be demonstrated by immunofluorescence and electron microscopy in fetuses as early as 9 to 10 weeks gestation. Expression of the disease's pathologic features depends on the fetus's ability to produce antibody to spirochetal antigen. Therefore, because young fetuses cannot mount a proper antibody response, the histopathologic changes cannot be seen in early infection.

Pathologic Features

The more severely the fetus is affected, the greater are the pathologic changes in the placenta. The placenta usually shows an *increase in weight*, which may be quite impressive. Placentas up to 2500 have been reported. Microcopically, *the villi tend to be "bulky" and enlarged.* Classically there is *endothelial and fibroblastic proliferation and chronic villitis with prominent plasma cells* (Figures 16.18, 16.19). The decidua also may show plasma cell infiltration with necrosis and perivascular fibroblastic proliferation (Figure 16.20). Chronic chorioamnionitis is uncommonly present. Abscesses or villous necrosis is seen in severe infections, but gummas or granulomas have never been reported in the placenta. *Necrotizing funisitis* may also be present (Figures 16.21, 16.22), which is a classic finding in syphilitic infection but is not considered pathognomonic as was previously thought.

Cytomegalovirus Infection

Clinical Features and Implications

Congenital **cytomegalovirus (CMV)** infection is a common disease, with 3000 to 4000 infected infants born in the United States each year. From 1.6% to 3.7% of seronegative women convert to seropositivity for CMV during pregnancy. The rate of transmission to the fetus after

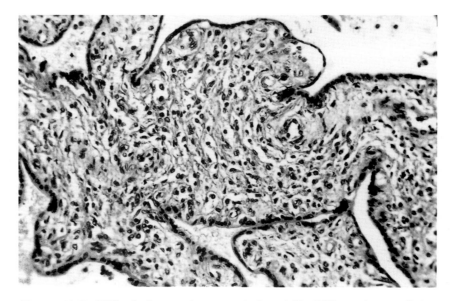

Figure 16.18. Villi of placenta in congenital syphilis. Villi are hypercellular, infiltrated with mononuclear cells. Note the focal necrosis and vascular obliteration. H&E. ×240.

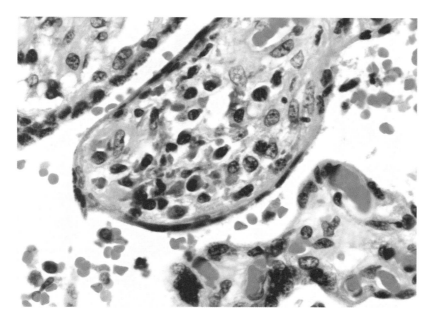

Figure 16.19. Plasma cell infiltration of chorionic villi in congenital syphilis. H&E. ×240.

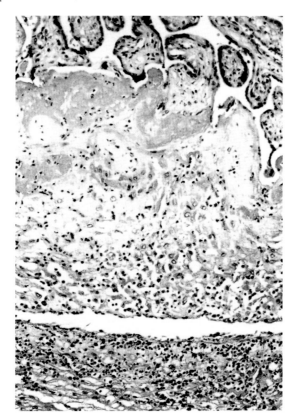

Figure 16.20. Chronic deciduitis of decidua basalis in an immature infant afflicted with typical congenital syphilis. The placenta was large (580 g). H&E. ×160.

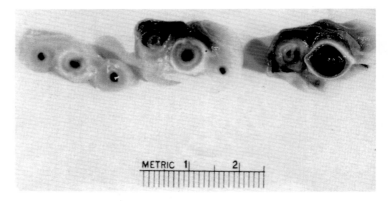

Figure 16.21. Concentric rings of perivascular exudate in necrotizing funisitis.

recent maternal infection is between 20% and 50%. Fetal infection is more serious when it occurs during a primary maternal infection than when it follows recurrent maternal disease and when it occurs during the first half of pregnancy. Fetal and neonatal infections have many manifestations, including *hearing loss, blindness, hydrops fetalis, obstructive uropathy, meconium peritonitis, growth restriction, hydrocephaly, stillbirth, and cerebral palsy.* The *hallmark of fetal infection is intracranial calcifications* and *perivascular echogenic signals in the basal ganglia*, both of which may be identified on ultrasound examination. Some of these manifestations may be ascertained only years later. Neonates with this infection may excrete virus for years and may become a major source for infection of pregnant mothers and toddlers in day care centers.

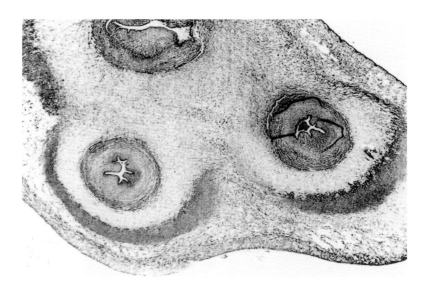

Figure 16.22. Necrotizing funisitis. The exudate is concentrically deposited around the vessels; the exudate is necrotic and beginning to calcify. A mural thrombus is present in the umbilical vein. von Gieson. ×12.

Pathogenesis

The virus is *often acquired by sexual contact.* Fetal infection is undoubtedly most often acquired during primary maternal infection from *maternal viremia and by the passage of virions through the trophoblast, which it infects and destroys.* Congenital infection is also *occasionally acquired from infected endometrium,* and CMV inclusions in endometrial glands have been demonstrated in abortion specimens.

Pathologic Features

The histologic hallmarks of CMV infection in the placenta are *chronic lymphoplasmacytic villitis* (Figure 16.23) with *inclusion-bearing cytomegalic cells.* The chronic villitis typically causes bulky enlargement of the chorionic villi. The inclusion bodies may be the typical nuclear "owl-eye cells," but cytoplasmic inclusions are also commonly seen (Figure 16.24). *Inclusions may be seen in villous capillary endothelium, villous stromal cells, the amnion, and even the decidua.* Vasculitis of chorionic vessels may occur leading to thrombosis and calcification in long-standing cases and leads to *hemosiderin deposits* in the adjacent stroma. Necrosis of villous tissue and trophoblast and villous fibrosis may also be present. The villitis is commonly *multifocal* with small foci widely scattered through the villous tissue. Thus, extreme scrutiny of many sections may be necessary to make the diagnosis from tissue sections.

When typical inclusions are not present, CMV can be detected by immunohistochemistry and in situ hybridization, which are both more sensitive than routine histology. Positivity in these cases is found to be mostly in the *villous stroma,* but also in *syncytiotrophoblast* and *endothelial cells.* Serologic studies, virus isolation, or PCR may also be used. However, even without typical inclusions, the presence of *plasma cells and hemosiderin deposition are virtually pathognomonic of CMV infection.*

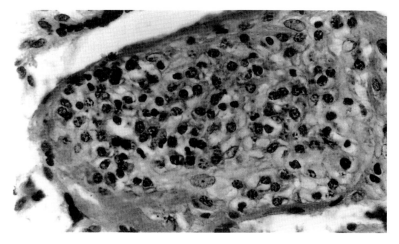

Figure 16.23. Congenital cytomegalovirus infection. Marked chronic villitis, composed almost entirely of plasma cells, is evident, as is focal necrosis of the trophoblast and capillary walls. H&E. ×650.

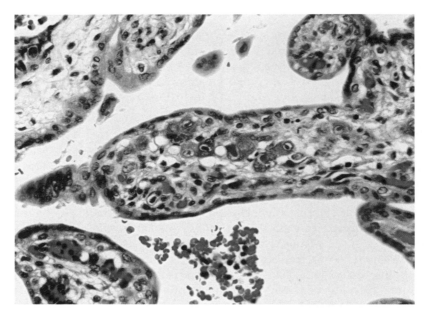

Figure 16.24. Owl-eye nuclear inclusion of a cytomegalic cell in the villus of a patient with cytomegalovirus (CMV) infection. This cell also contains many cytoplasmic inclusions. H&E. ×200.

Herpes Simplex Virus

Pathogenesis

The differences in severity and types of placental and fetal reactions in prenatal herpes infection suggest that *both transplacental and ascending infection* occur. *Herpetic endometritis* has been demonstrated, which is suggestive of direct spread as well. Infection with **herpes simplex virus (HSV)** occurs only occasionally, and this is likely due to the protective nature of transplacentally acquired maternal antibodies. The latter are common, and it is estimated that 16.4% of the U.S. population from 15 to 74 years of age has been infected with HSV-2. In addition, HSV is "silently" shed by 2.3% of pregnant women.

Pathologic Features

The placenta is usually *grossly unremarkable*. There is a *lymphoplasmacellular infiltrate* within the villous stroma. The characteristic *inclusion bodies and "ground-glass nuclei"* are diagnostic of a herpetic infection. The chronic villitis may be extensive or may be associated with necrosis. *Necrotizing deciduitis, amnion necrosis, chorionic vasculitis,* and *funisitis* may be present. *Necrotizing chorioamnionitis* with true "blisters," plasma cells, and inclusions bodies has also been described (Figure 16.25).

Clinical Features and Implications

Congenital herpes infection may develop without maternal illness or the presence of herpetic lesions. When infection occurs during the first

4 months of pregnancy, abortion is common, as is *stillbirth* in later gestation. At autopsy *ocular, renal,* and *cerebral anomalies* may be found including *massive destructive of the brain, resembling hydranencephaly.* Calcifications in fetal organs have also been described.

Parvovirus B19

Clinical Features and Implications

Infection with this highly contagious virus is an important cause of *second trimester abortion and hydrops fetalis.* Approximately 40% to 60% of adults have IgG antibodies from previous infection. The mother is asymptomatic in up to 75% of cases but may still transmit the virus to her fetus. Viral transmission from mother to fetus occurs in approximately 25% to 33% of women with acute infection during pregnancy and serious fetal disease occurs in 9% of these cases. Fetal infection is typically associated with *anemia,* and in some cases *hydrops* due to the predilection of the virus for erythrocyte precursors. It is estimated that

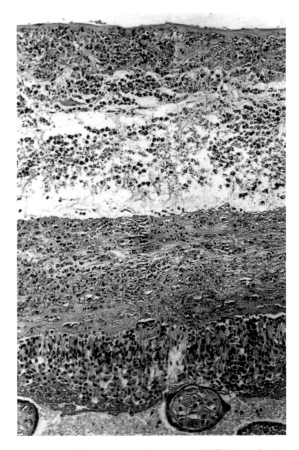

Figure 16.25. Congenital herpes simplex virus (HSV)-2 infection resulting in stillbirth. Note the subamnionic blister filled with plasma cells. The amnion and chorion are necrotic. H&E. ×160.

16% to 18% of fetal hydrops may be caused by infection with this organism. Although intrauterine transfusion therapy has been shown to be beneficial, recovery from this infection has also been witnessed without therapy. *Myocarditis and ocular anomalies* have also been described.

Pathologic Features

Macroscopically, the placenta is enlarged and, when fetal hydrops is present, is *pale, friable, and edematous.* Infection can usually be diagnosed by the *typical ground-glass inclusion bodies of nucleated red blood cells* it produces. The intranuclear inclusions are lightly stained and eosinophilic and are composed of crystals of the small, 20-nm virus particles. The infected cells are called **"lantern cells" because** they resemble Chinese lanterns (Figure 16.26). The inclusions are present in circulating normoblasts, in nucleated red blood cells, and in their precursors in fetal organs and the placenta. Chronic villitis may be present, and in this case the villi may be large and bulky. Additional findings include hemosiderin in chorionic macrophages, *villous destruction, necrosis, endothelial damage, and perivascular lymphocytic infiltrate.*

Many methods are available to identify the organism. Immunohistochemistry, DNA hybridization studies, and electron microscopy

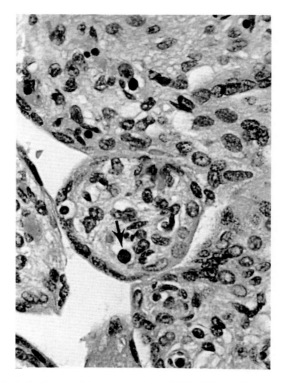

Figure 16.26. Infection with parvovirus B19. Normoblastic nuclei have smudged intranuclear inclusion bodies (arrow). H&E. ×240.

can demonstrate parvovirus in the placenta, and a rapid and sensitive PCR test for detection of the antigen has been developed for use on fetal blood and amniotic fluid. Serologic detection of the B19 antigen is also now widely available. As is true in many infections, elevated IgG titers in maternal blood denote former infection whereas an elevated IgM titer diagnoses recent or active disease.

Mycobacteria

Leprosy, caused by *Mycobacterium leprae*, is now an uncommon disease in the United States. Vertical transmission from mother to infant is either uncommon or does not occur. However, abortion has been associated with isolation of the organisms from the placenta and cord blood. Documented cases show *granulomatous lepromatous lesions in the chorionic villi* and *a few acid-fast bacilli*. The placentas tend to be relatively small. *Acid-fast organisms have been found in decidua, trophoblast,* and *villous stroma.*

In contrast to leprosy, congenital infection with *Mycobacterium tuberculosis* has been repeatedly demonstrated to occur. In fetal infection, *caseating granulomas in the lungs and acid-fast bacilli in the liver, spleen, and kidneys* are found. There may be difficulty in distinguishing transplacentally acquired tuberculosis from infection transmitted by inhalation of infected amniotic fluid and from neonatal disease acquired nosocomially. The placenta may be *grossly normal* or *may contain firm, white plaques*. Microscopically, typical but rare *granulomas with giant cells* in the chorionic villi or intervillous space may be seen. *The bacilli may be found in fetal vessels, intervillous fibrin, septa, or villous stroma.* Special stains for acid-fast bacilli will assist in identification of the rare organism. In some cases, congenital infection is present but the placenta is unaffected. *The decidua may contain areas of extensive necrosis and the placental floor may also contain granulomas.* Occasionally, acute granulomas occur, consisting of neutrophils in the intervillous space causing local villous destruction. In other cases, one may find isolated giant cells in the stem villi but no inflammation.

Toxoplasmosis

Pathogenesis
The *coccidian Toxoplasma gondii* is a pan-global parasite of cats, other felids, and many domestic animals. In infected cats, oocysts are shed in the stools. Rodents and other animals then ingest the oocysts and acquire the disease. Cats, preying on infected rodents, complete the life cycle. In humans, infection is acquired by two means: contamination with oocysts from feces of infected cats and ingestion of oocysts and tachyzoites in raw, infected meat, largely pork and mutton. Pregnant women are advised not to eat *undercooked or raw meat,* and should avoid having *contact with "wild" cats*. Cats raised solely on commercial diets are not infected. Emptying the litter box daily to prevent drying and dust-producing feces is recommended, but is best done by another member of the household.

It is generally assumed that almost all congenital *Toxoplasma* infections develop from a *primary infection* during pregnancy. Large prospective studies of toxoplasmosis in pregnancy have shown that in women with primary infection during pregnancy, 45% of the infants develop congenital toxoplasmosis. The rate of infection increases with gestation, and is 17%, 25%, and 65% in the first, second, and third trimesters, respectively. Fetal sequelae are the most severe when infection develops early in gestation.

Clinical Features and Implications

Transplacental toxoplasmosis can cause severe disease in the offspring. *Hydrops* and *hepatosplenomegaly* are common in infected neonates and *chorioretinitis, encephalitis, hydrocephaly,* or other organ involvement may cause crippling disease. Late onset of symptomatology is seen in children with congenital toxoplasmosis, and new lesions continue to appear well after the age of 5 years.

Pathologic Features

Placental infection with *Toxoplasma* is presumably produced by organisms circulating in the maternal blood, although the isolation of cysts from endometrium in chronic aborters makes direct infection from the endometrium possible. *Cysts are often present in the subamnionic/chorionic tissues* (Figure 16.27) unaccompanied by inflammation. They

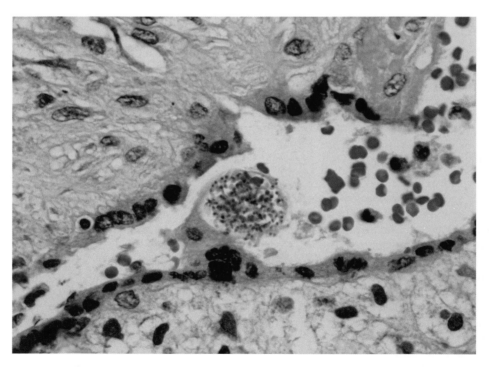

Figure 16.27. *Toxoplasma* cysts in syncytium in a child with congenital infection. H&E. ×240. (Courtesy of Dr. J. Hustin Loverval, Belgium.)

also may be identified in chorionic villi, trophoblast, or the umbilical cord. The villi show an *increase in Hofbauer cells, vascular proliferation, and an increase in circulating fetal normoblasts. Lymphocytic-plasmacellular villitis* is seen in only when cysts rupture and may be associated with *villous necrosis. Granulomatous villitis* has been described. *Thrombosis of chorionic or umbilical vessels* may occur, and the thrombi may become calcified. Identification is difficult in histologic sections and positive identification may require PCR, immunohistochemistry, fluorescence antibody technique, or electron microscopy. Without these techniques tachyzoites cannot be recognized with certainty. Handling and culturing this organism is often avoided because of the hazards of infection.

Malaria

Pathogenesis
Malaria, which is an infection with one of the four species of **Plasmodia**, is the most common infectious disease in the world. True congenital infection has been described only rarely, and the mechanism of fetal/neonatal infection is still uncertain. Although transplacental infection most likely occurs during delivery, some severely infected patients have died undelivered with an infected fetus still in utero. There is no agreement as to whether the organisms cross the placenta into the fetal circulation. It seems likely that the plasmodium does not cross by itself. When transplacental infection occurs, the parasites are probably transferred within red blood cells. Maternal to fetal transfer of red blood cells occurs, but is rare.

Clinical Features and Implications
Pregnancy substantially increases the severity of malaria in the mother and is associated with *premature births, low birth weight, and decreased placental weight*. Perhaps because of transferred immunity, symptomatic disease in the neonate is virtually never recognized at birth. It becomes evident only after several weeks.

Pathologic Features
On occasion the placenta has been described as *"diagnostically black at parturition"* owing to malarial pigment. In most cases, however, there is no macroscopic abnormality. Histologic studies of the placenta reveal *malaria-infected erythrocytes in the intervillous space* in 40% of cases, and an additional 35% of cases show evidence of malarial pigment without the presence of organisms (Figure 16.28). The *pigment*, which is a breakdown product of hemoglobin, may be present in *fibrinoid, macrophages, or free in the intervillous space.* Chronic intervillositis with accumulation of macrophages in the intervillous space is present to at least some degree in the majority of cases, and *massive chronic intervillositis* (see below) is seen in about 6% of cases. There may be a necrotizing villitis as well. An increased *amount of intervillous fibrinoid* and *thickening of the trophoblastic basement membrane* is often seen. Placentas may rarely have infarcts, abruptions, or fetal vascular thrombosis.

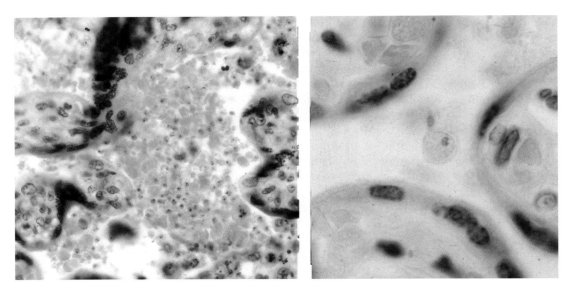

Figure 16.28. Malaria infection with presence of pigment and malarial organisms within the intervillous space. An intracellular organism is present in the right figure. H&E. Left ×200; right ×400.

> *Suggestions for Examination and Report: Specific Infections Causing Chronic Villitis*
>
> **Gross Examination:** If abnormalities in villous tissue are noted, or infection is suspected, additional section of villous tissue should be submitted.
>
> **Comment:** If the pattern of the villitis is consistent with a particular organism, based on the clinical history, one may do additional studies. With some organisms, such as CMV, definitive diagnosis of the organism can be made on histology alone or with the aid of immunohistochemistry. Specific infections in the differential diagnosis generally can not be ruled out on the basis of lack of pathologic findings.

Villitis of Unknown Etiology

Pathogenesis

Chronic villitis is frequent, occurring in 5% to 10% of all placentas. When placentas of complicated pregnancies, growth-restricted infants, and fetal deaths are studied, the incidence is much higher, up to 34%. At times, the infectious etiology of chronic villitis is apparent from the history or the pathologic features. In the majority of cases, however, despite much effort, no specific etiology is elicited, and then the term **villitis of unknown etiology (VUE)** is used. VUE is now a well-recognized entity but remains a significant challenge because of its frequency, high recurrence rate, and the associated poor outcome.

Two principal suggestions have been made with respect to the etiology of VUE. First, it is suggested that VUE is an *infectious disease* caused by a yet unrecognized agent or an agent that cannot be identified from placental examination. There is great histologic similarity of VUE to other known virus disorders that affect the placenta, and some common viruses are extremely difficult to recognize histologically or by electron microscopy (EM). They also may cause few symptoms in the mother and may not be detected. The second theory is that VUE is an immune reaction akin to placental *"rejection" or graft-versus-host disease*. This is supported by the histiocytic predominance of the inflammatory reaction, its frequent location in an area of maternal–fetal tissue interaction, its frequent recurrence, and its tendency to recur in families. Furthermore, 60% of the infiltrating immunocytes of VUE are maternal CD3-positive T cells from the intervillous space. An immunologic pathogenesis of VUE with maternal cells infiltrating the villi has long been championed. Whether this is tantamount to immune "rejection" mounted by the mother against the placenta needs further investigation. At this time, the only certain conclusion is that VUE is **not** the result of infection with common, known pathogens as no virus or other agent has been consistently identified.

Pathologic Features

Macroscopically the placentas of VUE have been described as *stiff*. The placentas are occasionally *smaller*, particularly in growth-restricted fetuses. If areas of villitis are large and associated with necrosis, the *villous tissue may appear mottled* (Figure 16.29). The mottling is a subtle finding and is only present when villitis is extensive. There are no specific changes that allow definitive macroscopic identification.

Microscopically, lesions have a wide spectrum, from focal to extensive involvement wherein virtually all villi have some pathologic reaction. The villitis is characterized by *infiltration primarily of histiocytes* with lesser numbers of *lymphocytes*. The chronic villitis may be *necrotizing* with *villous destruction* and secondary changes of *ischemia, infarction, fetal vascular thrombosis*, and *avascular villi* (Figures 16.30, 16.31). VUE is especially *frequent in the basal villi* in the maternal floor of the placenta. Associated findings in VUE include *villous dysmaturity, an increase in nucleated red blood cells, hemosiderin deposition*, and *chorangiosis*. All or none of these abnormalities may be found.

The similarity to known infectious causes of villitis, such as seen with CMV and rubella, is striking. However, VUE tends to be *more multifocal, is much less commonly associated with plasma cell infiltration, and tends to be concentrated in the basal plate*. There is, however, much overlap. One should also note that degenerative lesions simulating VUE occur peripheral to infarcts, and these should not be confused with typical VUE as discussed here.

Clinical Features and Implications

There is little doubt that VUE is able to eliminate a considerable amount of placental parenchyma from nutrient transfer. Therefore, the presence

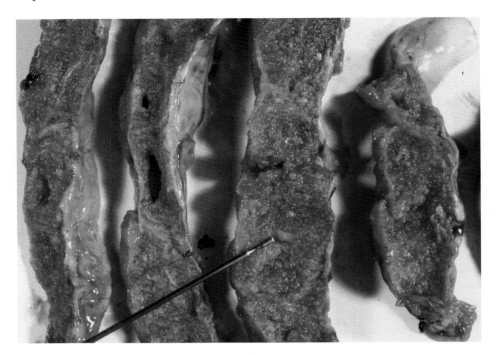

Figure 16.29. Placenta with diffuse villitis of unknown etiology (VUE). Note the mottling of the villous tissue. The probe indicates one area of subtle white discoloration which represents villitis and associated villous destruction.

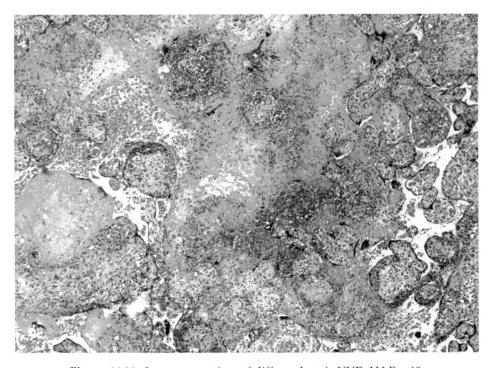

Figure 16.30. Low-power view of diffuse chronic VUE. H&E. ×40.

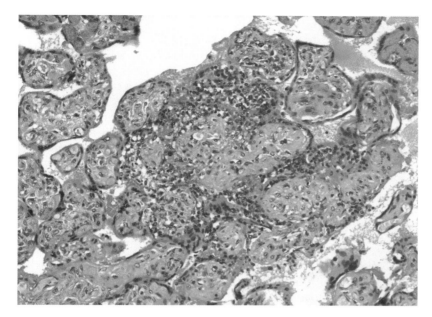

Figure 16.31. VUE with intense infiltration with lymphocytes and histiocytes. The vessels are obliterated. H&E. ×240.

of *fetal growth restriction* in as many as 33% of cases is not surprising. One must emphasize, however, that there is no absolute relationship between the severity of VUE and the severity of fetal growth retardation. VUE is also associated with *recurrent abortions*, *prematurity*, *abnormal neurologic development*, and *intrauterine fetal demise*. Of great interest is the frequently recurrent nature of this lesion with recurrence rates of 10% to 25%. Furthermore, the reproductive loss is 60% in patients with recurrent villitis in contrast to a 37% loss in nonrecurrent villitis. Recurrent VUE is also more often associated with autoimmune disease in the mother.

Suggestions for Examination and Report:
Villitis of Unknown Etiology

Gross Examination: If mottling of the villous tissue is identified, or there is a history of infection, growth restriction, or fetal demise, at least several additional sections of villous parenchyma should be submitted.

Comment: The diagnosis is consistent with VUE if the pattern is typical and there is no evidence of infectious etiology. Infectious etiologies generally cannot be ruled out.

Chronic Chorioamnionitis

Chronic chorioamnionitis is a recently described lesion in which the *inflammatory infiltrate in the fetal membranes consists predominantly of a mononuclear cells, lymphocytes and histiocytes* rather than acute inflammatory cells (Figure 16.32). The diagnosis should not be made if scattered chronic inflammatory cells in the membranes or greater numbers in the decidua are present. Chronic chorioamnionitis is found in association with VUE in approximately 79% of cases. Thus, its identification should alert the examiner to search for foci of chronic villitis. Clinically, chronic chorioamnionitis has been associated with *maternal hypertension, diabetes, fetal hydrops, growth restriction*, and *oligohydramnios*. If a mixed acute and chronic inflammatory infiltrate is present, subacute chorioamnionitis is likely present (see above).

Suggestions for Examination and Report:
Chronic Chorioamnionitis

Gross Examination: Chronic chorioamnionitis cannot be appreciated on gross examination.

Comment: Chronic chorioamnionitis may be associated with chronic villitis and adverse perinatal outcome.

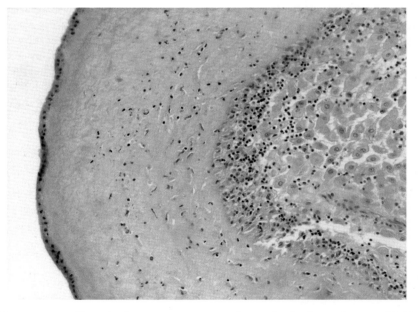

Figure 16.32. Chronic chorioamnionitis involving the fetal membranes. H&E. ×100.

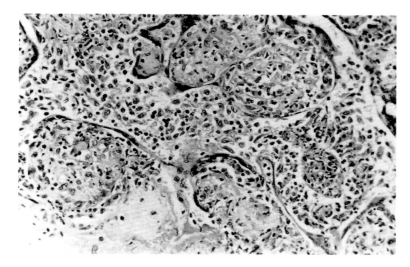

Figure 16.33. Severe chronic intervillositis associated with chronic villitis consisting of infiltrates of lymphocytes and histiocytes. H&E. ×250.

Chronic Intervillositis

Chronic intervillositis is an infiltrate of *mononuclear cells in the intervillous space* (Figure 16.33). The cells are predominantly CD68-positive macrophages, but lesser numbers of lymphocytes are also present. There is a *variable amount of intervillous fibrinoid deposition* as well, sometimes containing extravillous trophoblastic cells. This entity has most commonly been described in *recurrent abortion* specimens but also occurs in the second and third trimester where it is associated with *fetal growth restriction* and *intrauterine demise. Chronic villitis* is often also seen in association with chronic intervillositis. Because the macrophages are of maternal origin, it has been suggested that the etiology of the associated reproductive problems is of immunologic origin.

Suggestions for Examination and Report:
Chronic Intervillositis

Gross Examination: Chronic intervillositis is generally not recognized grossly.

Comment: Chronic intervillositis may be associated with recurrent abortion, fetal loss, or fetal growth restriction.

Table 16.1. Miscellaneous bacteria in ascending infection

Bacteria	Morphology and type	Pathologic features	Potential clinical sequelae	Other
Actinomyces	GP filamentous anaerobe	Foul-smelling placenta Severe ACA may be necrotizing Identifiable organisms	Preterm labor	May show massive invasion by organism
Bacteroides fragilis	GN anaerobe	ACA	Prenatal meningitis	Other neonatal infections described
Campylobacter	GN aerobe	ACA Villous necrosis Acute villitis	Recurrent abortions Fetal death	Common enteric pathogen
Corynebacteria	GP diphtheroids	ACA and AF gray-brown plaques on placental surface with invading organisms	Sepsis not described	Normal vaginal flora Occasional infection
Coxiella burnetii (Q fever)	GN obligate intracellular	Severe necrotizing villitis	Congenital infection Fetal death	Rare zoonosis Organisms may be identified in placenta
Ehrlichiosis	GN obligate intracellular	No lesions	Neonatal infection (of granulocytes)	Probable transplacental infection
Gardnerella	G variable	Occasionally mild ACA	Preterm delivery, fetal demise (rarely)	Common vaginal organism
Group A streptococcus (*S. pneumoniae, Enterococcus*)	GPC	ACA	Pneumonia	Common
Haemophilus influenzae	GNR	ACA	Preterm delivery, pneumonia Sepsis	Uncommon May mimic group B *Streptococcus* infection
Neisseria gonorrhoeae	GN diplococcus	ACA associated with cervical infection	Sepsis Ophthalmia neonatorum	
Rickettsia	GN obligate intracellular	No lesions	Full recovery	Very rare
Salmonella	GNR	ACA	Meningitis Pneumonia Fetal demise	Mothers are symptomatic or carriers
Shigella	GNR	ACA	Sepsis Enterocolitis	Uncommon
Staphylococcus	GPC	Severe ACA	Neonatal sepsis	
Streptobacillus	GNR	ACA		Causes "rat bite fever" or Haverhill fever

G, Gram; P, positive; N, negative; C, cocci; R, rods; ACA, acute chorioamnionitis; AF, acute funisitis.

Table 16.2. Miscellaneous organisms causing villitis

Organism	Category	Pathologic features	Potential clinical sequelae	Other
Blastomyces	Fungus	Granulomas Chronic villitis	No neonatal infection reported	
Borrelia (relapsing fever)	Spirochete	No lesions	Found in neonatal and placental blood	Follows bite of infected tick Geographically widespread
Borrelia burgdorfer	Spirochete	Rare plasma cells	Stillbirth	
Lyme disease (erythema migrans)		Increased nucleated red blood cells	Congenital anomalies	
Coccidioides immitis	Fungus	Fungal spherules Acute inflammatory response Fibrinoid deposition and necrosis Infarction and necrosis		
Cryptococcus	Fungus	Colonies of organisms in intervillous space Scant inflammation No villous invasion	Cryptococcosis or meningitis in mother Infants not affected	Associated with lupus and immunodeficiency
Leptospira	Spirochete	No lesions	Abortion	Rare
Coxsackie B	Virus	Villous necrosis Severe intervillositis	Fetal hydrops Myocarditis Meningitis	Rare fetal infection May not show placental lesions
ECHO	Virus	Chronic villitis Chronic intervillositis Mural thrombosis	Congenital infection	Rare
Epstein-Barr Virus	Virus	Deciduitis Lymphoplasmacytic villitis Trophoblastic necrosis Endothelial damage	Early abortion Congenital anomalies (rare)	Uncommon
Hepatitis	Virus	Yellow-green discoloration of placenta Bilirubin in Hofbauer cells and chorionic macrophages Relative villous immaturity Focal syncytial necrosis	Abortion Fetal ascites Meconium peritonitis	Usually hepatitis B
Human immunodeficiency virus	Virus	No lesions	Prematurity Endometritis	Transmission rate to fetus 24%
Influenza	Virus	No lesions		Transplacental infection occurs

(Continued)

Table 16.2. *Continued*

Organism	Category	Pathologic features	Potential clinical sequelae	Other
Mumps	Virus	Severe villous necrosis Small cytoplasmic inclusion bodies in decidua	Possible congenital anomalies	Virus isolated from placenta
Poliomyelitis	Virus	No lesions		Virus isolated from the placenta
Rubella	Virus	Endothelial damage in villi Obliteration of stem vessels Focal trophoblastic necrosis Villous inflammation and sclerosis Swollen Hofbauer cells (in early infection)	Congenital anomalies in early infection	
Robeola	Virus	Not described	Not teratogenic Fetal mortality	Rare
Smallpox	Virus	Villous, membrane, and trophoblastic necrosis Intervillous fibrinoid deposits Calcification	Fetal demise Early abortion	May occur with primary vaccination
Varicella	Virus	Chronic villitis Occasional multinucleated giant cells Rare granulomas Remote infection— occluded stem vessels	Cutaneous scars Limb hypoplasia Chorioretinitis Cataracts Hydrops Visceral calcifications	
Babesia microti	Protozoa	No lesions	Infection of neonatal red blood cells	Very rare
Leishmania major	Protozoa	Thrombosis of villous vessels Amastigotes within and outside macrophages Trophoblastic degeneration No inflammation		Occasional congenital infection
Trichomonas vaginalis	Protozoa	No specific lesions	Preterm delivery Low birth weight Neonatal infection Pneumonia	Rare

Table 16.2. *Continued*

Organism	Category	Pathologic features	Potential clinical sequelae	Other
Trypanosoma cruzi	Protozoa	Enlarged, pale placenta, Chronic destructive villitis Chronic intervillositis Amnionic epithelium, Hofbauer cells, or syncytium may contain amastigotes	Stillbirth Maternal myocarditis, esophagitis, and encephalitis	Transmitted by triatomid, the "kissing" bug
Enterobius vermicularis	Nematode	Embryo with worm in abdomen and no inflammation	One case reported	
Schistosomes	Trematode	Eggs with granulomas Occasional worms		

Selected References

PHP4, Chapter 20, pages 591–684 (Infectious Diseases), and Chapter 16, pages 477–482 (Parvovirus Infection).

Altshuler G. Placental infection, and inflammation. In: Perrin EVDK (ed) Pathology of the placenta. New York: Churchill Livingstone, 1984:141–163.

Altshuler G, Hyde SR. Fusobacteria. An important cause of chorioamnionitis. Arch Pathol Lab Med 1985;109:739–743.

Benirschke K, Mendoza GR, Bazeley PL. Placental and fetal manifestations of cytomegalovirus infection. Virchows Arch [B] 1974;16:121–139.

Doss BJ, Greene MF, Hill J, et al. Massive chronic intervillositis associated with recurrent abortions. Hum Pathol 1995;26:1245–1251.

Driscoll SG, Gorbach A, Feldman D. Congenital listeriosis: diagnosis from placental studies. Obstet Gynecol 1962;20:216–220.

Fojaco RM, Hensley GT, Moskowitz L. Congenital syphilis and necrotizing funisitis. JAMA 1989;261:1788–1790.

Hillier SL, Witkin SS, Krohn MA, et al. The relationship of amniotic fluid cytokines and preterm delivery, amniotic fluid infection, histologic chorioamnionitis, and chorioamnion infection. Obstet Gynecol 1993;81:941–948.

Jacques S, Qureshi F. Chronic chorioamnionitis: a clinicopathologic and immunohistochemical study. Hum Pathol 1998;29;1457–1461.

Kaplan C, Benirschke K, Tarzy B. Placental tuberculosis in early and late pregnancy. Am J Obstet Gynecol 1980;137:858–860.

Ohyama M, Itani Y, Yamanaka M, et al. Re-evaluation of chorioamnionitis and funisitis with a special reference to subacute chorioamnionitis. Hum Pathol 2002;33:183–190.

Popek EJ. Granulomatous villitis due to *Toxoplasma gondii*. Pediatr Pathol 1992;12:281–288.

Qureshi F, Jacques SM, Bendon RW, et al. *Candida* funisitis: a clinicopathologic study of 32 cases. Pediatr Dev Pathol 1998;1:118–124.

Redline RW, Patterson P. Villitis of unknown etiology is associated with major infiltration of fetal tissues by maternal inflammatory cells. Am J Pathol 1993; 143:473–479.

Russell P. Inflammatory lesions of the human placenta. III: The histopathology of villitis of unknown aetiology. Placenta 1980;1:227–244.

Samra JS, Obhrai MS, Constantine G. Parvovirus infection in pregnancy. Obstet Gynecol 1989;73:832–834.

Walter PR, Garin Y, Blot P. Placental pathologic changes in malaria: a histologic and ultrastructural study. Am J Pathol 1982;109:330–342..1, 16.2 removed for pencil edit.

Chapter 17

Maternal Diseases Complicating Pregnancy

General Considerations

In certain maternal diseases, placental findings may be confirmatory of the disease, while in others placental pathology may be the first indication of an abnormality. In many of the diseases complicating pregnancy, the associated placentas are often not examined, or are not reported. This is unfortunate because those placentas could aid in diagnosis and knowledge of the pathogenesis of these conditions and the mechanisms by which these conditions affect the fetus. The diseases covered in this chapter are summarized in Table 17.1, which also includes those disorders in which little information is known or has been reported.

Connective Tissue Disorders

Scleroderma, also called **systemic sclerosis**, is a disease of unknown etiology characterized by the production of autoimmune antibodies and the deposition of fibrous tissue in many organs. The disease has been reported on many occasions to occur in pregnancy, although the usually late onset of scleroderma makes it an uncommon association. *Stillbirths, abortions, and premature births* are common. Maternal deaths have also occurred. Pathologic features of the placenta include *infarcts, decidual vasculopathy, abruptio placentae, extensive fibrinoid deposits, X-cell (extravillous trophoblast) proliferation, and cysts*. These are findings often associated with disorders of placental malperfusion (see Chapter 18), including other autoimmune disorders. Interestingly, recent study has been shown that fetomaternal microchimerism, which is the transfer of small numbers of fetal cells to the mother during pregnancy, is implicated in the pathogenesis of autoimmune disorders, particularly scleroderma.

Dermatomyositis, an autoimmune disease with primarily cutaneous expression, has been reported during pregnancy uncommonly. Pathologic findings of reported cases include *subamnionic necrosis and hemorrhage, infarcts, and fibrinoid deposition* similar to maternal floor infarction (see Chapter 19).

Ehlers-Danlos syndrome is a heterogeneous disease. It occasionally occurs during pregnancy with an estimated incidence of 1 in 150,000 pregnancies. *Premature delivery and premature rupture of membranes* have been reported, suggesting that the membranes are exceptionally fragile in these patients. With the possible exception of increased fragility of the fetal membranes in affected offspring, the placenta has been reported to be normal.

Renal Disease

Patients in **acute renal failure** from any cause usually have normal infants when appropriately managed. In those cases, the placentas are found to be normal. This excludes, of course, when the renal failure is associated with pregnancy-induced hypertension and its frequently accompanying decidual vascular disease (see Chapter 18).

Pregnant women with **chronic renal failure** have a high perinatal mortality rate and have many placental lesions. Most notable among them is *diminished growth of the placenta*, presumably secondary to maternal decidual vascular disease and hypertension. The histologic findings may be similar to preeclampsia, but tend to be less pronounced. In particular, the *decidual vessels may show nonspecific thickening of the walls* (see Figure 18.6, page 337) without overt decidual vasculopathy or atherosis.

Patients with successful **renal transplantation** have a 30% incidence of preeclampsia during pregnancy and suffer occasional rejection of the transplant. Intercurrent infection is a serious hazard, but cyclosporin immunosuppression apparently does not interfere with placentation. The placenta, however, is rarely described.

Liver Disease

Acute fatty liver of pregnancy does not usually affect the placenta. It has a dismal prognosis with a survival rate between 18% and 23%. *Hemolysis, coagulation, and other disturbances occur clinically and preeclampsia* may result with its complications. It has recently been suggested that this disorder has a similar pathogenesis to preeclampsia and HELLP syndrome (see Chapter 18). When maternal bilirubin is high, *gross examination of the placenta can identify the pigment, particularly in the perivascular connective tissue of the fetal surface* (Figure 17.1). Microscopically, however, no abnormalities are detected, and visible pigment-laden macrophages are rare. **Cholestasis of pregnancy** has been associated with a high rate of *stillbirth* and other perinatal complications. *Meconium staining, preterm labor, and fetal distress* are common. Other than frequent meconium staining, no specific placental findings have been recorded.

Heart Disease

The effect maternal **heart disease** has on pregnancy, fetal outcome, and placental development is variable. Patients with valvular disease such as **aortic stenosis** or severe **rheumatic heart disease**, or those with **cardiomyopathies**, may have placentas with *infarcts* and *intervillous thromboses. The villous surface may be reduced*, and fetal growth restriction has also been described. Patients with less severe disease often have normal placentas.

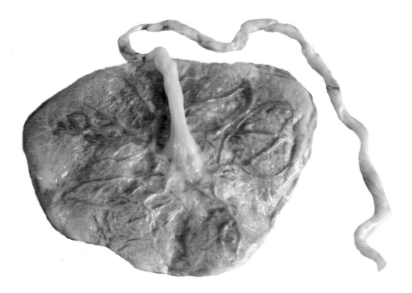

Figure 17.1. "Yellow"-stained placenta due to hyperbilirubinemia in the mother.

Hematologic Disorders

Sickle Cell Anemia

Clinical Features and Implications
Sickle cell anemia occurs predominantly in the African-American population. The heterozygous condition, **sickle cell trait**, occurs with a frequency of 9% in the United States African-American population and is as high as 45% in central Africa. Sickle cell anemia is characterized by the presence of *sickle-shaped red blood cells*, which result from crystallization of the abnormal hemoglobin S into "tactoids", particularly under conditions of reduced oxygen tension. Pregnant patients with sickle cell disease have many serious problems. *Urinary tract infection (45%), preeclampsia (25%), and puerperal sepsis (20%)* are the main complications. *Increased perinatal mortality, lower birth weights, and fetal growth restriction* have been reported. In heterozygotes, these complications are significantly less frequent and less severe. Prophylactic transfusion reduces the frequency of painful crises but does not secure a beneficial pregnancy outcome, presumably because the significant placental lesions are present before this therapy.

Pathologic Features
Macroscopically, placentas may be small and the associated fetuses have growth restriction. They may contain grossly visible infarcts. Formalin fixation usually allows the microscopic identification of *sickle cells in the intervillous space* in sections (Figure 17.2). It is thought that the hypoxia of postpartum placental separation induces sickling in the intervillous space. Of note, Bouin's fixation results in red blood cell

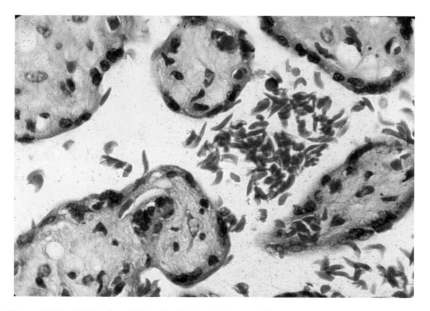

Figure 17.2. Sickled red blood cells in the intervillous space in a case of maternal sickle cell disease. H&E. ×400.

lysis and thus may compromise identification of sickle cells, while Zenker's solution causes reversal of the sickling phenomenon. Often, *nucleated red blood cells* can be found as well. *"Tenney-Parker" changes (increased syncytial knots), accelerated villous maturity, infarcts, increased fibrin, abruptios, and villous edema* have also been identified (see Figures 18.12, 18.17, pages 341, 345). Maternal sickle cells occasionally traverse the placenta to the fetal side and in about one-half of placentas, and sickle cells are found in aspirated cord blood. Doubtless, this is a traumatic feature of delivery of the placenta.

Other Hematologic Disorders

Mothers with β-thalassemia often have normal infants, but may have *growth-restricted infants or spontaneous abortions.* Placentas have not been found to have any associated abnormalities; however, in *infants* with sickle cell thalassemia (hemoglobin SC disease), placenta infarcts may be found. Maternal **anemia** may cause *significant placental enlargement.* It seems logical that the anemia leads to inadequate oxygenation of the fetoplacental unit, which in turn evokes a physiologic, compensatory placental hypertrophy. However, in severely anemic patients, the placentas are *small with pronounced morphologic changes of decreased uteroplacental perfusion* (see Chapter 18). Alternatively, in thalassemia trait, only mild placental enlargement with an increased placental to fetal ratio is seen. Simultaneously existing malnutrition is often associated with severe anemia, and this may explain differences in findings in the various studies.

The finding of placental hypertrophy with anemia has raised the question as to what changes may be observed in placentas of chronic oxygen deficiency at **high altitude**. Some studies have shown that the placenta at high altitude is considerably *larger than normal*, while other studies have found the placenta to be of normal size but the infants were smaller. Placentas at high altitude have shown histologic abnormalities. *The villous capillaries are more numerous and there is a larger capillary volume in these placentas.* This effect (presumably due to chronic hypoxia), leads to an altered capillary to villus ratio at high altitude. The capillaries are also more closely applied to the trophoblastic surface than is the case at sea level. At times, the increased capillaries are sufficient for a diagnosis of chorangiosis (see Chapter 19).

Idiopathic thrombocytopenia (ITP) is a rare complication of pregnancy. It carries with it the risk of *postpartum hemorrhage and, less commonly, neonatal hemorrhagic complications.* The latter is particularly an issue when obstetricians obtain fetal scalp samples for fetal pH determination or when cordocentesis is performed. On rare occasion, the placenta may have *intervillous thrombi, infarcts,* or *decidual vascular lesions.* It is not clear, however, whether these are caused by the ITP or are perhaps the result of preeclampsia.

Thrombotic thrombocytopenic purpura during pregnancy is a serious disease and carries a high mortality rate. Stillbirth has also been described. Often the disease is mistaken clinically for severe preeclampsia, perhaps because of the similarity of the vascular lesions.

The decidual arterioles may show "hyaline thrombi" or fibrin deposition that resembles atherosis.

Neonatal thrombocytopenia has many causes, including the *transfer of maternal HLA antibodies, maternal thiazide administration*, and *alloimmunization*. The latter condition has special dangers of fetal intracranial hemorrhage and is now being treated with prenatal platelet transfusions. Unfortunately, the placenta in these cases has not been well studied and, in the cases that *have* been described, the placenta was normal.

Thyroid Disease

Thyroid disease has *no known direct impact on placental structure and function* but many thyroid disorders enhance the probability of preeclampsia. Thus, *placental infarcts, decidual vasculopathy, and abruptio* are more common. Hyperthyroidism during pregnancy may be complicated by *hydramnios*, and *hydrops fetalis* has been reported in a number of patients with treated Graves' disease. Infants of hyperthyroid patients may be *growth restricted or hyperthyroid* and more frequently have *prenatal distress, meconium staining, and fetal demise*. Diabetes is also more frequent in hyperthyroid patients during pregnancy.

Untreated **hypothyroidism** renders most patients anovulatory. It is therefore not often encountered as a complication of pregnancy. *Abortions, congenital anomalies, anemia, preeclampsia, abruptio, and postpartum hemorrhage* are more common in those patients who do become pregnant. *Fetal death* occurs in 12% and *growth restriction* in 31%.

Diabetes Mellitus

Clinical Features and Implications

Abnormalities of glucose metabolism, including **gestational diabetes** and **insulin-dependent diabetes**, are among the most common medical complications of pregnancy. These conditions cause *increased fetal wastage, abortion, prematurity, macrosomia, and certain congenital anomalies*. Glucose passes the placenta readily, and the fetus responds to hyperglycemia with hyperplasia of the islets of Langerhans and increased insulin secretion, the primary reason for macrosomia in maternal diabetes. Periodic hyperglycemia is thought to cause fetal polyuria and resultant polyhydramnios. More severe disease, with vascular complications, may be associated with *fetal growth restriction*.

Pathologic Features

The placentas of diabetic women are often severely abnormal. Placental abnormalities are subject to many variations, mostly due to the degree of diabetic control during gestation. In addition, because of the high fetal mortality during the last 2 weeks of pregnancy, many pregnant diabetic patients are now delivered before term. The placenta of most poorly controlled diabetics is *enlarged, thick, and plethoric* (Figure

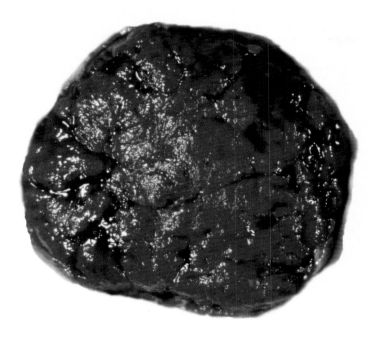

Figure 17.3. Placenta from a diabetic. The maternal surface shows congestion. Friability of the placental tissue leads to tears and depressions in the surface as seen here, even with careful handling. The placental disk was also markedly thick.

17.3), which is generally thought to be a manifestation of *fetal hypervolemia and maternal hyperglycemia*. There is a decrease in collagen content and mucopolysaccharide in diabetic placentas and they are therefore remarkably *friable*. They may also be edematous. The villous structure of the placenta in maternal diabetes may be focally *dysmature or immature* (Figure 17.4). *"Persistence" of the cytotrophoblastic layer* is often present and is evidence of relative immaturity, and there may be increased cytotrophoblastic mitoses. *Thickening of the trophoblastic basement membrane* may be present. There is frequently some degree of *villous hypervascularity, sometimes meeting the criteria for chorangiosis* (see Figure 19.8, page 359), and *nucleated red blood cells* are often present in villous capillaries. In contrast, when diabetes is well controlled during pregnancy, the placental weight does not usually deviate from that of normal organs and the villous tissue is usually normal.

Fetal and placental vascular thrombosis is more common in the infants of diabetic mothers. This problem is occasionally reflected in *fetal renal and adrenal vein thrombosis*. There is a slight increase in the frequency of *single umbilical artery* (3% to 5% in diabetic progeny compared to an

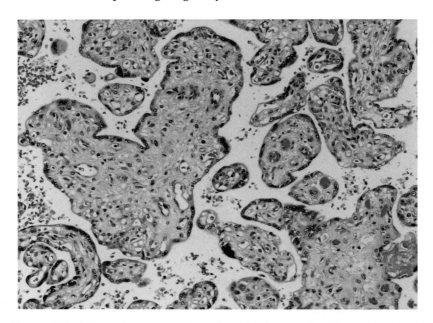

Figure 17.4. Villous dysmaturity in a diabetic placenta showing enlarged and immature-appearing villi and increased villous vascularity. H&E. ×100.

average incidence of less than 1%). The umbilical cord is usually more "edematous" or, more accurately, it contains more Wharton's jelly. No specific placental anomalies are associated with the one highly characteristic fetal anomaly of maternal diabetes, **sacral agenesis** (caudal regression syndrome).

When the pregnancy is complicated by **nephropathy (class F diabetes)**, fetal *growth retardation and placental infarcts* are found with increased frequency. *The decidua is also often unusually thick.* Infarcts are otherwise uncommon in diabetic mothers' placentas. In addition, the placental weight is not increased, as it is with diabetes not associated with renal disease. In some cases it may even be smaller than expected for that gestational age.

Miscellaneous Conditions

Pregnancy complicated by **hypercholesterolemia** or **hypobetalipoproteinemia** has resulted in entirely normal placentas but may be associated with fetal growth restriction. In one reported case, *numerous lipid-laden macrophages were present in the intervillous space*, concentrated in the maternal floor, but not within the placental villi. The infant was normal and the placenta had a normal gross appearance.

Pheochromocytoma complicating pregnancy has serious implications for the fetus and mother. It is estimated that pheochromocytoma is associated with fetal death in 45% of cases, abortions in 12%, and maternal mortality in 25%. *Thrombosis of the umbilical cord* has been found in one case and *abruptio placentae* in four cases. The disease is often mistaken for preeclampsia because of the hypertension and albuminuria.

Maternal Drug Use

Tobacco

Clinical Features and Implications
Smoking during pregnancy has been the topic of numerous studies, which unfortunately have yielded contradictory results. Smoking is often considered the cause of an increased frequency of *low birth weight infants*. It has also been associated with *abortions, premature rupture of membranes, stillbirth, and abruptions. Passive smoking* may also have a similar deleterious effect on fetal development.

Pathogenesis
The adverse effects of smoking may be mediated through reduced blood flow to placenta and fetus. When umbilical and uterine blood flow velocities have been studied, the effect on fetal growth appears to result from a significant rise in fetal placental vascular resistance. The relative hypoxia has been incriminated as the cause of the significant elevation of fetal erythropoietin levels with maternal smoking.

Pathologic Features
There is an increase in the placental to fetal ratio in smokers, which is due to the lower fetal weights rather than to larger placentas. An increased frequency of *single umbilical artery* (SUA) and *abnormal cord insertions* is seen in smokers. Smokers' placentas have *more calcifications, more subchorionic fibrin deposits,* and an increased incidence of abruptions. **Electron microscopy** of the placenta has also yielded significant changes induced by smoking. Alterations and damage to the endothelium of the umbilical arteries and vein have been identified, as well as a reduction in the microvillous surface of the syncytial cells and other changes that adversely affect oxygen exchange from mother to fetus.

Alcohol

A direct effect of **alcohol** on the placenta is disputed, although fetal growth restriction and other consequences of the fetal alcohol syndrome are well delineated in the offspring of patients with alcohol abuse during pregnancy. Several studies have shown that the placenta is smaller than that of controls and there is an *increased incidence of chorioamnionitis, chronic villitis, meconium staining, chorangiomas, abruptio placentae, and embryologic remnants in the umbilical cords.* The significance of these lesions is unknown.

Cocaine

The use of **cocaine** (benzoylmethylecgonine) and "**crack**" (the free base smokable form of cocaine) during pregnancy has increased appreciably. Consuming cocaine in pregnancy has been linked to *abruptio* *placentae, prematurity, preeclampsia, fetal growth restriction, transient hypertension, and severe placental vasoconstriction.* Much of the effect of cocaine, at least during pregnancy, seems to be mediated through its known hypertensive and vasoconstrictive activity. Following cocaine exposure, there is a rise of maternal arterial pressure combined with a reduction of uterine blood flow. The frequency of abruptio placentae is, in our experience, not as excessive as given in the many reports. It must be admitted that cocaine abuse is often combined with alcohol and other drug abuse and with maternal cigarette smoking, which may confound the issue. The vasoconstriction caused by these agents may be transmitted to the fetus, in which *cerebral infarction* has occasionally been observed.

Miscellaneous Therapeutic Medications

Few other drugs have shown well-recorded effects on placental structure, the notable exception being **methotrexate** in which there is *severe trophoblast toxicity.* This is apparently the reason it is used successfully in the eradication of early ectopic pregnancies and treatment of trophoblastic disease. A number of other chemotherapeutic agents have been used on pregnant women in the treatment of malignancies, generally with little ill effect. Severe fetal growth restriction occurred with a patient who attempted to cause abortion by taking **aminopterin**; the placenta was not described. **Cyclophosphamide** is considered teratogenic and therefore is generally not used in the first trimester. The data on **6-mercaptopurine** and **azathioprine** suggest that the risk for congenital anomalies early in pregnancy is low. **Alkylating agents** have been used successfully and have been attended without ill effect. Neither fetal toxicity nor placental abnormalities have been described with use of a variety of cytotoxic drugs. In general, malignancy and the need for administration of chemotherapy are not considered an indication for termination of pregnancy.

Irradiation during pregnancy is usually avoided, of course, because of the known deleterious effects it has on the fetus. Occasional reports of the effect of therapeutic irradiation on fetuses have shown variable findings including fetal anomalies (such as hydronephrosis) and placental abnormalities including decidual inflammation and necrosis, necrosis of the fetal membranes and nonspecific degenerative changes.

Suggestions for Examination and Report: Maternal Diseases and Conditions

Gross Examination: In the setting of maternal disease, gross examination is relatively routine. Any gross lesions identified should be sampled.

Comment: Correlation of findings with those typical for the specific maternal disease should be attempted. Diagnosis of maternal disease from placental pathology can only be suggested.

Table 17.1. Reported features of maternal disorders

Disorder	Clinical features	Pathology
Connective tissue disorders		
Dermatomyositis	—	Subamnionic necrosis, infarcts, ↑fibrinoid
Ehlers-Danlos	PM, PROM	?Fragile membranes
Myositis ossificans	PROM	NR
Periarteritis nodosa	—	NL
Rheumatoid arthritis	IUGR	Small infarcts, calcification
Scleroderma	IUFD, Ab, PM, Abruptio, maternal death	Infarcts, DV, ↑fibrinoid
Takayasu's arteritis	—	NR
Renal, liver, and heart disease		
Chronic renal disease	—	Small, abnormal decidual vessels
Acute fatty liver of pregnancy	PEC, coagulation abnormalities	Gross bilirubin staining
Cholestasis of pregnancy	IUFD, PM	Meconium macrophages
Heart disease	↓Fetal/placental weight ratio, IUGR	Infarcts, intervillous thrombi
Hyperlipidemia	IUGR	Rare foam cells in intervillous space
Miscellaneous inherited disorders		
Cystic fibrosis	—	NR
Cytsinosis	—	Vacuolization of decidual cells
Cytsinuria	IUGR	NR
Gaucher's disease	Thrombocytopenia	NL
Gordon's syndrome	—	NL
Impetigo herpetiformis	IUFD	"Placental insufficiency"
Niemann-Pick disease	—	NL
Phenyketonuria	—	NL
Pruritus gravidarum	Cholestasis, PM, IUFD	Meconium macrophages
Sarcoidosis	—	Granulomas
Smith-Lemli-Opitz	—	NL
Wilson's disease	—	NL
Hematologic disorders		
β-Thalassemia	Ab, IUFD	Occasional infarcts
Factor VII deficiency	—	NR
Folate deficiency	Ab, abruptio	Retroplacental hematoma
Hemorrhagic hereditary telangiectasia	—	NR
High altitude	—	Placentomegaly, increased syncytial knots, chorangiosis
ITP	Postpartum hemorrhage	Intervillous thrombus, infarcts, decidual vasculopathy
Leukoagglutinins	—	NR
Maternal anemia	—	Placentomegaly or small placenta with increased syncytial knots
SC disease (sickle thalassemia)	Ab, IUFD	Infarcts
Sickle cell disease	PEC, sepsis, perinatal mortality, IUGR, abruptio	Small placenta, sickle cells in intervillous space, increased syncytial knots, infarcts, increased fibrin, villous edema, retroplacental hematoma
Sickle cell trait	Similar to disease but less severe	Similar to sickle cell disease but less severe
TTP	IUFD, high mortality	Hyaline thrombi in decidual vessels
Von Willebrand's disease	—	NR

Table 17.1. *Continued*

Disorder	Clinical prenatal features	Pathology
Endocrine disorders		
Cushing's disease	Ab, IUFD, PM	NL
Diabetes insipidus	Severe oligohydramnios	NR
Diabetes mellitus	Macrosomia, PM, Ab, IUGR, congenital anomalies, fetal vascular thrombopathy	Placentomegaly, dysmature villi, hypervascular villi, NRBCs, thrombosis
Thyroid disease (general)	PEC, abruptio, IUGR, IUFD	Infarcts
Thyroid, hyperthyroidism	Polyhydramnios, fetal distress	Meconium macrophages
Thyroid, hypothryoidism	Ab, congenital anomalies, postpartum hemorrhage	—
Zollinger-Ellison	—	NL
Maternal drug use		
Alcohol	IUGR, fetal alcohol syndrome, abruptio	Acute chorioamnionitis, meconium macrophages, chorangioma, umbilical cord remnants
Cocaine	Abruptio, IUGR, maternal hypertension, PM, PEC	Retroplacental hematoma
Heroin	IUGR	Acute chorioamnionitis, meconium macrophages
LSD	Ab, chromosome breakage	NL
Tobacco	IUGR, Ab, PROM, IUFD, abruptio	Single umbilical artery, abnormal cord insertions, calcifications
Marijuana	—	NR

Ab, abortion; IUFD, intrauterine fetal demise; IUGR, intrauterine growth restriction; NL, normal; NR, not reported; PEC, preeclampsia; PM, prematurity; PROM, premature rupture of membranes; DV, decidual vasculopathy; NRBC, nucleated red blood cells.

Selected References

PHP4, Chapter 19, pages 523–542.

Baldwin VJ, MacLeod PM, Benirschke K. Placental findings in alcohol abuse in pregnancy. Birth Defects 1982;18:89–94.

Beischer NA, Sivasamboo R, Vohra S, et al. Placental hypertrophy in severe pregnancy anaemia. J Obstet Gynaecol Br Commonw 1970;77:398–409.

Davis LE, Leveno KJ, Cunningham FG. Hypothyroidism complicating pregnancy. Obstet Gynecol 1988;72:108–112.

Davis LE, Lucas MJ, Hankins GDV, et al. Thyrotoxicosis complicating pregnancy. Am J Obstet Gynecol 1989;160:63–70.

Dombrowski MP, Wolfe HM, Welch RA, et al. Cocaine abuse is associated with abruptio placentae and decreased birth weight, but not shorter labor. Obstet Gynecol 1991;77:139–141.

Fox H. Pathology of the placenta in maternal diabetes mellitus. Obstet Gynecol 1969;34:792–798.

Haust MD. Maternal diabetes mellitus: effects on the fetus and placenta. In: Naeye RL, Kissane JM, Kaufman N (eds) Perinatal diseases. Baltimore: Williams & Wilkins, 1981:201–285.

Naeye RL. Relationship of cigarette smoking to congenital anomalies and perinatal death: a prospective study. Am J Pathol 1978;90:289–294.

Naeye RL, Blanc W, Leblanc W, et al. Fetal complications of maternal heroin addiction: abnormal growth, infections and episodes of stress. J Pediatr 1973; 83:1055–1061.

Shanklin DR. Clinicopathologic correlates in placentas from women with sickle cell disease. Am J Pathol 1976;82:5a.

Singer DB. The placenta in pregnancies complicated by diabetes mellitus. Perspect Pediatr Pathol 1984;8:199–212.

Wurzel JM. TTP lesions in placenta but not fetus. N Engl J Med 1979;301: 503–504.

Chapter 18

Placental Malperfusion

General Considerations

"Placental insufficiency" is often a term used in connection with placental malperfusion and is sometimes defined as a critical reduction of the placental exchange membrane. It is a most difficult term to define precisely. Ratios of placental to fetal weight have been used to correlate with placental function, but alterations of this ratio are so frequent that one cannot deduce placental dysfunction from an abnormal ratio (see Table 3.8, page 42). "Placental insufficiency" may be due to a variety of factors including abnormal fetal genome, chronic infection, maternal disease, localization of the placenta in the uterus, cord insertion, preeclamptic changes, chorangiosis, tumors, fetal thrombotic vasculopathy, excessive fibrinoid deposits, and so on. We prefer to specify the lesions that are present rather than to embrace them all in the imprecise terminology of "placental insufficiency."

The classic disorder of placental malperfusion and "placental insufficiency" is preeclampsia. The constellation of placental findings, however, is also seen in the syndrome of lupus anticoagulant, systemic lupus, and occasionally in coagulation disorders. This suggests that there is a common thread in the underlying pathophysiology of these disorders, which is not fully understood.

Preeclampsia and Gestational Hypertension

Clinical Features and Implications

The diagnosis of preeclampsia (PEC) is made clinically based on three criteria:

- **Increased blood pressure** associated with pregnancy
- **Proteinuria**
- **Edema**

Hypertension associated with pregnancy and not associated with the clinical findings of proteinuria and edema is frequently referred to as **pregnancy-induced hypertension**, and more recently as **gestational hypertension**. Eclampsia is merely preeclampsia with seizures. It is important to note that preeclampsia is a pregnancy-induced disease and that, typically, after delivery, the disease ceases. In rare cases, sequelae persist into the early postpartum period. Inasmuch as preeclampsia occurs in the absence of a fetus, as it occurs in increased frequency in hydatidiform moles, it is clearly dependent upon the presence of placental tissue. The ultimate pathogenesis, however, has yet to be fully defined.

Preeclampsia is a common complication of pregnancy, occurring in 7% to 10% of primigravidas. If untreated, it may result in eclampsia. *The disease is much more frequent in primigravidas, in very young gravidas, and in multiple pregnancy*. The fetus is commonly *growth restricted* because of characteristic placental alterations (see below). It has serious complications, such as *abruptio placentae and fetal demise*. Maternal demise can also ensue due to *cerebral hemorrhage or disseminated intravascular coagulation*. Preeclampsia is thought to be associated with the **HELLP syndrome** *(hemolysis, elevated liver enzymes, low platelets)*. Indeed, approximately 80% of patients who develop HELLP syndrome were previously diagnosed with preeclampsia.

Pathologic Features
The principal pathologic changes of the placenta in preeclampsia are:

- **Decidual vasculopathy**,
- **Infarcts**,
- **Abruptio placentae**,
- **Villous maldevelopment**, and
- **Diminished growth**.

These pathologic features do not necessarily correlate with the clinical disease. Even in severe clinical disease, they are not always present. Severe placental changes may also occur when no maternal symptoms are present, and placental lesions may occur long before clinical manifestations. Finally, these lesions are not pathognomonic for preeclampsia as they may be found in other disorders such as lupus anticoagulant and thrombophilias (see below). They are, however, indicative of abnormal uteroplacental perfusion.

Decidual Vascular Changes: Various changes occur in the decidual arterioles, which are collectively referred to as **decidual vasculopathy**, **decidual arteriopathy**, and **decidual arteriolopathy**. These lesions are the underlying cause of the other placental changes such as infarcts and abruptios. Vascular changes include:

- **Lack of physiologic conversion**,
- **Thrombosis**,
- **Atherosis**, and
- **Fibrinoid necrosis**.

Under physiologic conditions, trophoblast of the placental shell infiltrate the arterial beds of the decidua and superficial myometrium, destroy the walls of the arterioles, and replace them with fibrinoid. This infiltration of the implantation site ultimately opens the lumens and renders the vessels incapable of a vasoconstrictive response to the various vasoactive mediators. Therefore, in normal *physiologic conversion*, the arteries are transformed into *enlarged, tortuous, but rigid channels*. In preeclampsia, on the other hand, the invasion of trophoblast is more superficial and there is *failure of trophoblastic invasion of the proximal, myometrial branches. Invasion of decidual vessels is also impeded* to some degree. This is referred to as **lack of physiologic conversion** (Figure 18.1).

Fatty infiltration can be observed in endothelial cells and later by the presence of *macrophages containing phagocytosed fat from degenerating lipid-laden myogenic foam cells*. This change is called **atherosis** or, sometimes, acute atherosis (Figures 18.2, 18.3). Proliferative activity of intimal and muscle cells along with damage to the vascular endothelium leads to **decidual vascular thrombosis** (Figure 18.3). Eventually, **fibrinoid necrosis** of the media occurs (Figure 18.4). Inflammatory changes such as *chronic inflammation of the decidual tissue and decidual*

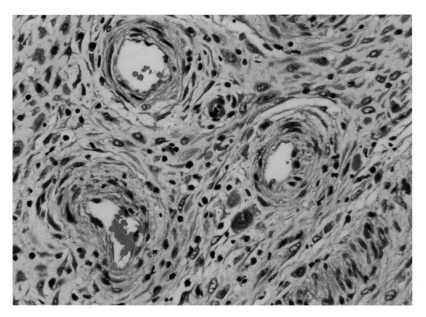

Figure 18.1. Lack of physiologic conversion of decidual vessels. The arterioles retain their thick muscular coat and small lumens in spite of abundant extravillous trophoblast in the implantation site. H&E. ×360.

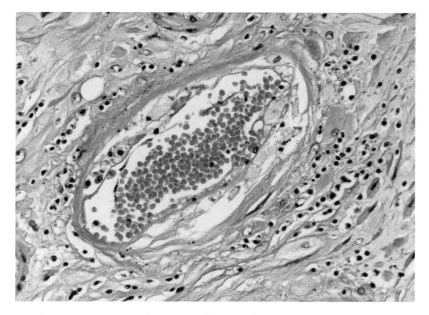

Figure 18.2. Acute atherosis and fibrinoid degeneration. H&E. ×360.

vessels are also found in association with the vascular lesions, some-times referred to as **decidual vasculitis** (Figure 18.5). Although lymphoid cells may be present, plasma cells are conspicuously absent. There is often necrosis of the decidual tissue as well (Figure 18.4).

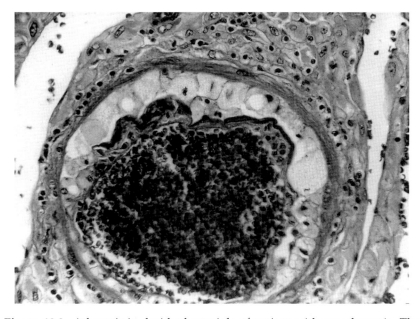

Figure 18.3. Atherosis in decidual arteriole of patient with preeclampsia. The vessel wall has been replaced by fibrin, the intima is replaced by cholesterol-laden macrophages, and there is mural thrombosis. H&E. ×250.

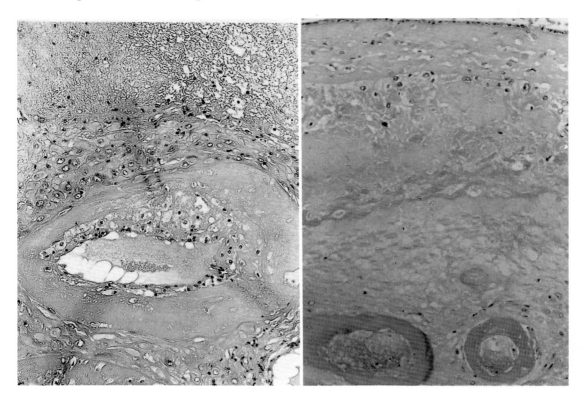

Figure 18.4. Hyalinized decidual vessels with adjacent decidual necrosis. H&E. ×60.

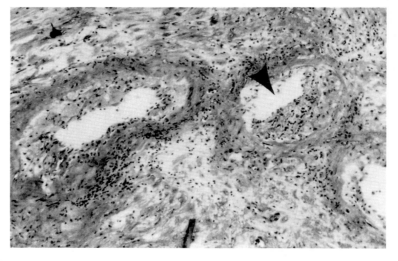

Figure 18.5. Decidual vessels show lymphocyte and macrophage infiltration and an old mural thrombus (arrowhead). H&E. ×250.

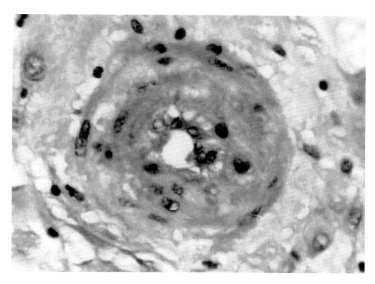

Figure 18.6. Myometrial vessel from the implantation site of a patient with hypertensive disease. Note the thickened vascular wall, which may be secondary to spasm. H&E. ×220.

The vascular changes are not easily found in the delivered placenta. For that reason, it has been suggested that *en face* sections of the maternal floor be prepared to obtain more cross sections of maternal arterioles. Although this makes intuitive sense, we have not found that it enhances our ability to diagnose atherosis or other lesions. Depending on the skill of the histotechnologist preparing the section, variable success is achieved. However, the vessels in the decidua capsularis that accompany the membranes are often pathologically altered and so in some respects may be superior for diagnosis. Sections of the membranes from the placenta margin are particularly good in showing these changes. *Vascular thickening or "spasm" has also been described, but this is more common in chronic hypertension without pregnancy-induced hypertension or preeclampsia* (Figure 18.6).

Infarcts: **Placental infarcts** are the most common and conspicuous lesions observed by the pathologist. They represent *villous tissue that has died because of deficient intervillous (maternal) circulation.* Infarcts are firm, condensed, dead areas of villous tissue that often encompass the entire thickness of the placenta (Figures 18.7, 18.8). Frequently, they involve the base of the placenta and are particularly common at the placental edge. Generally, small marginal infarcts at term usually represent atrophy of placental tissue rather than true infarcts, although they are histologically indistinguishable. *When infarcts are found away from the placental margins, and particularly when they are randomly distributed, conditions of malperfusion almost invariably exist.* Infarcts in any location in first and second trimester placentas are always abnormal.

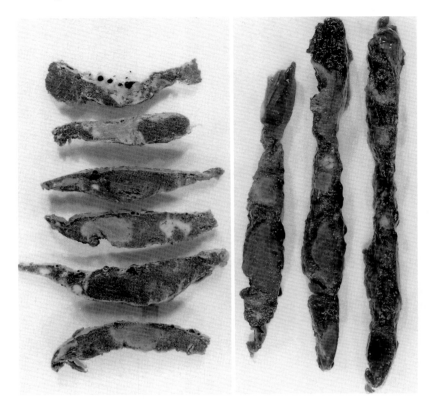

Figure 18.7. Placental sections from a patient with severe preeclampsia and stillbirth. Infarcts of varying ages are present. The recent infarcts are dark red, intermediate infarcts are gray, and old infarcts are white.

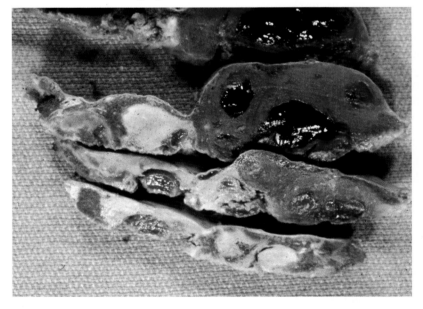

Figure 18.8. Placental sections from a patient with preeclampsia and infarcts of varying age. Recent infarcts show dark discoloration, which gradually changes to pink, tan, and then white in the oldest infarcts. Recent hemorrhage represents retroplacental hematomas.

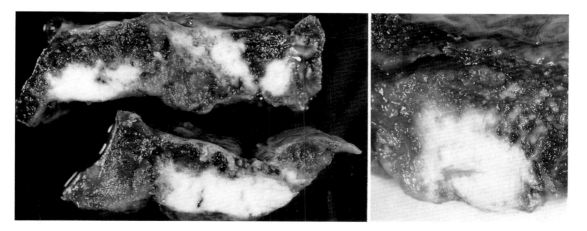

Figure 18.9. Multiple old infarcts involving primarily the placental floor.

Macroscopically, infarcts are *firmer than the surrounding villous tissue and have a granular surface.* Early infarcts are initially dark red and congested and can be distinguished from normal tissue by their firmness and by their lack of a spongy texture (Figure 18.8). *As they age, infarcts become yellow, then tan-gray, and finally white and firm* (Figure 18.9). Microscopically, the earliest change is congestion of villous capillaries and intravillous hemorrhage followed by *villous agglutination,* or collapse of the intervillous space (Figure 18.10). Shortly thereafter, there is *loss of distinct nuclear basophilia of the syncytium with "smudging" of nuclei* (Figure 18.11). *Pyknosis and karyorrhexis then follow.* The endothe-

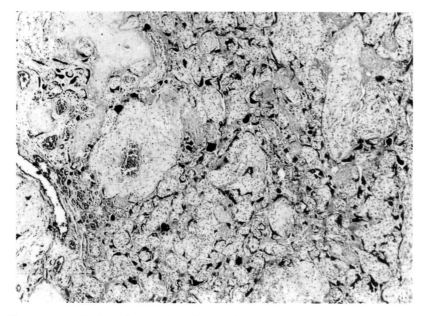

Figure 18.10. Early infarct with ischemic change, collapse of villi, and loss of the intervillous space. H&E. ×16.

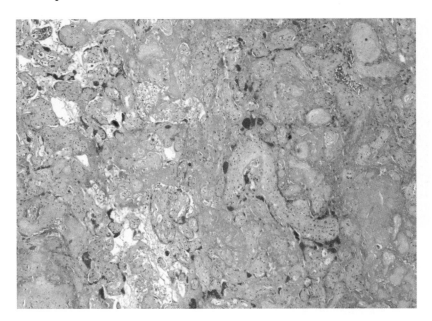

Figure 18.11. Intermediate-age infarct with smudging and early karyorrhexis of trophoblastic nuclei. H&E. ×20. (From Kaufmann P, Luckhardt M, Schweikhart G, Cantle SJ. Cross-sectional features and three-dimensional structure of human placental villi. Placenta 1987;8:235–247.)

lium and intravascular erythrocytes then lose staining and become pale and ghostlike. Occasionally, acute inflammatory cells are seen at the edge of the infarct. With time, the trophoblast and villous stromal cells completely lose their staining characteristics. The ghost villi are completely collapsed, interspersed only with a thin layer of fibrinoid material (Figure 18.12). The periphery of the infarct often shows less well developed changes. Unlike infarcts of other organs, such as the spleen or kidney, placental infarcts do not "organize" and are never invaded by "organizing" fibrous tissue; in their subsequent evolution, they only become atrophic. The number of infarcts, and more importantly, *the percentage of the placental mass involved*, has important clinical significance for the fetus. It has been stated that a minimum of 190 g placental tissue is needed for fetal survival. Thus, large infarcts, or multiple small infarcts involving a substantial portion of the placenta, may be fatal.

Abruptio Placentae: **Abruptio placentae** is defined as *detachment of the placenta from its decidual seat*. The most common predisposing cause is preeclampsia. Here, the hemorrhage begins with the decidual vascular lesions described above. Particularly, *thrombosis of the decidual arterioles leads to necrosis and subsequent venous hemorrhage*. Pathologically, this results in a **retroplacental hematoma** (Figures 18.13, 18.14). Ultimately, the villous tissue underlying the hematoma will become infarcted, as it has lost its blood supply. Abruptios are discussed in more detail in Chapter 19.

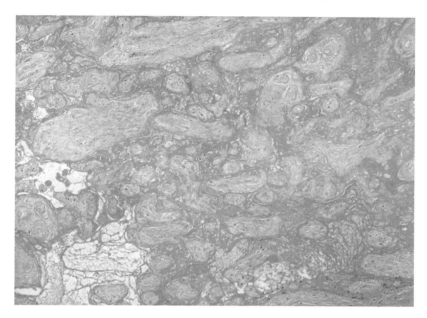

Figure 18.12. Old infarct with ghostlike villi showing virtually no basophilic staining. The villous are collapsed on one another with a thin layer of fibrinoid interposed. H&E. ×20.

Villous Maldevelopment and Syncytial Knotting: Reconstructions of serial paraffin sections show that most "syncytial knots" are in fact tangential sections of irregularly shaped villous surfaces. Correct interpretation of syncytial knots is of considerable importance as increased syncytial knotting is widely accepted as a diagnostic indicator of placental ischemia. Even though most knots are artifacts, evaluation is still useful because they represent a characteristic deformation of the terminal villi (see below). When *more than 30% of terminal villi possess syn-*

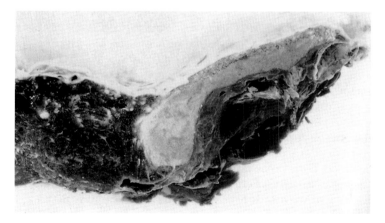

Figure 18.13. Abruptio with a layered retroplacental clot (right) and adjacent old infarct.

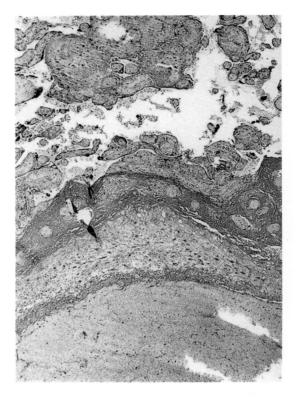

Figure 18.14. Fresh abruptio with early infarction of villous tissue. The clot below is elevating the decidua basalis. H&E. ×60.

cytial knots, especially in the premature placenta, *it is diagnostic of perfusional compromise.* Even so, diagnosis is particularly difficult for inexperienced observers as recognition of this finding is dependent on precise knowledge of what is normal for a specific gestational age.

Villous Maldevelopment and Hypoxia: Several different patterns of villous maldevelopment emerge that are associated with preplacental, uteroplacental, or postplacental hypoxia. **Preplacental hypoxia** *may be associated with maternal anemia, pregnancy at high altitude, maternal cyanosis, or other conditions in which the mother experiences hypoxia.* The classic example of **uteroplacental hypoxia** is *pregnancy-induced hypertension* and *preeclampsia* in which the placenta experiences hypoxia. **Postplacental hypoxia** is seen with *intrauterine growth restriction associated with absent or reversed end-diastolic umbilical flow.* It may or may not be associated with preeclampsia. The resulting histologic appearance in each case is due to several aspects of villous development. The first is the degree **of maturation**. Accelerated maturation results in a developmental shift from immature intermediate villi toward mature intermediate and then terminal villi. Second is the **degree and type of**

fetoplacental angiogenesis. This is controlled by intraplacental oxygen level, which in turn influences the *numbers and shapes* of terminal villi (Figure 18.15).

In postplacental hypoxia, there are high oxygen levels, which induces nonbranching angiogenesis resulting in *poorly developed, long, slender, or filiform terminal villi with minimal branching, minimal syncytial knots, and long, largely unbranched capillary loops* (Figure 18.15). In the past, this has been referred to as **terminal villus deficiency** (Figure 18.16). In preplacental hypoxia, the low oxygen levels induce branching angiogenesis, resulting in clusters of *richly capillarized, short, highly branched and notched terminal villi, showing increased syncytial knots or*

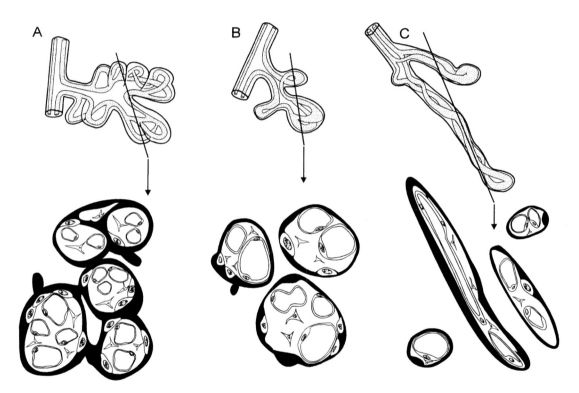

Figure 18.15. Capillary branching patterns and their effect on shapes of terminal villi in histologic section. (A) Predominance of branching angiogenesis resulting in highly branching capillaries and short, knoblike, multiply indented terminal villi, which on section show increased syncytial knotting. This is seen in both preplacental and uteroplacental hypoxia. (B) Groups of grapelike terminal villi with smooth surfaces are the result of a balanced mixture of branching and nonbranching angiogenesis. The resulting histologic sections reveal less trophoblastic knotting than in (A), and the terminal villi contain sinusoidally dilated capillaries. This is the pattern in normal pregnancy. (C) Prevalence of nonbranching angiogenesis causes long, poorly branched, and minimally coiled capillaries in long, filiform terminal villi. Due to the absence of parallel capillary loops within the villi, they have unusually small diameters, ranging between 30 and 40 μm. Histologically, these features result in small-caliber villous cross sections and a few longitudinal sections. This is terminal villus deficiency and is seen in postplacental hypoxia associated with absent or reduced end-diastolic umbilical flow.

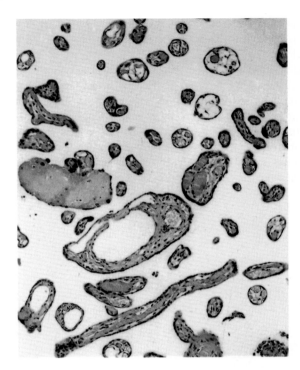

Figure 18.16. Placenta from a patient with intrauterine growth restriction and absent end-diastolic flow (postplacental hypoxia) at the 40th week of gestation. There is a striking predominance of small villous calibers and filiform longitudinal profiles and an unusually wide intervillous space. H&E. ×55.

Tenney-Parker changes (Figure 18.17). The highly branched, netlike capillary beds are easy to perfuse, as their structure provides less flow resistance than comparably large capillary beds composed of longer, less-branched capillaries. Placentas from cases of uteroplacental hypoxia are similar to those with preplacental hypoxia irrespective of whether they are complicated by preeclampsia.

Terminal Villus Deficiency: **Terminal villus deficiency** is associated with *postplacental hypoxia and intrauterine growth restriction (IUGR) with absent or reversed end-diastolic flow.* Terminal villus side branches of the mature intermediate villi are largely missing. *The terminal capillary loops, resulting from nonbranching angiogenesis, are long, slender, and usually unbranched,* thus explaining the high Doppler resistance index. The straight course of the largely unbranched, filiform terminal villi results in *predominance of small, round, villous cross sections of minimum diameters (30 to 60 μm) with admixture of some longitudinal sections* (see Figure 18.16). The prevalence of smallest villous diameters, in combination with occasional unbranched, filiform low-caliber villous sections, absence of syncytial knotting, and an unusually wide intervillous space, make this an easily identifiable condition. The abnormalities in end-diastolic flow in the umbilical arteries by Doppler measurement provide evidence that the resulting blood flow impedance is considerably increased. Clinically the Doppler findings are considered evidence of fetal compromise, often with the need for immediate delivery.

Other Placental Changes in Preeclampsia: Aside from the liability of infarcts, abruptio, villous maldevelopment, and the nearly invariable decidual vascular alterations, the placenta in PEC undergoes some additional and mostly minor structural changes. More often than not, the placenta is *smaller and "drier"* than expected for that gestational age. When sectioned, the placenta is much *darker than normal organs*, reflecting the hemoconcentration of the fetus. In preeclampsia, and particu-

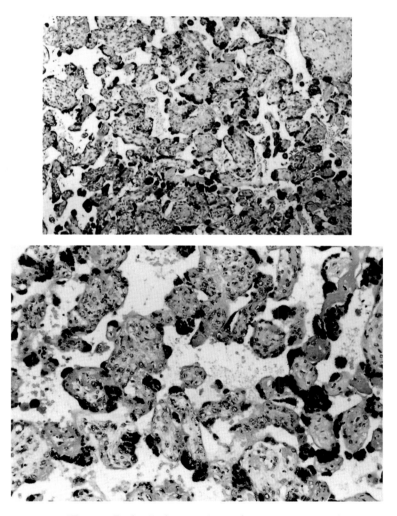

Figure 18.17. "Tenney-Parker" changes in a placenta at 25 weeks gestation. There is obvious acceleration of villous maturation and increased syncytial knots, which appear enlarged and bulbous in shape compared to syncytial knots seen in cross sections of a mature placenta. H&E. Top ×64; bottom ×160.

larly in eclampsia, there is enhanced pulmonary embolization of syncytial cells. Occasional authors have even suggested that excessive pulmonary embolization with syncytial buds may cause maternal death. It is probably fortunate that these cells are swiftly disposed of in the lung.

Pathogenesis

The principal cause of preeclampsia is still unknown. Preeclampsia is more likely to develop in *primigravidas, in women with increased placental tissue (moles and multiple gestation), and in women with preexisting vascular disease or with a predisposition to vascular disease.* While it is certain that the disease relates to the presence of placental tissue, the proximate cause is obscure. Theories involving immunologic mechanisms, genetic predisposition, environmental and dietary factors, vasoactive mediators, endothelial dysfunction, and activation of complement have all been suggested. The pathophysiology of preeclampsia is complex, but **vasospasm** and **diffuse endothelial injury** are key events. Small vessels in affected organs undergo *vasoconstriction, which causes increased resistance to flow and subsequent arterial hypertension.* The associated endothelial damage has serious sequelae, including vascular thrombosis and end-organ ischemia and damage. Placental injury and ischemia also appear to play a role.

Lupus Erythematosus

Clinical Features and Implications

Systemic lupus erythematosus (SLE) occurs primarily in young women (M:F ratio, 10:1), and it often complicates pregnancy. Fetal survival is reduced due to *an increased number of abortions, maternal renal insufficiency,* and *preeclampsia.* Pregnancy itself does not constitute a risk to patients with SLE, and some patients with SLE have essentially normal placentas and normal infants.

The disease is accompanied by a variety of **circulating antibodies**, of which the best known is the **antinuclear antibody** (ANA). It must be remembered, however, that up to 50% of clinically normal, pregnant women have antinuclear antibodies at least once during the course of their pregnancy. **Lymphocytotoxic antibodies** possessing antitrophoblastic activity have been found in about 80% of patients with SLE. Fluorescent antibodies (fibrinogen, IgG, IgM, IgA, and C3) have been found localized to the trophoblastic basement membranes, which show thickening on electron microscopy. **Anticoagulant antibodies** also occur in SLE patients, and patients with these antibodies have more spontaneous abortions (58.7%) than those who do not (24.7%).

Some antibodies of patients with SLE are transferred to the fetus. These antibodies may cause *thrombocytopenia, leukopenia, hemolytic anemia, skin lesions, discoid lupus, fetal growth restriction,* and a variety of other conditions, including the LE phenomenon. LE cells may be observed in the neonates of mothers with SLE, but these usually disappear within 7 weeks after delivery, and there is subsequent normal development of the infant. In infants of mothers with discoid lupus, neonatal skin lesions develop but disappear within 5 months, leaving only small scars. *Congenital heart block* has recently been described to occur in an estimated 1 of 60 SLE pregnancies. The constellation of congenital heart block with fetal hydrops and skin lesions is now considered part of the **neonatal lupus syndrome**.

Pathologic Features

Although the placentas of patients with SLE may be normal, more often they show changes that are frequently impossible to differentiate from the lesions of preeclampsia. Preeclampsia is also more frequently seen in patients with SLE. When both are present, it is thus difficult to know whether the placental pathology is due to preeclampsia or to SLE. Histologic study of placentas with SLE reveals *decidual vasculopathy* and/or *atherosis* (17%), *villitis of unknown etiology* (28%), and *infarcts* (18%), which are principally associated with the simultaneous presence of antiphospholipid antibodies. *Thrombosis of decidual vessels and ischemic/hypoxic changes are also prominent* (see Figure 18.3). One may see intensive chronic deciduitis with infiltration of the decidual vascular walls by abundant chronic inflammatory cells in which, unlike preeclampsia, *plasma cells predominate*. The decidual vascular lesions result in *placental* infarcts and abruptios, which in turn result in retarded placental and fetal growth (see Figures 18.10 to 18.14). The villous tissue displays *Tenney-Parker changes*, the increased syncytial knotting that is best known in preeclampsia and is due to reduced maternal perfusion (see Figure 18.17). Although Tenney-Parker change, infarcts, and other lesions are usually not seen until the third trimester in preeclampsia, in SLE they are seen in the second trimester as well. Thus the presence of decidual vasculopathy and infarcts in the second trimester, whether in association with preeclampsia or not, suggests the possibility of undiagnosed SLE.

Lupus Anticoagulant and Antiphospholipid Antibodies

Clinical Features and Implications

Lupus anticoagulant is the most commonly observed of several **antiphospholipid antibodies**. Others include **anticardiolipin** and **antiphosphatidylserine**. Lupus anticoagulant was first described in patients with SLE who had thrombotic complications. Since then it has been recognized that women with histories of *repeated abortion and premature births* often possess circulating lupus anticoagulants that may indirectly be responsible for this excessive fetal wastage. The term anticoagulant is clearly a misnomer because lupus anticoagulant is more frequently encountered in patients **without** lupus, and it is **not** associated with abnormal bleeding in most patients. In some patients, however, thrombotic sequelae may occur, especially in the arterial circulation. Recent studies suggest that pregnancy losses may occur from abnormal activation of complement rather than thrombosis.

Antiphospholipid antibodies correlate with *early spontaneous abortions, fetal demise, IUGR, and rarely with neonatal stroke. Vascular occlusions, aortic thrombosis, carotid artery thrombosis,* and *CNS lesions* have also been observed. Prednisone and aspirin administration has been advocated for treatment. but studies of the efficacy of various modes of treatment have shown that low-dose aspirin is preferable and that fewer placental infarcts occur with heparin therapy.

The antibodies are heterogeneous but generally prolong phospholipid-dependent coagulation tests by binding to epitopes on the phospholipid portion of prothrombinase (factors Xa and Va, calcium, and phospholipid). Laboratory test results may be discordant, necessitating measurements of specific coagulation factors to establish the diagnosis. The antibodies are usually IgG molecules, but may be also be IgM and IgA, or combinations. When abnormal immunologic findings are present in pregnant patients, such as an unexpectedly positive VDRL, further investigation is required, particularly a search for the presence of lupus anticoagulant and anticardiolipins.

Pathologic Features
The placenta is morphologically indistinguishable from that of patients with severe preeclampsia or SLE. Anticoagulants have a coagulative ability in the placenta, leading to the *thrombosis in the intervillous space. Abruptios are also seen.* There is often *extensive placental infarction* and *decidual vascular lesions,* which are found at much younger gestational ages than in preeclampsia. The lesions may occur before the 20th week of pregnancy. When present in the early second trimester in patients with no history of preeclampsia or pregnancy-induced hypertension, the likelihood of the presence of an antibody or other procoagulant condition is increased. The degree of infarction and compromise of the intervillous circulation adequately explain resultant stillbirth and growth retardation.

Thrombophilias

Clinical Features and Implications
Inherited thrombophilias include **activated protein C resistance, prothrombin mutation, deficiency of antithrombin III, protein C deficiency, protein S deficiency,** and **hyperhomocysteinemia** (homozygous deficiency of methylene tetrahydrofolate reductase, MTHFR). The most common defect is "activated protein C resistance," which is usually due to a point mutation in the factor V gene **(factor V Leiden mutation)**. The allele frequency is highest in Europeans, while it is absent from many non-European populations. *Increased spontaneous abortions, fetal loss, IUGR, and preeclampsia* have all been reported to be increased in maternal thrombophilias. Maternal deep vein thrombosis is uncommonly reported, but often women with these defects have no history of thrombotic events and present with an unexplained pregnancy loss. Peripartum thrombosis in the fetus has been reported in protein C deficiency, and neonatal stroke has also been described.

Pathologic Features

The placentas of such pregnancies have been reported to show an increased incidence of thrombosis, including *intervillous thrombi, intervillous fibrinoid deposition, abruptio, and fetal thrombotic vasculopathy*. Placentas have occasionally shown changes similar to that seen in preeclampsia, including *atherosis, infarcts, and increased syncytial knots*, but placental lesions are not found in all women with these disorders. There is also some controversy about the etiology of the placental lesions and the reproductive losses in these women. Although the assumption has been that abnormal coagulation was responsible, other factors such as the activation of complement may be implicated.

Suggestions for Examination and Report: Conditions of Placental Malperfusion

Gross Examination: The presence of infarcts and abruptios should be noted, and, importantly, the percentage of placental tissue involved. Location of the infarcts (central versus peripheral) and age of the lesions should also be recorded. It is not necessary to record the location, size, and age of each infarct, but an overall comment in the report should be made, for example, "multiple central infarcts, recent and remote, comprising 20% of the villous tissue." This is also true for abruptios. Representative sections of the infarcts and abruptio should be taken along with routine sections. Extra sections to evaluate decidual vessels are also advised. These may be additional sections of maternal surface, membranes, or en face sections.

Comment: A comment on the extent of the infarcts and/or abruptio is helpful. Decidual lesions may be all listed individually or included under the category of "decidual vasculopathy." If there is no history of hypertensive disease, preeclampsia, or other systemic disease associated with these findings, workup for the disorders noted above may be suggested.

Selected References

PHP4, Chapter 7, pages 143–147 (Villous Development); Chapter 14, pages 419–436 (Villous Alterations); Chapter 15, pages 437–460 (Villous Maldevelopment); and Chapter 19, pages 542–571 (Hypertensive Disorders, Lupus Erythematosus).

Baergen RN, Chacko SA, Edersheim T, et al. The placenta in thrombophilias: a clinicopathologic study. Mod Pathol 2001;14:213A.

Dizon-Townson DS, Meline L, Nelson LM, et al. Fetal carriers of the factor V Leiden mutation are prone to miscarriage and placental infarction. Am J Obstet Gynecol 1997;177:402–405.

Infante-Rivard C, David M, Gauthier R, et al. Lupus anticoagulants, anticardiolipin antibodies and fetal loss. A case-control study. N Engl J Med 1991;325:1063–1066.

Khong TY, Pearce JM, Robertson WB. Acute atherosis in preeclampsia: maternal determinants and fetal outcome in the presence of the lesion. Am J Obstet Gynecol 1987;157:360–363.

Kingdom JCP, Kaufmann P. Oxygen and placental villous development: origins of fetal hypoxia. Placenta 1997;18:613–621.

Kupferminc MJ, Eldor A, Steinman N, et al. Increased frequency of genetic thrombophilia in women with complications of pregnancy. N Engl J Med 1999;340:9–13.

Magid MS, Kaplan C, Sammaritano LR, et al. Placental pathology in systemic lupus erythematosus: a prospective study. Am J Obstet Gynecol 1998;179:226–234.

Preston FE, Rosendaal FR, Walker ID, et al. Increased fetal loss in women with heritable thrombophilia. Lancet 1996;348:913–916.

Rand JH, Wu XX, Andree HAM, et al. Pregnancy loss in the antiphospholipid-antibody syndrome: a possible thrombogenic mechanism. N Engl J Med 1997;337:154–160.

Robertson WB, Brosens I, Dixon HG. The pathological response of the vessels of the placental bed to hypertensive pregnancy. J Pathol Bacteriol 1967;93:581–592.

Salmon JE, Girardi G, Holers VM. Activation of complement mediates antiphospholipid antibody-induced pregnancy loss. Lupus. 2003;12(7):535–8.

Tenney B, Parker F. The placenta in toxemia of pregnancy. Am J Obstet Gynecol 1940;39:1000–1005.

Wiener-Megnagi Z, Ben-Shlomo I, Goldberg Y, et al. Resistance to activated protein C and the Leiden mutation: high prevalence in patients with abruptio placentae. Am J Obstet Gynecol 1998;179:1565–1567.

Yoon BH, Lee CM, Kim SW. An abnormal umbilical artery waveform: a strong and independent predictor of adverse perinatal outcome in patients with preeclampsia. Am J Obstet Gynecol 1994;171:713–721.

Chapter 19

Miscellaneous Placental Lesions

Intervillous Thrombi

Pathogenesis

Intervillous thrombi are common lesions, occurring in approximately one-fifth of term placentas. They are defined as localized clots in the intervillous space and were previously known as Kline's hemorrhages. Intervillous thrombi may occur secondary to *leakage from the fetal capillaries* and thus may be a manifestation of **fetomaternal hemorrhage**. If they are large or numerous, they may be an indication of significant hemorrhage (see Chapter 20). Immunohistochemistry for fetal hemoglobin has identified fetal red blood cells in intervillous thrombi, and in fact a good correlation exists between the presence of fetal red blood cells in the maternal circulation and intervillous thrombi. It should also be mentioned that when the maternal and fetal bloods are compatible clotting might not take place even in a significant fetal hemorrhage. In many cases, intervillous thrombi have no clinical impact on mother or infant.

Alternatively, intervillous thrombi may develop due to *increased thrombosis in the maternal circulation* in the setting of **maternal thrombophilias** or **preeclampsia**. When associated with the latter, they are often found in the maternal floor in relation to decidual vasculopathy. Intervillous thrombi are also seen in cases of **erythroblastosis fetalis**

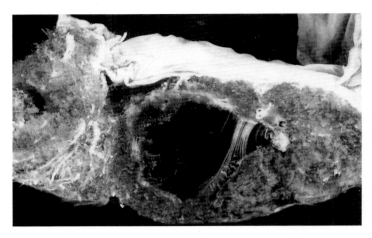

Figure 19.1. Intervillous thrombus in a term placenta shows recent clot with laminated fibrin on the right.

and in **hydatidiform moles**. In these situations, the edema so alters the intervillous blood flow as to cause local eddying and stasis, with thrombosis the end result. Fresh intervillous thrombi may also simply be the result of **local stasis of blood flow during labor**. Finally, small breaks may occur, perhaps from fetal movement, injuring the villi in some way. This may explain the frequency of fetal bleeding in otherwise normal placentas.

Pathologic Features

The maternal "jet" of blood enters in the center of the cotyledon. In this region, the villous tissue is usually composed of larger, more immature villi, which are separated by wide intervillous clefts. This is the most common site of intervillous thrombi. Gross examination of fresh intervillous thrombi reveals *red, shiny lesions with sharp, angular outlines* (Figure 19.1). At times one can see that their triangular shape originates from vessels in the placental floor. They are *often laminated with light tan-gray and red alternating lines*. Older intervillous thrombi tend to be more white-tan (Figure 19.2).

Microscopically, intervillous thrombi *displace adjacent villous tissue* and form a clot in the intervillous space (Figure 19.3). Older clots may contain macrophages that have engulfed fetal red blood cells. *If intervillous thrombi become large, or if they are of longer duration, the compressed adjacent villous tissue will become infarcted.* Thus, older lesions may be difficult to differentiate from infarcts. They may also be found in the subchorionic region, forming because of eddying of the intervillous blood as it is reflected beneath the chorion. This type of intervillous thrombus is common and increases with gestational age. It is of parenthetic interest here to note that intervillous thrombi *never undergo the repair process known to pathologists as "organization"* and so do not show the fibrous tissue ingrowth and neovascularization that occurs in other organs.

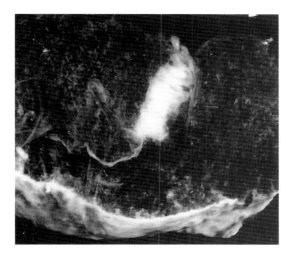

Figure 19.2. Layered fibrin is present in this older intervillous thrombus.

Suggestions for Examination and Report: Intervillous Thrombi

Gross Examination: Description of the number and size of the intervillous thrombi is important in evaluating the clinical significance. Representative sections are recommended, but in the case of multiple lesions, not all lesions need to be sampled.

Comment: If intervillous thrombi are large or numerous, the possibility of a fetomaternal hemorrhage should be raised and a Kleihauer-Betke test recommended (see Chapter 20). This is particularly important in the case of a fetal demise.

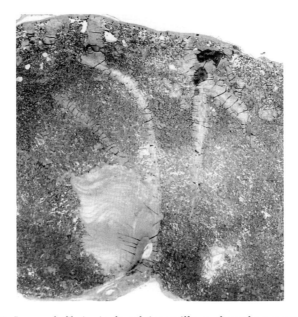

Figure 19.3. Layered fibrin in basal intervillous thrombus associated with decidual necrosis. H&E. ×6.

Intravillous Hemorrhage

Intravillous hemorrhage is most commonly due to sudden placental ischemia with disruption of the capillaries. Trauma to the placenta, particularly abruptios resulting from motor vehicle accidents, leads to this type of "bruising" of the villous tissue. Histologically, it consists of extravasation of red blood cells from the villous capillaries into the stroma (Figure 19.4). There is no associated alteration of the villous structure. This is an acute change and precedes evidence of the early ischemic change of the villi following an abruption or an infarction, for example, collapse of the intervillous space.

Suggestions for Examination and Report:
Intravillous Hemorrhage

Gross Examination: This lesion is not usually visible grossly.

Comment: Intravillous hemorrhage is seen in conditions of early ischemia, trauma, or acute hypoxia.

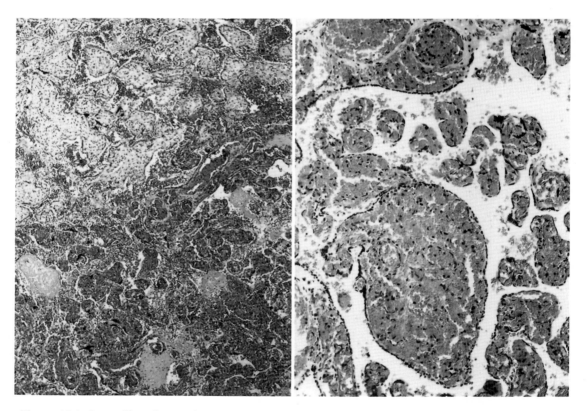

Figure 19.4. Intravillous hemorrhage in an immature placenta 14 hours after an automobile accident. H&E. Left ×40; right ×160.

Retroplacental Hematoma and Abruptio Placentae

Pathogenesis

An **abruptio placentae** is defined as the *detachment of the placenta from its decidual seat*. There are many causes of abruptio, including *maternal vascular disease, trauma from accidents, amniocentesis, uterine anomalies, placenta previa, folic acid deficiency, grand multiparity, and rarely pheochromocytoma*. Most abruptios are the result of either *maternal vascular disease or trauma*, preeclampsia being the cause in 13% and eclampsia in 35%. Automobile accidents are the commonest cause of *traumatic* placental hemorrhages.

Clinical Features and Implications

The frequency of abruptio placentae is estimated to be between 0.96% and 3.75%. With a total abruptio, or with a large acute abruptio, there may be pain due to sudden stretching of the uterine peritoneal covering, sometimes accompanied by vaginal bleeding or backache. More often, abruptio is partial and painless. Because not all abruptios bleed externally ("concealed abruptio"), nor produce the classical clinical signs of a painful, rigid abdomen, the clinical diagnosis is bound to be made less frequently. Clinical "abruptio" is also mimicked by *active peripheral bleeding that ultimately leads to circumvallation, bleeding from placenta previa, and by marginal hemorrhage associated with severe ascending infection*. Therefore, placental examination is essential in these cases to determine the cause of the symptomatology.

When pregnant women are involved *in car accidents, fetal loss occurs in 25%*, with 50% of these due to maternal death. When one-half or more of the placenta detaches suddenly, the fetus dies. If placental detachment takes place over a long period, in stages and with infarcts ensuing, then the fetus may survive but will suffer from deficient transplacental oxygen and nutrient supply. This may result in *neonatal shock from anemia or hypoxia, growth restriction, or neurologic injury. Vaginal bleeding, uterine rupture, fetal brain damage, and skull fractures* also have been reported. Exsanguination into the amniotic sac from a complete placental tear sometimes occurs. Transplacental bleeding often accompanies the trauma. Delayed abruptio may occur up to 5 days after an automobile accident, but if it leads to fetal demise this usually occurs within 48 hours. In these cases, there is a smaller intial abruptio which extends over time.

Pathologic Features

Premature placental separation, or abruptio, is diagnosed pathologically by the presence of a **retroplacental hematoma**. Abruptio placentae and retroplacental hematoma are similar but not equivalent diagnoses. *A retroplacental hematoma is the pathologic lesion that results from the clinical condition of abruptio.* They are most common at the margin of the placenta. Grossly, fresh retroplacental hematomas, those less than 2 hours or so old, may not be distinguishable from the normally present postpartum maternal blood clot that is loosely adherent. *After several hours, however, the retroplacental clot will become adherent to the maternal surface* and identifiable on gross examination. *Compression* *of the underlying villous tissue then follows* (Figures 19.5) in a few hours. With time, the blood dries, becomes firmer and stringy, and then changes color to brown and eventually may become greenish. The placental tissue underneath the clot becomes compressed and will ultimately become infarcted (Figures 19.6, 19.7). Over time, *the blood cells begin to degenerate and there is laminated fibrin present. Hemosiderin-laden macrophages will be present after approximately 4 to 5 days.* The decidua

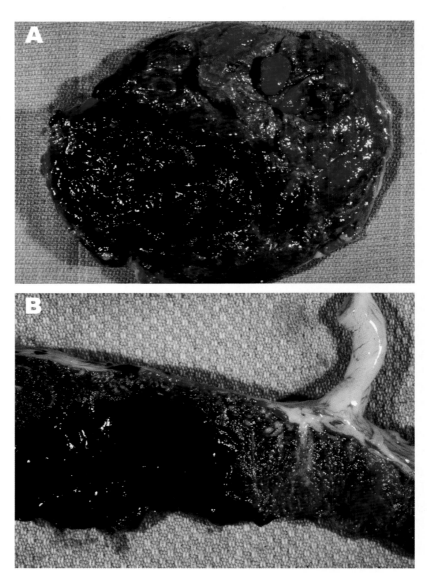

Figure 19.5. (A) Maternal surface of a the placenta with a recent retroplacental hematoma showing recent adherent blood clot. (B) Cross section of the placenta shows that the recent clot compresses the underlying villous tissue, which shows no alteration.

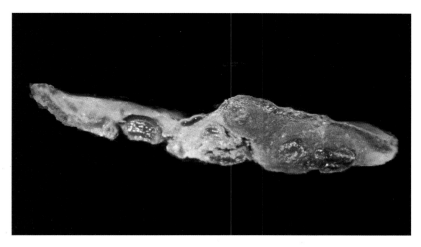

Figure 19.6. Several retroplacental hematomas are seen in this cut section of a placenta from a woman with severe preeclampsia. The fetal surface is at the top of the figure and the maternal surface is at the bottom. The hematoma on the left is old with infarction of the underlying villous tissue presenting as white, firm tissue. A more recent hematoma is seen on the right with mild discoloration of the underlying villous tissue consistent with a more recent infarct.

basalis becomes degenerated and necrotic and is often replaced by the hematoma. Depression of the villous tissue disappears as the overlying placenta becomes infarcted and then atrophies.

Because most abruptios are the result of maternal vascular disease or trauma, assessment of the decidual spiral arterioles is desirable. In the locale of the abruption, this is usually impossible as the vessels here are often

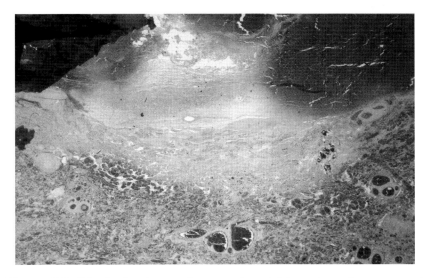

Figure 19.7. Histologic picture of a retroplacental hematoma from a recent abruption. The maternal surface is at the top and shows a recent clot with some compression of the villous tissue but no obvious infarction. H&E. ×20.

destroyed by the process or have remained behind during the delivery of the placenta. One must therefore look in adjacent portions of decidua and, especially, in the decidua capsularis. *Atherosis and thrombosis* are often well displayed in these vessels. It is frequently impossible to rule out vascular changes as cause of abruption, and in some cases the etiology of the abruptio remains obscure.

Suggestions for Examination and Report:
Retroplacental Hematoma

Gross Examination: Identification of the retroplacental hematoma, the percentage of the placenta involved, and the age of the hematoma is essential. The presence of adherent clot and villous compression should specifically be noted. Representative sections of the clot and underlying villous tissue should be taken.

Comment: The presence of the retroplacental hematoma, percentage of the surface involved, and the findings of maternal vascular disease or other associated lesions should be included in the report.

Chorangiosis and Chorangiomatosis

Chorangiosis, chorangiomas, and chorangiomatosis are related lesions and can be generally defined as:

* **Chorangiosis**—a diffuse increase in the number of villous capillaries
* **Chorangioma**—a benign neoplastic proliferation of capillaries and stroma within a villus forming an expansile nodular lesion
* **Chorangiomatosis**—a multifocal lesion characterized by an increase in villous capillaries that tends to permeate the normal villous structures

Chorangiosis and chorangiomatosis are discussed in the following sections, and chorangiomas are discussed with other neoplasms in Chapter 22.

Chorangiosis

Pathologic Features
Chorangiosis is diagnosed principally by low-power lens inspection of histologic sections. It is defined specifically as *10 or more capillaries in each of 10 villi in 10 fields inspected with a 10× objective in three different, noninfarcted areas of the placenta* (Figure 19.8). Three or more areas may be interpreted as separate sections from three different areas of the placenta. A grading system has been developed but is seldom used. The increase in capillary lumen cross sections seen in this lesion comes about through endothelial proliferation. It thus takes *weeks to develop full-blown chorangiosis*. Villous congestion should not be misinterpreted

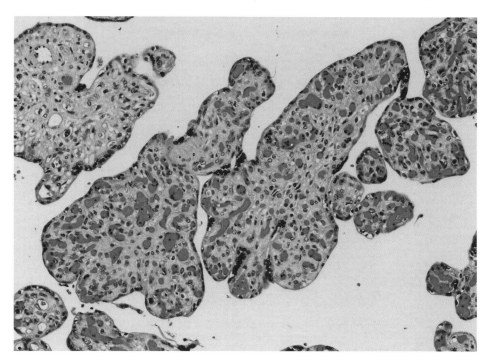

Figure 19.8. Chorangiosis showing a marked increased in the number of villous capillaries. H&E. ×100.

as chorangiosis (Figure 19.9). Congestion of the terminal villi may occur when the cord has been clamped soon after delivery of the neonate, from cord compression, knots, torsion, and cord entanglements, and in placentas of diabetic mothers.

Pathogenesis

At term, the terminal villi comprise nearly 40% of the villous volume and about 60% of villous cross sections. These figures explain why a remarkable reduction of terminal villi, as in terminal villus deficiency (see Chapter 18), may lead to fetal hypoxia. *There is a clear-cut inverse relation between the area of villous vasculosyncytial membranes and fetal hypoxia.* Conversely, the proliferation of villous capillaries seen in chorangiosis is an adaptation to chronic oxygen deficiency. This is supported by the fact that chorangiosis occurs in placentas of women *at very high altitude*, *in preeclampsia*, and in *severely anemic mothers*. Further support comes from experiments in guinea pigs in which an increase in capillaries can be demonstrated when they are chronically (45 days) deprived of oxygen. Thus, *an altered capillary to villus ratio is characteristic of hypoxic placentas.*

Clinical Features and Implications

Chorangiosis is presently underrated as an indicator of chronic prenatal hypoxia. In an unselected population, chorangiosis is relatively rare but it is found with increasing frequency in the placentas of infants

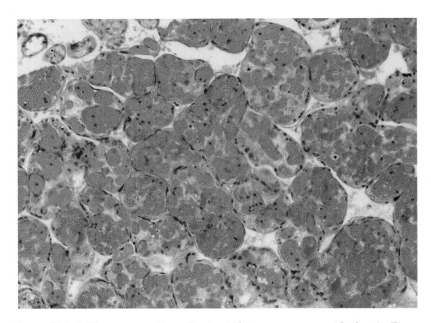

Figure 19.9. Villous congestion. Contrast this appearance with that in Figure 19.8. Here the capillaries are enlarged and distended with blood but their number is not increased. H&E. ×200.

admitted to neonatal intensive care units. It is strongly correlated with *perinatal mortality*, and a wide variety of pregnancy and placental disorders, including *perinatal circumstances that suggest long-standing hypoxia*. It is more commonly observed in the placentas of babies who develop *cerebral palsy* and in infants with *cord problems* of one kind or another. Its presence betrays a deleterious intrauterine environment for the fetus and a manifestation of an attempt (teleologically speaking) of the placenta to enlarge its diffusional surface.

> **Suggestions for Examination and Report: Chorangiosis**
>
> **Gross Examination:** Chorangiosis is not diagnosed grossly.
>
> **Comment:** Chorangiosis is associated with conditions of chronic hypoxia and is strongly correlated with perinatal morbidity and mortality. If the increased vascularity does not fully meet the diagnostic criteria, the terms mild, focal or borderline chorangiosis may be used.

Chorangiomatosis

Like chorangiosis, **chorangiomatosis** is characterized by an increase in the villous capillaries. However, chorangiosis involves terminal villi, whereas in chorangiomatosis the process involves immature intermediate or stem villi and the terminal villi are generally spared. In chorangiosis, the capillaries are surrounded by basement membranes only, while in chorangiomatosis the vessels are surrounded by loose bundles of reticular fibers that blend into the surrounding stroma. Chorangiomatosis also has many features in common with chorangiomas, namely the presence of *perivascular cells around vessels, increased cellularity, and stromal collagen.* Chorangiomas are also thought to arise from immature intermediate or stem villi.

Chorangiomatosis may be divided histologically into two main patterns: **localized (focal or segmental)** and **diffuse multifocal**. **Focal** and **segmental chorangiomatosis** involve focal areas of contiguous villi, with segmental chorangiomatosis involving more than five villi and focal chorangiomatosis involving fewer than five. Microscopically, small clustered groups of *stem villi or immature stem villi show increased cellularity of the stroma as well as increased vessels.* Perivascular cells are present but are not easily identified on routine tissue stains. **Diffuse, multifocal chorangiomatosis** involves multiple independent areas of the placenta. Although it is not considered a gross lesion, occasionally it may be identified as multiple nodules within the villous parenchyma (Figure 19.10). In this pattern, there are *multiple nodules of expanded chorionic villi, which contain numerous small capillaries* (Figure 19.11). While localized chorangiomatosis is associated with prematurity, preeclampsia, and multiple gestation, diffuse multifocal chorangiomatosis is associated with extreme prematurity, preeclampsia, intrauterine growth restriction (IUGR), placentomegaly, and congenital anomalies. It has been suggested the diffuse multifocal form of chorangiomatosis may be a developmental abnormality of the villi.

Suggestions for Examination and Report: Chorangiomatosis

Gross Examination: If nodules are identified grossly, generous sampling of the villous tissue is recommended.

Comment: A comment on the clinical associations may be made including preeclampsia, prematurity, and multiple births for localized chorangiomatosis and IUGR, extreme prematurity, preeclampsia, placentomegaly, and congenital anomalies for diffuse multifocal chorangiomatosis.

Fibrinoid Deposition

Normal Perivillous Fibrinoid

Perivillous fibrin or fibrinoid deposition is a normal feature of term placentas. It likely develops secondary to damage of the syncytiotrophoblast with subsequent clotting in the intervillous space and closure of the trophoblastic defect by a fibrinoid plug. It is particularly prominent in stem villi, whose trophoblastic surface is largely replaced by fibrinoid at term. One normally finds some increase in fibrinoid encasing larger groups of villi below the chorionic plate (*subchorionic laminated fibrin or fibrinoid*) and in the *marginal zone*. The amount of fibrinoid increases with advancing pregnancy. Although modest amounts are considered normal, a diffuse increase may be interpreted as reflecting *chronic intervillous perfusional problems* as it is seen in *preeclampsia and abnormal maternal coagulation*. If the perivillous fibrinoid is excessive, it is referred to as maternal floor infarction (see below). In foci of more significant fibrinoid deposition, *shiny, white irregular deposits* may be grossly visible in the villous tissue. Microscopically, fibrinoid is *pink and lamellar in structure*. Perivillous fibrinoid either *fills gaps in the syncy-*

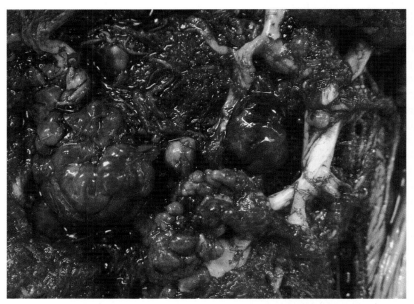

A

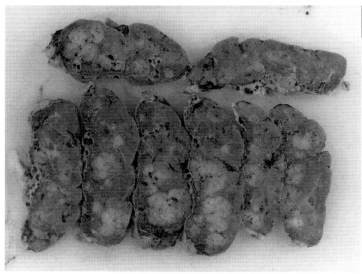

B

Figure 19.10. (A) Multifocal chorangiomatosis may be visible grossly as nodular areas in the placenta. (B) Cross sections of villous tissue may show pale nodules.

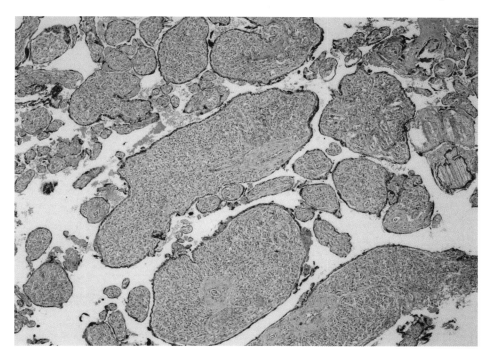

Figure 19.11. Diffuse, multifocal chorangiomatosis. Note the multiple, nodular foci of villi with increased capillaries. H&E. ×100.

tiotrophoblastic cover of villi, or encases villi or small groups of villi (Figure 19.12). The syncytiotrophoblast of these villi is often degenerated and may be absent.

Maternal Floor Infarction

Pathogenesis
Maternal floor infarction is a placental lesion with specific pathologic features and particular clinical associations. The incidence has been reported to be as high as 1 of 200 placentas, but that figure is much higher than is our experience. The cause is unknown but suggested etiologies have included *congenital infection, immune-mediated rejection, and abnormal extravillous trophoblastic proliferation.* It appears to be a specific entity, in part because of its frequently recurrent nature. It may be related to an *abnormal host–placental interaction*, but the interaction may not necessarily be an immunologic one. Some investigators have separated cases in which the maternal floor was primarily involved from those with diffuse fibrinoid deposition, hence the designation of **"massive perivillous fibrin deposition."** At this time, there is no convincing evidence that these are two different entities.

Pathologic Features
Excessive fibrinoid deposition is the main diagnostic feature of **maternal floor infarction**. In this condition, the decidual floor heavily is infiltrated by fibrinoid, which also disseminates throughout the villous

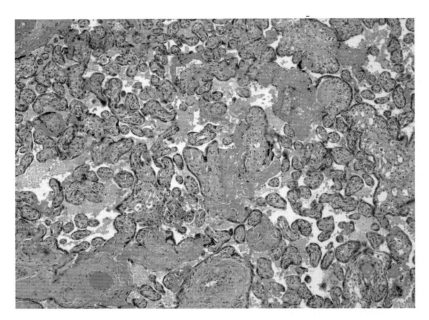

Figure 19.12. Mature placenta with typical amount of perivillous fibrinoid. H&E. ×40.

tissue. The maternal surface loses its normal cotyledonary development and shows a corrugated appearance. The *floor of the placenta is thick, stiffened, and often yellow* (Figure 19.13). The villous tissue is diffusely penetrated with gray fibrinoid (Figure 19.14), but the process is not always completely expressed. Thus, in some placentas, the

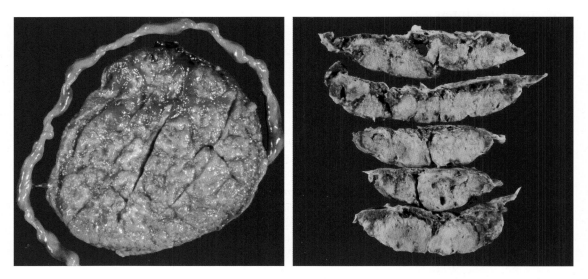

Figure 19.13. Maternal surface of a placenta with maternal floor infarction. On the left, the maternal surface of the placenta shows loss of normal cotyledonary structure with yellow discoloration of the surface. On the right, cross sections of the placenta demonstrate the typical "net-like" deposition of fibrinoid maternal throughout the parenchyma.

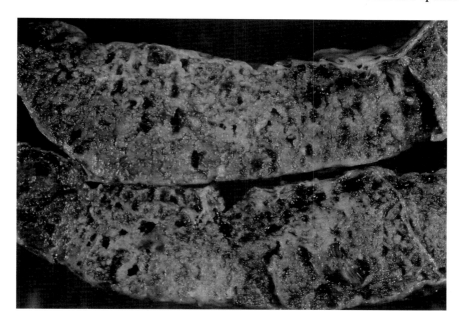

Figure 19.14. Another placenta showing grossly identifiable fibrinoid deposition consistent with a maternal floor infarction.

characteristic fibrinoid deposition does not involve the entire floor or portions of the villous tissue are inexplicably spared.

Microscopically, *fibrinoid encases villi in a netlike pattern* while intervening villi are normal. Initially the encased villi appear viable (Figure 19.15). Over time, the syncytiotrophoblast degenerates and eventually

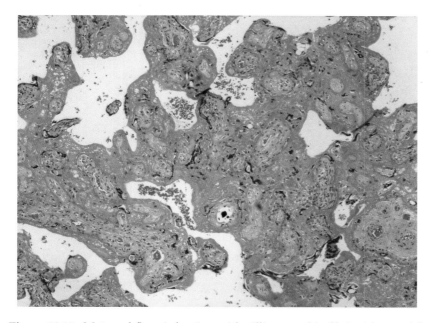

Figure 19.15. Maternal floor infarction with villi encased in fibrinoid material. Here, the villi are still visible and have begun to show only minimal degenerative change. H&E. ×100.

disappears completely. A thickened trophoblastic basal lamina then surrounds the fibrotic villous stroma. In some cases, chronic villitis may be associated with the lesion. The fetal vessels sometimes remain intact, but ultimately become obliterated. The villi are literally strangled by the fibrinoid. Therefore, older lesions appear quite similar to true villous infarcts. However, the *diffuse pattern of fibrinoid infiltration, the lack of confluence of infarcted villi, and the fact that the process is often confined to the placental floor favors the diagnosis of maternal floor infarction* (Figure 19.16). *Proliferation of extravillous trophoblast* is occasionally associated with this lesion and, in some cases, the proliferation may be quite striking (Figure 19.17). In most cases, extravillous trophoblastic cells are present in *strings or as single cells deep within the fibrinoid.*

Clinical Features and Implications

In maternal floor infarction, the excessive fibrinoid deposits reduce blood flow in the intervillous space, obstructing maternofetal exchange. If a large enough area is involved, fetal growth and survival may be endangered. Typically, the pregnant patient who develops maternal floor infarction is clinically normal, and a dropoff of fetal growth or decreased fetal movements in the late second or third trimesters is the only indication of problems. Maternal floor infarction *strongly correlates with IUGR, intrauterine fetal demise (IUFD), and neurologic impairment. Microcephaly* has also been described. Importantly, the condition recurs frequently in subsequent pregnancies at rates of 30% or more. One patient had nine consecutive losses due to maternal floor infarction. With other patients in whom the lesion had previously

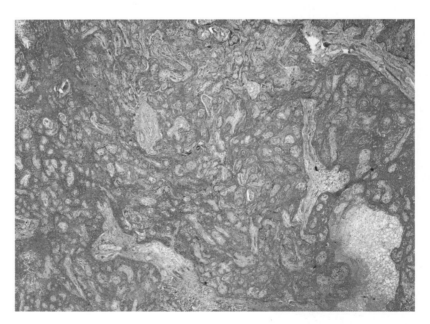

Figure 19.16. More advanced maternal floor infarction with almost complete infarction of villous tissue. The vague net-like pattern can still be appreciated and strands of fibrinoid are present. H&E. ×20.

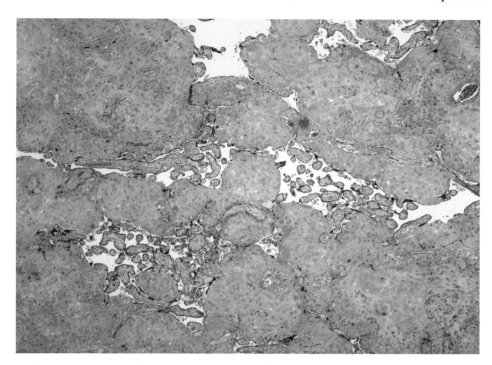

Figure 19.17. Maternal floor infarction with excessive fribrinoid associated with a more prominent proliferation of extravillous trophoblast. H&E. ×20.

occurred, the anticipation of its recurrence has led to intense fetal monitoring and improvement in outcome. *Elevations in maternal serum alpha fetoprotein*, likely due to disruption of the maternal–fetal interface, may be detected from the second trimester on. Major basic protein (MBP) levels in maternal serum are also significantly elevated in some patients with maternal floor infarction. Ultrasonographic criteria for the diagnosis of maternal floor infarction have been established and are useful in anticipating the disease.

Suggestions for Examination and Report:
Maternal Floor Infarction

Gross Examination: Recognition and description of the gross pathologic features is essential. These include firmness and discoloration of the maternal surface and deposition of fibrinoid in the placental parenchyma. An estimate of the percentage of involvement of the placental tissue by fibrinoid is also important. Sections should be taken of any grossly "normal" tissue as well as abnormal tissue.

Comment: Maternal floor infarction has been associated with IUGR, IUFD, and poor neurologic outcome as well as recurrence in subsequent pregnancies.

Mesenchymal Dysplasia

Clinical Features and Implications

Mesenchymal dysplasia is a rare condition of unknown etiology with specific gross and microscopic placental abnormalities. Approximately half of the 30 or so reported cases have been associated with Beckwith-Wiedemann syndrome. Mesenchymal dysplasia has also been associated with *preeclampsia, maternal hypertension, IUGR, IUFD, polyhydramnios, macrosomia, omphalocele, and kidney abnormalities*. Most commonly, the fetus has a 46,XX karyotype. Clinically, mesenchymal

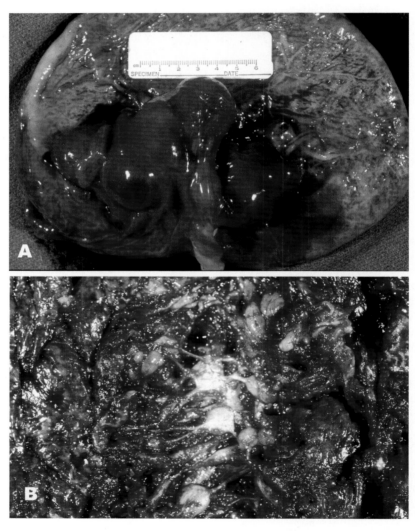

Figure 19.18. (A) Fetal surface of a placenta with mesenchymal dysplasia demonstrating large, dilated and tortuous vessels surrounded by gelationous material and blood. (B) Maternal surface of the same placenta with enlarged, grossly identifiable, chorionic villi similar to those seen in partial hydatidiform moles. The remaining villous tissue is grossly normal.

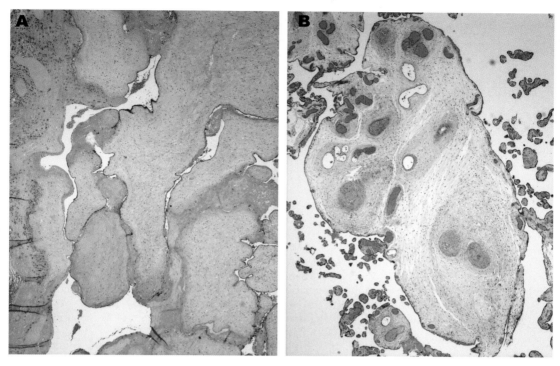

Figure 19.19. (A) Mesenchymal dysplasia showing dilated and hydropic villi underneath the chorionic plate. In contrast to moles there is no trophoblastic proliferation. Myxoid stroma is present in some villi. H&E ×20. (B) Enlarged villi are present with persistence of fetal vessels that appear thick walled and abnormal. H&E. ×20.

dysplasia may be misdiagnosed as a partial hydatidiform mole as it has a similar appearance on prenatal ultrasound examination. Imaging may also reveal large vascular areas with features consistent with both arterial and venous signals under the chorionic plate.

Pathologic Features

Grossly, there is significant *placentomegaly* with an increase in both placental size and weight. The *surface chorionic vessels are markedly dilated, and somewhat tortuous and gelatinous material may be visible around the vessels* (Figure 19.18 A). *Grossly enlarged and cystic villi* may also be visible (Figure 19.18 B). These changes are usually focal with more grossly normal areas intervening. Histologically, the *stem villi are enlarged and contain loose connective tissue and cistern-like formations* (Figure 19.19 A). Some stem villi may measure up to 1.5 cm in diameter. The enlargement and hydropic change of the villi is the basis for confusion with partial moles. However, there is no trophoblastic proliferation and the *hydropic villi are well vascularized*. In fact, there is often a concentration of vessels under the trophoblastic cover. *The vessels tend to be abnormally small and thick walled* and may show *thrombosis or aneurysmal dilatation*. Occasionally, *some villi have a more fibromatous stroma with a myxoid core* (Figure 19.19 B). The grossly normal areas usually show immature-appearing villi, which are occasionally hydropic.

Suggestions for Examination and Report:
Mesenchymal Dysplasia

Gross Examination: Sections of the abnormal vessels and cysti-
cally dilated villi should be submitted.

Comment: Mesenchymal dysplasia is a disorder of unknown etiology, which may be associated with fetal anomalies and adverse
perinatal outcome.

Selected References

PHP4, Chapter 9, pages 196–202 (Fibrinoid), pages 242–248 (Maternal Floor
    Infarction); Chapter 17, pages 501–506 (Intervillous Thrombi); Chapter
    19, pages 551–557 (Abruptio); Chapter 14, pages 786–787 (Chorangiosis,
    Chorangiomatosis).

Adams-Chapman I, Vaucher YE, Bejar RF, et al. Maternal floor infarction of
    the placenta. Association with central nervous system injury and adverse
    neurodevelopmental outcome. J Perinatol 2002;22:236–241.

Altshuler G. Chorangiosis: an important placental sign of neonatal morbidity
    and mortality. Arch Pathol Lab Med 1984;108:71–74.

Benirschke K, Gille J. Placental pathology and asphyxia. In: Gluck L (ed)
    Intrauterine asphyxia and the developing fetal brain. Chicago: Year Book
    Medical, 1977.

Fox H. Perivillous fibrin deposition in the human placenta. Am J Obstet
    Gynecol 1967;98:245–251.

Jauniaux E, Nicolaides KH, Hustin J. Perinatal features associated with pla-
    cental mesenchymal dysplasia. Placenta 1997;18:701–708.

Ogino S, Redline RW. Villous capillary lesions of the placenta: distinctions
    between chorangioma, chorangiomatosis and chorangiosis. Hum Pathol
    2000;31:945–954.

Pearlman MD, Tintinalli JE, Loren, RP. Blunt trauma during pregnancy. N Engl
    J Med 1990;323:1609–1613.

Reshetnikova OS, Burton GJ, Milovanov AP. Effects of hypobaric hypoxia on
    the fetoplacental unit: the morphometric diffusing capacity of the villous
    membrane at high altitude. Am J Obstet Gynecol 1994;171:1560–1565.

Sander CM. Angiomatous malformation of placental chorionic stem vessels
    and pseudo-partial molar placentas. Pediatr Pathol 1993;13:621–633.

Vernof KK, Benirschke K, Kephart GM, et al. Maternal floor infarction: rela-
    tionship to X cells, major basic protein, and adverse perinatal outcome. Am
    J Obstet Gynecol 1992;167:1355–1963.

Chapter 20

Placental Abnormalities in Fetal Conditions

Hydrops Fetalis

Hydrops fetalis is defined as severe, diffuse edema of the fetus. It has an overall incidence of 0.02% to 0.07% and is usually divided into immune and nonimmune hydrops. The majority of cases are nonimmune hydrops, the etiology of which is extremely varied. Nonimmune hydrops may be separated into the general categories of *congenital anomalies, infections, genetic disorders, hematologic disorders, fetomaternal hemorrhage, trauma, and miscellaneous.* Cardiac abnormalities are the most common, comprising approximately 40% of cases of nonimmune hydrops. About 35% of cases can be ascribed to genetic diseases; chromosomal anomalies make up 10% to 15%, hematologic disorders about 10%, and miscellaneous causes make up the remaining cases (Table 20.1).

Immune Hydrops

Pathogenesis

Erythroblastosis fetalis, **hemolytic disease of the newborn** or **immune hydrops**, is a condition caused by *maternal antibodies directed* *against fetal red blood cell antigens.* The antibodies form due to "sensitization" from previous exposure to the antigen, usually from a previous pregnancy. These antibodies cause destruction of fetal red blood cells with resultant severe fetal anemia. These are largely Rh-(D) antigens, but unusual cases of sensitization against other antigens such as Kell or ABO have been described. Hemolytic disease due to other antibodies does not differ *histopathologically* from anti-D-caused erythroblastosis, but clinical disease due to ABO-incompatibility and many other blood groups is mild compared to Rh disease. Fetal hemolysis may rarely result from *G-6-PD (glucose-6-phosphate dehydrogenase) deficiency or virus infections,* and it is important to differentiate these causes for prognosis and treatment. As Rhogam prophylaxis has become more widespread, Rh incompatibility disease has become relatively uncommon in this country, except in immigrant patients.

In typical erythroblastosis, there is transplacental transfer of maternal Rh antibodies leading to hemolysis in the fetus. The fetus attempts to replace this loss of red blood cells by overproduction and premature dissemination of immature red cell precursors (nucleated red blood cells, NRBCs). Fetal hematopoiesis becomes increasingly activated, and the peripheral blood thus contains a markedly increased number of **NRBCs** and **erythroblasts**. Over time, the severe anemia leads to *cardiomegaly and high-output congestive heart failure.* With extensive hemolysis, the fetus becomes *progressively anemic and large iron stores may be present in the liver and spleen.* When the fetal hematocrit falls much below 15%, severe edema, ascites, and anasarca develop; the condition known as **hydrops fetalis**.

Pathologic Features

The pathologic features of the placenta in erythroblastosis fetalis are not specific. They develop largely because of the fetal anemia and cardiac failure, and therefore the intensity of the findings is related to the severity of those conditions. The most striking feature of the placenta in erythroblastosis fetalis is the *pallor and marked uniform enlargement,* a condition referred to as **placental hydrops**. The villous tissue is diffusely *pale, boggy, and friable* (Figure 20.1). Rarely, one observes gross icteric staining of placental surface vessels and umbilical cord.

Microscopically, the most striking feature is *villous enlargements and edema* (Figure 20.2). *Bone marrow elements and hematopoietic cells* are present in the fetal circulation (Figure 20.3). Fetal NRBCs are particularly prominent. Additional histologic features in the placenta are *villous immaturity* (Figure 20.4), *a marked decrease in the number of fetal vessels, and an increased number and size of Hofbauer cells* (Figure 20.5). On occasion, one may find *small amounts of hemosiderin* deposited in chorionic *macrophages* betraying the long-standing hemolysis, but this is usually not a prominent finding. *Intervillous thrombi* are also common in erythroblastosis fetalis (see Figure 19.3, page 353). It is likely that the villous edema so alters the intervillous blood flow as to cause local eddying and stasis, with thrombosis the end result. Nevertheless, because NRBCs are often found in the thrombi, *fetal bleeding must occur at times* due to local villous hypoxic injury.

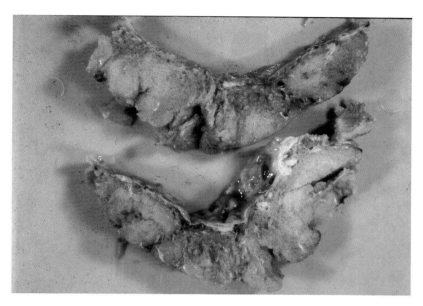

Figure 20.1. Cut sections of a placenta with hydrops in an infant with ery-throblastosis fetalis. Note the extreme pallor of the villous tissue.

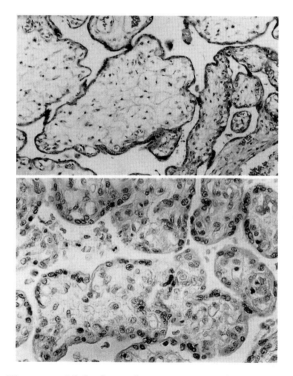

Figure 20.2. Placenta with hydrops demonstrating enlarged villi with edema. H&E. ×160.

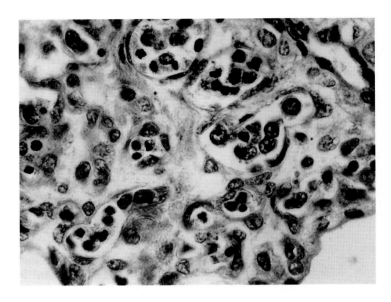

Figure 20.3. Placenta in fetal hydrops. Note the abundant hematopoietic cells in the fetal capillaries. H&E. ×640.

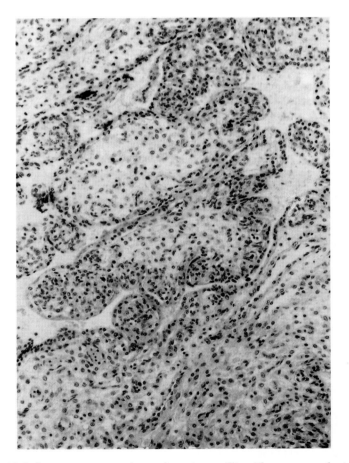

Figure 20.4. Immature-appearing, edematous villi with many nucleated red blood cells (NRBCS) in fetal hydrops. H&E. ×100.

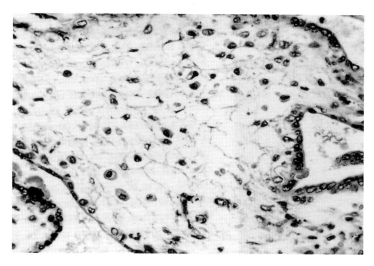

Figure 20.5. Stillborn with typical erythroblastosis fetalis showing edema, abundance of Hofbauer cells, and persistent cytotrophoblast. Because of fetal demise, the fetal vessels are obliterated. H&E. ×250.

Clinical Features and Implications

Fetal hydrops is now readily diagnosed sonographically. If the hydrops is caused by hemolysis, it may be quickly reversed through prenatal transfusion (transabdominally or by cordocentesis), thus restoring oxygenation. Although intrauterine transfusions are not without significant risk, the morbidity and mortality of untreated infants is very high. *Hepatosplenomegaly* is prominent and usually infants have some degree of *hypoproteinemia, thrombocytopenia,* and *increased beta-cell activity of the islets of Langerhans* (due to insulin binding by the circulating hemoglobin). Elevated serum levels of human chorionic gonadotropin (hCG), human placental lactogen (hPL), and placental protein 5 (PP5) may be present which are presumably due to the increased placental mass. Occasionally one sees large *maternal ovarian lutein cysts* and *fetal ovarian cysts* due to the elevated hCG.

Hematologic Disorders

Clinical Features and Implications

Normal adult hemoglobin molecules contain two pairs of polypeptide (globin) chains, **α-chains** and **β-chains**. In embryonic and fetal life, special forms of hemoglobin are prevalent at carefully scheduled times. *Abnormal construction of the globin chains results in altered hemoglobins that may be deficient in oxygen-carrying capacity.* This, in turn, can lead to abnormal red blood cell shapes, as in sickle cell disease. In α- and β-**thalassemias**, *anemia results from a decreased **production** of normal hemoglobin.*

Homozygous **alpha-thalassemia** is inherited as an autosomal *recessive*, and therefore has a recurrence rate of one in four. The pathology in the newborn is essentially identical to that of Rh disease, and it is lethal unless intrauterine blood transfusions are performed. The abnormal gene for alpha thalassemia (α-thal$_1$) is common in Indonesians, Filipinos, Thais, Chinese, Germans, African-Americans, and Canadian Asians. It is also common in Kurdish and Ashkenazi Jews, but in those populations, it has not been associated with hydrops. The frequency of this deletion of alpha-chain genes is greatest in Indonesians and Chinese.

Bart's hemoglobin disease occurs when the *alpha chains are replaced by gamma chains*. The gamma chains are often heterogeneous, and different chain compositions cause different severities of the disease. *Hydrops occurs when the gamma chain gene is homozygous and the four α-chains are replaced by four τ-chains.* The defective hemoglobin is unable to release its oxygen effectively, causing tissue hypoxia, fetal cardiac failure, and hydrops. It is lethal at birth or very shortly thereafter. The fetal red blood cells are frequently *misshapen* and may even be *sickled*. *Cardiac hypertrophy* is often striking, as is the extensive, widespread *extramedullary hematopoiesis*.

In **hemoglobin-H disease**, the hemoglobin molecule consists of *four β-chains*. This particular hemoglobinopathy is prevalent in Asians and, although it causes neonatal anemia, hydrops has not been described. The same is true of **sickle cell anemia** and **sickle cell β-thalassemia**. Both are associated with poor reproductive outcome, but do not feature hydrops as a complication.

Hemoglobin electrophoresis is perhaps the simplest and most widely available tool for the differential diagnosis of the various types of hemoglobin. Chorionic villus sampling has made possible the accurate diagnosis of sickle cell disease and thalassemia by direct globin gene analysis. In a demise, *appropriate samples of blood should be saved for such studies at autopsy when the etiology of hydrops is uncertain.* The aforementioned methods also much facilitate the diagnosis of heterozygotes.

Pathologic Features

The placentas in these disorders do not differ very much from those with classical erythroblastosis. *Histology alone cannot make the correct differential diagnosis.* The placental enlargement may be massive and is usually *even more enlarged than in erythroblastosis*. Placentas weighing up to 3500 g have been described. The placenta is also *pale, friable, and edematous*. Microscopically, the *cytotrophoblast is prominent* and, in the much-enlarged fetal circulation, large numbers of *red cell precursors* are found. Pigment is occasionally seen within *chorionic macrophages*, representing either hemosiderin or bilirubin from bilirubinuria and liver damage. Preeclampsia is a frequent corollary of this condition, presumably because of the massive placental enlargement.

Trauma

Fetal hemorrhage with resultant hydrops may occur due to various traumatic events. An example is **cordocentesis**, which is usually a benign procedure, but rarely hemorrhage has led to exsanguination. Thrombosis of umbilical vessels due to cordocentesis has also been described. It also carries a risk of *transplacental hemorrhage* and, thus, the possibility of *maternal alloimmunization.* **Retroplacental hematoma** (abruptio), although usually associated with maternal bleeding, may sometimes be associated with fetal hemorrhage. Blunt abdominal trauma to the mother without abruption may also be associated with fetal hemorrhage. It is thought that trauma from fetal movement, such as "kicking" the placenta, may cause hemorrhage. Cases of totally unexplained acute exsanguinations have also occurred.

Miscellaneous Causes of Fetal Hydrops

Occasionally, *tumors or tumor-like lesions may lead to significant fetomaternal hemorrhage, fetal hemorrhage, or hydrops.* For example, placental **choriocarcinomas** (see Chapter 24) may invade villous tissue and cause fetal vascular discontinuity. Discovery of placental choriocarcinomas is usually fortuitous, and perhaps other "unexplained" transplacental hemorrhages would yield similar lesions, if the placenta were examined in more detail. **Chorangiomas** may also be the source of transplacental hemorrhage (see Chapter 22), and hydrops may develop secondary to sequestration of fetal blood cells and due to obstructed venous return from the placenta. **Hemangiomas** of the umbilical cord have also led to hydrops. Other fetal tumors associated with hydrops are listed in Table 20.1.

Fetal hydrops may be associated with various congenital syndromes, in particular, the **Beckwith-Wiedemann syndrome**. *Placentomegaly* is quite common in this disorder and *hydrops* has been described. The placenta often shows *villi with lacunar, hydropic expansion and focal chorangiomatosis* (Figure 20.6). Venous thrombi have been described, as have edematous and excessively *long umbilical cords*. The placental and cord

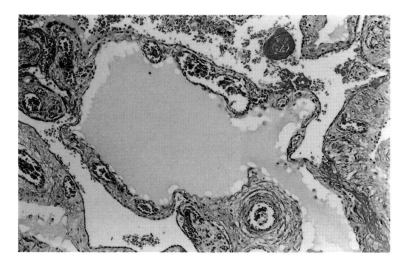

Figure 20.6. Villous alteration in the placenta of a case of Beckwith-Wiedemann syndrome shows a massive cistern and congestion. Placentomegaly was also present, and the cord was 69 cm in length with a true knot. Masson Trichrome. ×160.

enlargement may be secondary to the dysregulation of normal growth control seen in this syndrome. Hydrops may also be associated with a number of metabolic storage disorders (see below).

Finally, hydrops may be **idiopathic**. However, as more cases are being investigated, the number of cases that cannot be explained is diminishing. The indications are that, with careful prenatal sonographic surveillance and with the help of more sophisticated autopsy and molecular techniques, this entity may vanish in future. Some of the rarer entities that cause fetal hydrops should be considered before evoking this diagnosis.

Suggestions for Examination and Report:
Fetal or Placental Hydrops

Gross Examination: A description should be made of the pale, hydropic nature of the placenta. If a fetal demise has occurred, and the etiology is unknown, blood should be submitted for hemoglobin analysis. It is also prudent to fix a small amount of tissue for electron microscopy in the event the hydrops is due to a metabolic disorder (see below).

Comment: The histologic features are consistent with hydrops. Hydrops has a varied etiology and clinical correlation is necessary for diagnosis.

Fetomaternal Hemorrhage

Pathogenesis
Despite the anatomical separation of the fetal and maternal circulations, transplacental transfer of blood occurs. Transfer of blood from mother to fetus is rare, but the fetus often bleeds into the maternal circulation. The reason for this fetal bleeding is usually obscure. Etiologic factors that have been implicated include *cesarean section delivery, external fetal version, amniocentesis, trauma, certain fetal tumors, subchorionic hematomas, tight nuchal cord,* and *tumultuous labor*. In the majority of cases, hemorrhage is of a minor degree, but rarely is it a cause of fetal death (approximately 1 in 2000 deliveries). The prenatal diagnosis of a **fetomaternal hemorrhage** may be suggested by a sinusoidal rhythm of the fetal heart tracings.

Pathologic Features
One should suspect transplacental bleeding when placenta and villous tissue *is unusually pale*. This observation presupposes that the examiner is familiar with the "normal" color of the placental tissue at different stages of gestation. The presence of *intervillous thrombi* may be another clue signaling that hemorrhage has occurred through the placenta and may even signify the point of origin of hemorrhage. Intervillous thrombi may, of course, occur for other reasons. The villous tissue is also unusually *thick as well as pale*, but not so overtly hydropic as in tha-

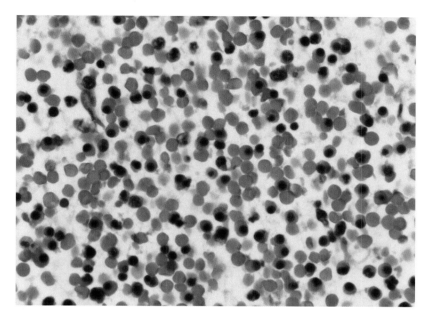

Figure 20.7. Numerous nucleated red blood cells within fetal capillaries. H&E. ×200.

lassemia or erythroblastosis. A marked increased in the NRBCs in the fetal circulation of the placenta are also an important pathologic finding (Figure 20.7).

Clinical Features and Implications

Significant **fetomaternal hemorrhage** may cause *severe fetal anemia, hemorrhagic shock, hydrops fetalis, maternal isoimmunization, fetal cardiac arrhythmias*, and *fetal or neonatal death. Cerebral palsy, cerebral infarcts, and microcephaly* have also resulted, presumably due to acute hypotension.

In a massive, chronic fetomaternal hemorrhage, hydrops may result from cardiac failure, and brain injury is common. In an acute, massive fetomaternal hemorrhage, fetal death is more often the result.

In the event of an *unexplained stillbirth, marked placental pallor, or significant neonatal anemia, the maternal blood should be examined for fetal cells.* This may be done using the **Kleihauer-Betke test**. This technique depends on the fact that fetal hemoglobin is less soluble than maternal (adult) hemoglobin in an acid milieu. Air-dried maternal blood films are fixed, eluted in buffer, and stained. Fetal red blood cells maintain their color but, because the maternal hemoglobin is largely eluted, the maternal cells appear as mere shadows (Figure 20.8). Ten fields at 250× magnification are reviewed and fetal and maternal cells are counted. The results are reported as a percentage of fetal red blood cells in the maternal circulation. Thus, based on a maternal blood volume of approximately 5000 to 6000 mL, one can calculate:

___% **fetal cells** × **5000 mL** = ___ **ml of fetal blood in maternal circulation.**

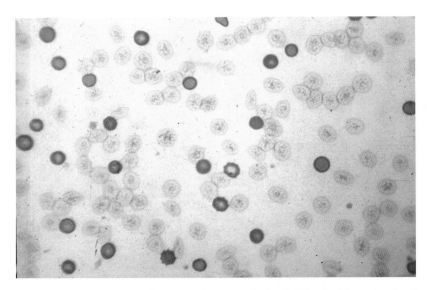

Figure 20.8. Kleihauer-Betke stain of maternal blood. The darkly stained cells are fetal erythrocytes, and there are approximately 5% of cells staining. Eosin; Kleihauer. ×1000.

The blood volume of the infant can be estimated to be approximately 80 mL per kilogram of body weight. Therefore, the volume of hemorrhage relative to the total fetal blood volume can also be determined. It is important to realize that if a *large quantity of fetal blood* is present in the mother, particularly if it is *equal to or greater than the blood volume of the infant,* a chronic hemorrhage must have occurred.

Although the lifespan of fetal cells in the maternal circulation is somewhat shorter than that of normal cells, transplacental bleeding may be ascertained for as long as *4 to 6 weeks after delivery* by Kleihauer-Betke tests alone. All the cells will be gone 3 months after delivery. Unfortunately, the test is, at times, inaccurate. Falsely high values may result from maternal sources of hemoglobin F (present in 25% of pregnant women), for instance in β-thalassemia minor. On the other hand, there will be an *underestimation of fetal blood loss* or false negative results for the following reasons:

- Only 90% of the fetal cells will stain as 10% already contain hemoglobin A.
- Some fetal cells die; the number being dependent on the time since the hemorrhage.
- ABO incompatibility between mother and fetus clears fetal cells rapidly.
  - For example: if the mother is blood group O and the fetus is A, the fetal cells will be rapidly cleared by maternal anti-A antibody.

Other tests used in the determination of the presence and/or quantification of fetomaternal hemorrhage are **α-fetoprotein**, the **Apt test**, and **flow cytometry**. These tests have also been used after Rh-negative women give birth to Rh-positive infants to determine the amount of Rhogam prophylaxis necessary.

> *Suggestions for Examination and Report: Suspected Fetomaternal Hemorrhage*
>
> **Gross Examination:** If the placenta is markedly pale, fetal anemia should be suspected.
>
> **Comment:** If there is placental hydrops and the presence of numerous NRBCs, a fetomaternal hemorrhage should be suspected, and there should be a suggestion for a Kleihauer-Betke test.

Fetal Nucleated Red Blood Cells

It is known that **nucleated red blood cells (NRBCs)** appear in the circulation of *anemic fetuses*, and this is best exemplified in erythroblastosis fetalis (Figure 20.7). Similarly, there is an increase in NRBCs with *acute blood loss* and in fetuses experiencing *hypoxia*. This feature plays an important role in current medicolegal decisions. One of the most important aspects to the presence of elevated NRBCs in the fetal circulation is how rapid the response is to the loss of red cells and hypoxia, and whether this response is quantitatively reflected in the number of the NRBCs in the circulation.

Studies have shown that NRBCs disappear by the end of the third month of pregnancy. In the histologic evaluation of placentas *only rare NRBCs should be observed in the term placenta*. When NRBCs are present in the fetal blood, and thus in the fetal vessels in the placenta, it is a distinctly abnormal finding. The pathologist should then try to find the reason for their presence. A value *greater than $1 \times 10^9/L$ should be considered as a potential index of intrauterine hypoxia*. Normally there are about 200 to 600 NRBCs/mm^3 and 10,000 to 30,000 white blood cells (WBC). However, *infants of diabetic mothers have increased numbers, as do growth-restricted infants*. NRBCs that have already formed may be released initially, but because of the complex sequence of signals to initiate erythropoiesis and release of NRBCs, many hours must pass from the initiation of a hypoxic stimulus to the appearance of *significant* numbers of NRBCs in the circulation.

> *Suggestions and Examples for Report: Nucleated Red Blood Cells*
>
> **Gross Examination:** NRBCs are not evident on gross examination.
>
> **Comment:** The presence of increased NRBCs is indicative of intrauterine hypoxia.

Transplacental Passage of Cellular Elements

Although transplacental red blood cell passage has the most serious consequences due to anemia and immunization, **transplacental white blood cell transfer** is also of interest. Fetal lymphocytes pass to the mother in most normal pregnancies and may be found years postpartum in the maternal blood or bone marrow. Of course, **deported syncytiotrophoblast** traveling to the maternal lung has long been known. **Transplacental passage of tumor cells** from mother to fetus has been described many times. Chimerism, induced by prenatal **maternal lymphocyte transfer**, has also been reported. A few additional reports of 46,XX cells in the circulation of male fetuses have been forthcoming. Such passage is clearly exceptional. There have also been occasional reports of fetal plethora that were apparently due to **mother-to-fetus blood transfer**; however, numerous studies have affirmed the transfer of small numbers of maternal red blood cells to the fetus without fetal plethora or abnormal placentas.

Fetal Metabolic Storage Disorders

Many of the **metabolic storage disorders** produce inclusions or vacuoles in the tissues of affected individuals. In some, involvement of placental tissues enables prenatal diagnosis via chorionic villus biopsy or from material obtained at amniocentesis. Many of these diseases may cause fetal *hydrops*, the etiology of which remains obscure. Nevertheless, because of the association with storage disorders, *cases of nonimmune hydrops fetalis warrant special attention*. Many of the inclusions are highly water and/or lipid-solvent soluble and can only be identified with proper fixation. *Electron microscopy* and *special enzyme studies* are often necessary to make the definitive diagnosis. Therefore, consideration should be given to fixation of tissue for electron microscopy when one of these disorders is suspected. Importantly, there are numerous cases in which a *storage disorder was suspected only after placental examination* revealed characteristic features. Even without clinical suspicion or evidence of disease, the presence of **foam cells**, **trophoblastic vacuolization**, and **irregular calcification** *are all indicative of an unidentified fetal storage disorder*. Further work-up is then warranted.

Pathologic Features
Macroscopically, the placenta is often *enlarged, pale, and/or soft*. On microscopic examination, intracellular accumulation of material is revealed as *vacuolization of the cytoplasm* of certain cells, the distribution of which is particular to that storage disorder. Because the cellular glycolipids are highly water soluble, the empty appearance of the vacuoles is the usual finding in many fetal storage disorders. In the majority of the disorders with placental manifestations, it is primarily the *syncytiotrophoblast* that shows the typical vacuolated cytoplasm (Figure 20.9). Other trophoblastic cells may show vacuolation as well, including *cytotrophoblast and extravillous trophoblast*. Furthermore, *villous fibroblasts, Hofbauer cells, villous capillary endothelial cells, and, rarely, the amnion*

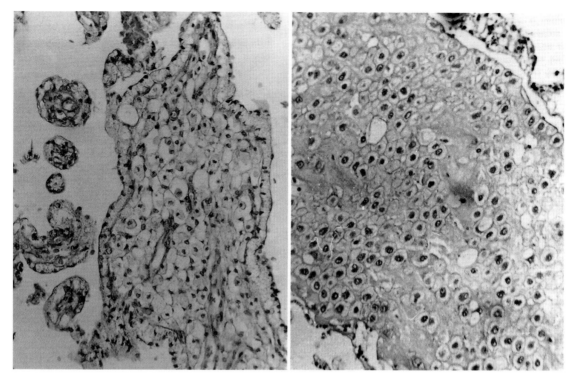

Figure 20.9. Villus (left) and X-cell column of placenta, affected by mucolipidosis II (I-cell disease). Note the abundance of vacuoles in the syncytium and Hofbauer cells. H&E. ×240.

may show vacuolization. Endothelial damage, perhaps secondary to lipid accumulation, is seen in a number of storage diseases leading to *thrombosis* of chorionic or fetal stem vessels.

If vacuolization of cells in the placenta is identified, a metabolic storage disorder may be tentatively diagnosed. Based on which cells contain the vacuolization, whether the infant or fetus has hydrops and other clinical information, a differential diagnosis may be compiled. Table 20.2 lists selected storage disorders and the particular placental cells in which vacuolization can be identified. Histochemical stains can be helpful in differentiating some of these disorders, but this has not been studied on placental tissue in every disorder. After making the tentative diagnosis of storage disorder, diagnosis and/or confirmation of the specific disease must be made via enzyme or other special studies.

Specific Disorders

A few specific disorders are mentioned here as they show some unique features. For instance, **Morquio disease** or **mucopolysaccharidosis type IV**, unlike many of the storage diseases, only rarely has histologic evidence of storage products in trophoblast but rather shows *granularity in Hofbauer cells*. The absence of β-galactosidase defines **type 1 G_{M1} gangliosidosis**. Typical inclusions or *zebra bodies* may be ultrastructurally identified in the fetal ganglion cells. Fetal cells will be unremarkable in paraffin sections, but *"empty vacuoles" in the syncytial cytoplasm, the amnionic epithelial cells, and Hofbauer cells* are present. Occasionally, vacuolization has been demonstrable in endothelial cells in villous stem vessels, and *calcified thrombi* in large fetal vessels have also been identified. As membrane-bound inclusions are present in amnionic cells, diagnosis can be made from cells cultured from the amniotic fluid. **Tay Sachs' disease (G$_{M2}$-gangliosidosis type I)** produces *vacuolization of syncytiotrophoblast*. In **G$_{M2}$-gangliosidosis type II, Sandhoff's disease,** vacuolation is seen in *stromal* as well as the *syncytial* cells. Ultrastructurally, the most striking feature is the occurrence of *parallel membranous arrays in occasional lysosomes* in stromal cells.

Niemann-Pick disease type A, which is caused by sphingomyelin diphosphodiesterase deficiency, can be diagnosed from the absence of the enzyme in amniotic fluid. Unusual *echogenic densities in the placentas* of several cases have been demonstrated sonographically, and these placentas have had *thick chorionic plates. Vacuolated syncytium, Hofbauer cells,* and *fibrocytes* contain accumulations of sphingomyelin, which is also present in the umbilical cord and the chorion laeve.

Gaucher's disease is a heterogeneous disease that may cause *fetal hydrops.* The placenta is *large* and *edematous* with macroscopic features similar to that of erythroblastosis fetalis. In the absence of hydrops, there are generally no placental findings. However, some cases may show *Hofbauer cells with minimal vacuolization.* Uncommonly, characteristic histiocytes, or *Gaucher cells,* may be found in fetal vessels in the placenta. Absence of α-galactosidase A results in **Fabry's disease**, a disorder of glycosphingolipid metabolism. The tissues accumulate ceramide trihexose. Although the syncytiotrophoblast does not show vacuolization, the *decidual cells* and *decidual vessels* contain *argyrophilic granules,* which by electron microscopy have an appearance similar to zebra bodies. The fetal portions of the placenta are normal.

Mucolipidosis type II or **I-cell disease** is a rare and fatal disorder whose genetic transmission is autosomal recessive. *Periodic acid-Schiff (PAS)-positive lysosomal inclusions* are present in the cells of affected children, including kidney cells, leukocytes, and fibroblasts. The typical "inclusions" cannot be seen in paraffin embedded sections, but are obvious in epoxy-embedded material. Placental involvement with inclusion-bearing cells in the *villous fibroblast* has also been demonstrated. In paraffin sections of the placenta, the *vacuoles of formerly mucolipid-containing lysosomes* are readily apparent in the *syncytium* and in *Hofbauer cells* (Figure 20.9). The features are much enhanced by processing the tissues in epoxy resin. In some cases vascular lesions have been present in the *villous stem arteries ranging from fibrinoid necrosis to complete obliteration.* Focal *villous calcification* is also a common finding. As with many of these disorders, diagnosis may be made with electron microscopy.

Unusual placental findings in **Pompe's disease** or **glycogen storage disease type II** consist of *cytoplasmic vacuolation of syncytium, cytotrophoblast, fibroblast,* and *amnionic connective tissue cells.* By electron microscopy, typical *membrane-bounded, glycogen-filled inclusions in capil-*

lary endothelial cells and villous fibroblasts are found. These inclusions may be found in cells obtained via CVS as early as 10 weeks. In **type IV glycogen storage disease**, vacuoles are only present in the *amnionic epithelium.*

> ### Suggestions for Examination and Report: Storage Disorders with Vacuolization of Trophoblast or Other Cell
>
> **Gross Examination:** Generally, the placentas in these disorders are grossly unremarkable, but may be pale, enlarged, and soft, particularly if hydrops is present. If a disorder is suspected, tissue should be fixed for electron microscopy.
>
> **Comment:** Vacuolization of trophoblast or other placental cells is highly suggestive of a fetal metabolic disorder and further testing should be suggested.

Placental Changes in Intrauterine Fetal Demise

After death in utero, the fetal tissue begins to undergo autolysis. Certain placental changes also occur that are attributable to fetal death, which are different from the pathologic changes that are the cause of death. Macroscopically, the *fetal surface and fetal membranes may be discolored red-brown* due to hemolysis. Microscopically, the pathologic changes in the placenta that are directly caused by the fetal demise mostly relate to the *cessation of fetal circulation*. This causes *progressive sclerosis of the fetal vessels* and ultimately their *obliteration*. This is particularly true of the villous capillaries. Studies have shown that these and other changes occur after fetal death in a relatively predictable manner such that they time of fetal death may be roughly estimated by the presence of absence of particular features.

One of the first changes that occur is **intravascular karyorrhexis**. This consists of particles of nuclear debris, predominantly derived from leukocytes, stained deeply with hematoxylin, present within villous capillaries and small villous vessels (Figure 20.10). This change is not present if fetal death has occurred less than 6 hours before delivery. Another early change is **degeneration of the umbilical vascular smooth muscle cells**. This finding may be present within a few hours but is present in virtually all cases by 12 hours. It consists of some *loss of nuclear basophilia* and *nuclear pyknosis*. In addition, the *smooth muscle cells become thin and spindled*, also taking on a *"wavy"* appearance (Figure 20.11). The loss of fetal circulation also causes **luminal abnormalities of the fetal stem vessels** consisting of *septation of the lumen and obliteration by fibromuscular sclerosis* (Figure 20.12). The septation commonly appears as the presence of *multiple irregular lumens connected by thin fibrous tissue* containing degenerated blood and occasionally thrombi. In fibromuscular sclerosis there is *thickening of the muscular wall of the vessel with progressive obliteration of the lumen and loss of*

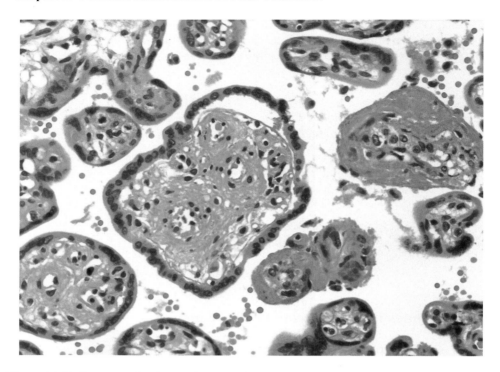

Figure 20.10. Intravascular karyorrhexis with nuclear debris in fetal capillaries. H&E. ×200.

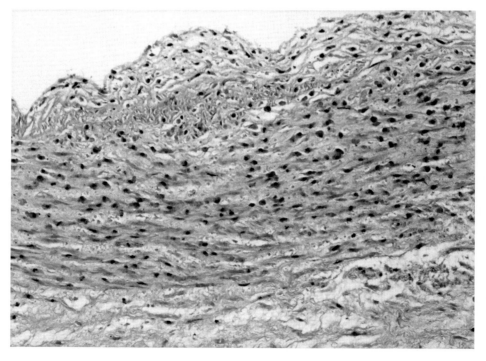

Figure 20.11. Degeneration of vascular smooth muscle of umbilical cord after demise. H&E. ×320.

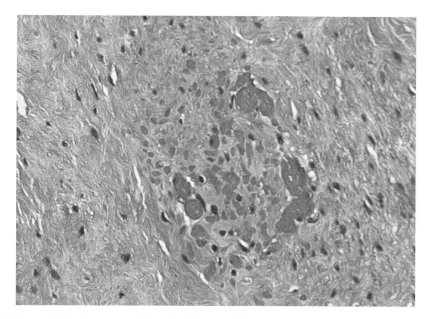

Figure 20.12. Stem vessel luminal abnormalities, septation, and fibromuscular sclerosis with partial obliteration. H&E. ×400.

endothelial lining. If these changes are multifocal and present in 10% to 25% of stem villi, then the time from fetal death is at least 48 hours. The changes do not become extensive, involving more than 25% of the stem villi, until approximately 2 weeks after fetal death. *Sclerosis and fibrosis of the villous stroma* often accompanies obliteration of the fetal vessels. This change is also seen when cessation of fetal blood flow is secondary to fetal vascular thrombosis and has been termed **avascular villi** (see Chapter 21). Extensive avascular villi, involving at least 25% of the terminal villi, also occur roughly 2 weeks after fetal demise.

Other changes also occur but in a less predictable manner. Some authors have suggested that **increased syncytial knots** are associated with fetal death, while others do not find this association. It is, however, important to note that although there is some decrease in maternal blood flow after fetal death, flow does not completely stop nor does it impair the viability of the trophoblast. Thus, weeks and even months after fetal death when the villous stroma is completely avascular and hyalinized, the trophoblastic cover continues to be viable. After fetal death, **villous stromal microcalcification** may be present consisting of fine, *granular calcification of the trophoblastic basement membrane* or fine, punctate granules within the stroma (Figure 20.13). It is likely that calcium is not the sole mineral that deposits within the villi in this situation. Normally, the fetal vessels transport these minerals away from the placenta, but with the loss of fetal circulation, there is accumulation and deposition within the villous stroma and the trophoblastic basement membrane. Other changes that may occur with fetal death include **thickening of the trophoblastic basement membrane** and **degeneration or necrosis of Wharton's jelly**.

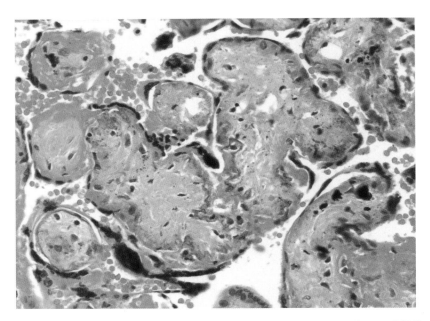

Figure 20.13. Microcalcification of trophoblastic basement membrane. H&E. ×200.

Suggestions for Examination and Report: Fetal Demise

Gross Examination: The cord and fetal surface may be hemolyzed and discolored red. No additional gross examination or sections need to be submitted if the cause of demise is known. If it is not, four to five additional random sections of villous tissue should be submitted to identify possible causes of demise.

Comment: The change seen will be consistent with fetal demise and may potentially give an approximating of the time of uterine retention after demise.

Table 20.1. Etiology of nonimmune hydrops fetalis

Cardiovascular: Congenital heart disease including
   Coarctation of the aorta
   Hypoplastic left heart
   Cardiac arrhythmias, particularly supraventricular tachycardia
   Premature closure of the foramen ovale
   Endocardial fibroelastosis
   Ebstein's anomaly of the tricuspid valve

Chromosomal (see Chapter 11)
   Turner's syndrome, 45 XO
   Trisomy 13, 15, 16, 18, and 21
   Duplications of the long arms of chromosomes 15 or 17
   Triploidy

Anemia
   Twin-to-twin transfusion syndrome (see Chapter 10)
   Thalassemia (see Chapter 17)
   Fetomaternal hemorrhage
   Hemolytic anemia

Thoracic: space-occupying lesions
   Cystic adenomatoid malformation and pulmonary sequestration
   Diaphragmatic hernia
   Cystic hygroma
   Chylothorax
   Lymphangiectasias

Infection (see Chapter 16)
   Parvovirus
   Cytomegalovirus
   Toxoplasmosis
   Herpes simplex virus
   Syphilis
   Rubella

Congenital tumors (see Chapter 22)
   Congenital neuroblastoma
   Hepatoblastoma
   Sacrococcygeal teratoma
   Leukemia
   Mesoblastic nephroma
   Hemangioma
   Chorangioma

Miscellaneous
   Malformations of the genitourinary tract
   Fetal storage disorders
   Thyrotoxicosis
   Small bowel volvulus
   Intussusception
   Trauma
   Beckwith-Wiedemann syndrome
   Idiopathic

Table 20.2. Summary of placental findings in metabolic storage diseases

Disorder	Deficiency	Hydrops
Mucopolysaccharidoses		
MPS I (Hurler disease)	α-1-Iduronidase	+
MPS III (San Filippo disease)	Various	
MPS IV (Morquio disease)	Various	+
MPS VII (Sly disease)	β-Glucuronidase	+
Sphingolipidoses		
GM1 gangliosidosis	β-Galactosidase	
GM2 gangliosidosis		
Type I (Tay-Sachs disease)	β-Hexosaminidase, α-subunit	
Type II (Sandhoff disease)	β-Hexosaminidase, β-subunit	
Niemann-Pick disease, type A	Sphingomyelinase	+
Niemann-Pick disease, type B	Sphingomyelinase	
Gaucher disease	β-Glucosidase	+
Fabry disease	α-Galactosidase	
Other lipidoses		
Wolman disease	Acid lipase	+
Cholesterol ester storage disease	Acid lipase	+
Niemann-Pick disease, type C	Unknown	
Neuronal ceroid lipofuscinosis	Unknown	
Mucolipidoses		
Type I, sialidosis	Sialidase	
Type II, I cell disease	N-Acetylglucosamine-1-phosphotransferase	+
Type IV	Unknown	
Oligosaccharidoses		
Galactosialidosis	β-Galactosialidase	+
Sialic acid storage disease (Salla disease)	Sialic acid transporter	+
Glycogen storage disease		
Type II, Pompe disease	α-1,4-Glucosidase	
Type IV	Amylopectinase	

ST, syncytiotrophoblast; ET, extravillous trophoblast or X-cell; FB, villous stromal fibroblast; HC, Hofbauer cell; EN, endothelium; AE, amnionic epithelium; PAS, periodic acid-Schiff; ORO, oil red O; M, minimal vacuolization.
[a] Granularity and *not* vacuolization can be seen in Hofbauer cells.

Selected References

PHP4, Chapter 16, pages 461–491 (Hydrops); Chapter 17, pages 492–515 (Transplacental Hemorrhage, Trauma); Chapter 18, pages 516–522 (Fetal Storage Disorders).

Bouvier R, Maire I. Fetal presentation of 23 cases of lysosomal storage disease. A collaborative study of the French Society of Fetal Pathology. Pediatr Pathol Lab Med 1997;17:675.

Bowman JM, Lewis M, de Sa DJ. Hydrops fetalis caused by massive maternofetal transplacental hemorrhage. J Pediatr 1984;104:769–772.

Fox H. The incidence and significance of nucleated erythrocytes in the foetal vessels of the mature human placenta. J Obstet Gynaecol Br Commonw 1967; 74:40–43.

Genest DR. Estimating the time of death in stillborn fetuses: II. Histologic evaluation of the placenta; a study of 71 stillborns. Obstet Gynecol 1992; 80:585–592.

Hellman LM, Hertig AT. Pathological changes in the placenta associated with erythroblastosis of the fetus. Am J Pathol 1937;14:111–120.

Higgins SD. Trauma in pregnancy. J Perinatol 1988;8:288–292.

Intracellular vacuolization						Histochemistry			
ST	ET	HC	FB	EN	AE	PAS	Alcian blue	Colloidal Ee	ORO
								+	
+		+	+						
+									
		a							
		+							
+	+	+			+	+	+	+	+
+		+			+				
+			+						
+	+	+	+			±			+
		M				+			
						+			+
+									+
+			+						
+				+	+				
+		+	+						
+	+	+			M	±	±	±	±
			+						
+			+						
+	+	+		+	+		+	+	
+			+	+		±			
					+				

Jones CJP, Lendon M, Chawner LE, et al. Ultrastructure of the human placenta in metabolic storage disease. Placenta 1990;11:395–411.

Kleihauer E, Braun H, Betke K. Demonstration von fetalem Hämoglobin in den Erythrocyten eines Blutausstriches. Klin Wochenschr 1957;35:637–638.

Lage JM. Placentomegaly with massive hydrops of placental stem villi, diploid DNA content, and omphaloceles: possible association with Beckwith-Wiedemann syndrome. Hum Pathol 1991;22:591–597.

Machin GA. Hydrops revisited: literature review of 1,414 cases published in the 1980s. Am J Med Genet 1989;34:366–390.

Mostoufi-Zadeh M, Weiss LM, Driscoll SG. Nonimmune hydrops fetalis: a challenge in perinatal pathology. Hum Pathol 1985;16:785–789.

Potter EL. Intervillous thrombi in the placenta and their possible relation to erythroblastosis fetalis. Am J Obstet Gynecol 1948;56:959–961.

Roberts DJ, Ampola MG, Lage JM. Diagnosis of unsuspected fetal metabolic storage disease by routine placental examination. Pediatr Pathol 1991;11: 647–656.

Santamaria M, Benirschke K, Carpenter PM, et al. Transplacental hemorrhage associated with placental neoplasms. Pediatr Pathol 987;7:601–615.

Schröder J. Review article: transplacental passage of blood cells. J Med Genet 1975;12:230–242.

Stonehill LL, LaFerla JJ. Assessment of fetomaternal hemorrhage with Kleihauer-Betke test. Am J Obstet Gynecol 1986;155:1146.

Chapter 21

Fetal Thrombotic Vasculopathy

General Considerations

The umbilical vessels insert onto the placental surface, branch, and then at the periphery turn abruptly toward the maternal surface, branching repeatedly to finally become villous capillaries. Blood is returned from the capillary loops to the umbilical cord by veins that merge. In the overwhelming majority of cotyledons, there is *a 1:1 relation between artery and vein* at the periphery and each artery "supplies" a single cotyledon (placentone). It is remarkable that at least *the larger arteries always cross over the veins on the placental surface*. They can thus be readily identified by macroscopic examination, while histologically it is nearly impossible to make this distinction. It is interesting to note that the circumferential architecture of the placental surface vessels is asymmetric. This is the result of hemodynamic thinning in that the pressure buckles and thins the superficial portions of the vessels, whereas the "fixed" portions resist this pressure. This phenomenon of thinning of the superficial aspect of chorionic vessels is also shared with cord vessels.

Thrombosis in the Fetal Circulation

Pathologic Features
Thrombosis: **Mural and occlusive thrombi** occur frequently in the superficial placental vessels and their villous ramifications. They are

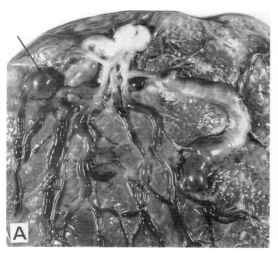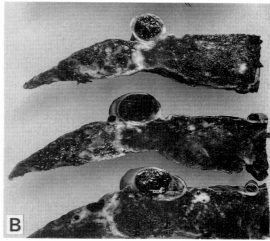

Figure 21.1. (A) Distended surface chorionic vessel (arrow) and a distended and thrombosed vein (at right). (B) Layered thrombi are apparent on cut section of the same placenta.

more commonly present in the veins and are variably located across the fetal surface and within the placenta. They are only occasionally accompanied by thrombi in the umbilical cord. *Surface thrombi can be recognized by careful gross examination.* When the vessel is hugely distended (Figure 21.1), the identification of thrombosis is easy. Much more frequently overlooked are such thrombi as seen in Figure 21.2. When thrombi are fresh, their *gross appearance is that of a slightly enlarged vessel that may have an unusual color, usually tan or white* (Figure 21.3). The vessel is not so shiny and blue as normal vessels. One is also unable to move the blood mechanically in thrombosed vessels.

Mural thrombosis is much more frequent than complete obliteration of the vessel (Figures 21.4, 21.5). Thrombosis may even *calcify* (Figures

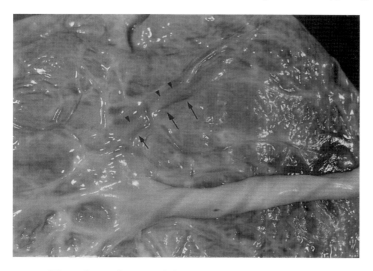

Figure 21.2. Thrombus of an umbilical vein tributary (arrows). The infant developed cerebral palsy.

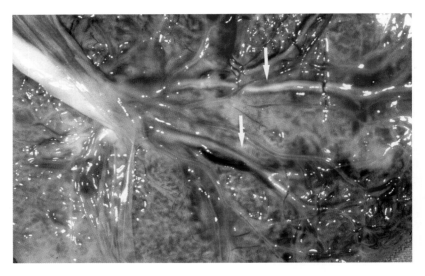

Figure 21.3. Thrombi in chorionic vessels are visible as tan-white streaks (arrows).

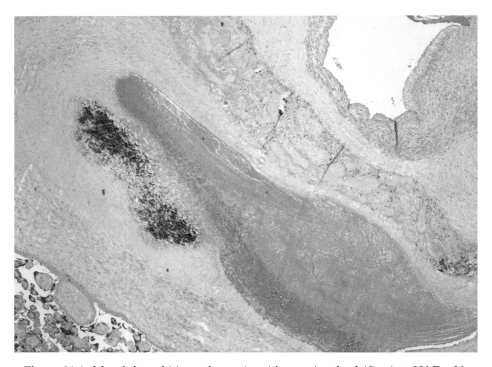

Figure 21.4. Mural thrombi in surface vein with associated calcification. H&E. ×20.

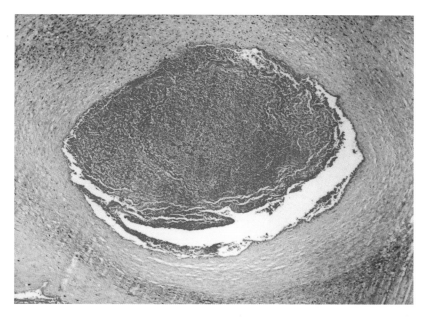

Figure 21.5. Nearly occlusive thrombus in a dilated chorionic vein associated with long cord and stillbirth. H&E. ×20.

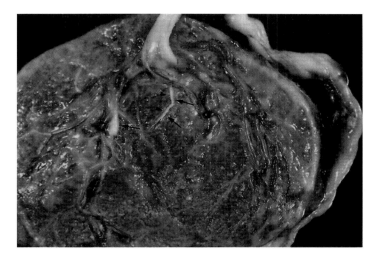

Figure 21.6. Partially calcified thrombi (arrows) associated with a long (77 cm) umbilical cord.

21.6, 21.7) but variations are frequent; and when thrombosis has occurred a *long time before examination, the vessel may obliterate completely. They then appear as a rounded fibromuscular structure without a lumen* (Figure 21.8). True organization of dead tissues, as the pathologist knows it from renal or splenic infarcts, is rare in all placental degenerative lesions. That is, removal of debris by phagocytes and ingrowth of

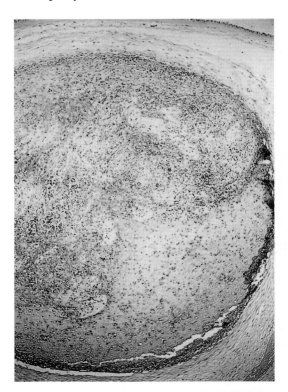

Figure 21.7. Occlusive thrombus with partial calcification (right margin) of surface vein. H&E. ×26.

granulation tissue and fibrous tissue are phenomena not seen in true placental infarcts, nor do these occur in thrombosed placental vessels. Rather, these lesions shrink, and some phagocytes may appear, but eventually they become calcified or the vessel atrophies. It may eventually disappear completely, becoming unrecognizable as a former vessel.

Avascular Villi: If the thrombi have been *occlusive for a prolonged time, particularly if the thrombi are present in the arterial circulation*, the villous tree may become avascular and atrophy (Figure 21.9). These villi then become **avascular villi**. Avascular villi are considered direct evidence of thrombosis in the fetal circulation, even without the presence of frank thrombi within vessels. Larger foci of avascular villi may be visible *grossly as a triangular area of pallor with the consistency of villous tissue*. The base is usually at the basal plate, and may be easier to visualize in a fixed specimen. Microscopically, the area is *sharply demarcated* from the surrounding normal villous tissue. Avascular villi differ from true infarction in that the trophoblast is viable because it is still being perfused by the maternal blood in the intervillous space. There may, however, be increased syncytial knotting. The villous vessels and stroma essentially atrophy over time due to loss of the fetal circulation. *The stroma is usually pink and hyalinized without vessels. Occasional hemo-*

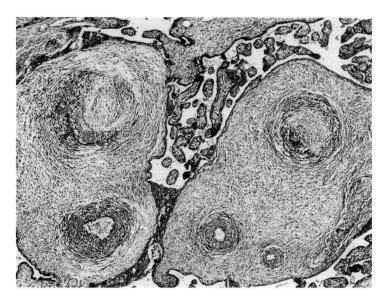

Figure 21.8. Muscular hypertrophy and old occlusions in stem vessels. H&E. ×260.

siderin deposits may be present. At the apex of the lesion, one may occasionally find the supplying artery with thrombosis. In older lesions, the distal stem vessels may show thickening of the vascular walls, ultimately with obliteration of the lumen. Caution must be used in cases of stillbirth, as loss of the entire fetal circulation will cause a similar but diffuse change.

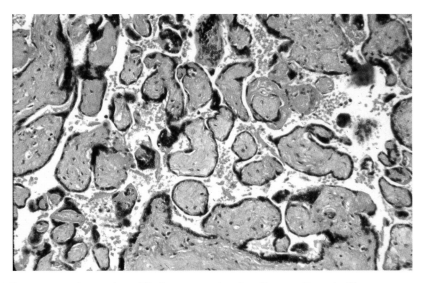

Figure 21.9. Avascular villi demonstrating hyaline quality of villous stroma, which is devoid of vessels. Extensive thrombosis was also present in surface vessels. H&E. ×100.

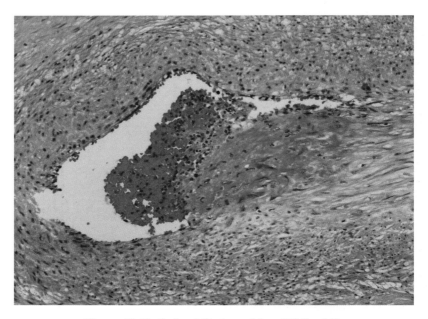

Figure 21.10. Intimal fibrin cushion. H&E. ×100.

Intimal Fibrin Cushions: **Intimal fibrin cushions** or intimal vascular cushions are microscopically similar to those that pathologists find in the pulmonary vessels of patients with pulmonary hypertension. *Laminated fibrin is deposited in the intima of the vessel and bulges out into the lumen like a "cushion"* (Figure 21.10). The lumen is often not obstructed to a significant degree. At times, one may see *accumulation of what appears to be mucopolysaccharide or ground substance within the intima as well*. This appears as pale, blue material separating the vascular smooth muscle from the endothelium. Calcifications may occur in older lesions (Figure 21.11).

Fibromuscular Sclerosis: A vascular lesion of small vessels called **fibromuscular sclerosis** has been found to be associated with abnormal Doppler flow. It is often seen in conjunction with terminal villus deficiency. In this lesion, there is *an increase in the smooth muscle and fibrous tissue of the stem arteries leading to narrowed lumens*. Occasionally, complete occlusion may occur.

Hemorrhagic Endovasculitis: Finally, a group of lesions referred to as **hemorrhagic endovasculitis** or **HEV** have been described. The lesions are divided into two groups, bland and active lesions. **Bland lesions** consist of *extravasated red blood cells in the stroma, karyorrhexis of the nuclei of endothelial and blood cells, and septation* (Figure 21.12). The integrity of the vascular walls is lost, and they may be hard to identify on histologic section. Similar to avascular villi, some of the bland lesions may be present in the setting of fetal demise. In the latter case, they tend to be more diffuse, but the differences are often subtle. **Active lesions** are those with *evidence of inflammatory infiltrates in the villi, which is called*

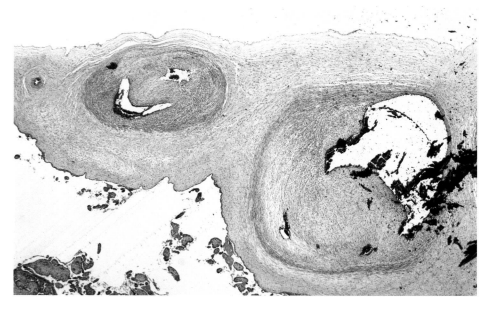

Figure 21.11. Intimal fibrin cushion from same case with calcification in the vessel wall. H&E. ×20.

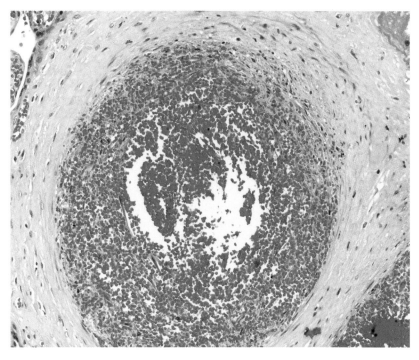

Figure 21.12. Bland hemorrhagic endovasculitis (HEV). Extravasated blood cells are present around this vessel in a stem villus. H&E. ×100.

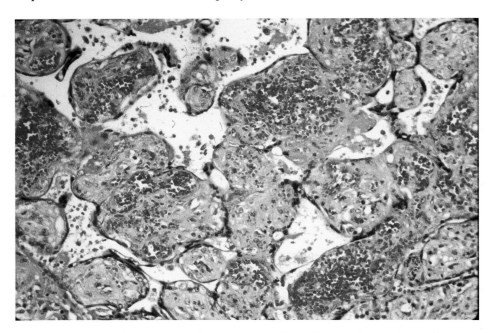

Figure 21.13. Active HEV demonstrating hemorrhagic villitis. There is destruction and necrosis of the vessel wall and karyorrhexis. H&E. ×200.

hemorrhagic villitis, or necrosis and destruction of the vascular walls (Figure 21.13). Active lesions may involve all types of vessels, from the large stem vessels down to the villous capillaries. Associations with poor neonatal outcome are stronger with active lesions. HEV also has a recurrence rate of 28% in subsequent pregnancies.

Pathogenesis

Thrombosis clearly bespeaks a pathologic prenatal environment. Thrombotic lesions may form in the venous or arterial circulation and may involve umbilical vessels (see Figure 15.24, page 271), chorionic vessels, large and small stem vessels, and villous capillaries. Arterial thrombosis is much less common than thrombosis in the venous circulation. *Significant obstruction in the arterial circulation* will rob the "downstream" villi of their vascular supply. Whenever the fetal circulation is lost but the maternal circulation is maintained, there will be loss of the fetal vasculature but the trophoblastic cells will be left intact. The villi then become sclerotic or **avascular** (see Figure 21.9). The presence of avascular villi can be considered direct evidence of the presence of thrombosis.

Thrombi may develop when blood flow through the umbilical cord is compromised, and here the problem is *primarily in the venous circulation*. Cord accidents such as *excessively long cords, excessive spiraling, true umbilical cord knots, cord entanglement, and velamentous cord insertion* are common antecedents. Mechanical obstruction of the cord will initially lead to compression of the umbilical vein, as it is more pliable than the umbilical arteries. *Occlusion of blood flow in the venous circula-*

tion leads to congestion, venous stasis, and increased intraluminal pressure, which in turn results in endothelial injury and subsequent thrombosis. Venous stasis also may lead to vasospasm, further compromising the circulation. Thrombosis may also be seen in the arterial circulation, and in this case it is more likely to be associated with abnormal coagulative states in the mother or the fetus.

The origin of **intimal fibrin cushions** is not completely clear, but it is thought that they either are *"organized" mural thrombi or are an early stage of thrombosis.* The fact that they may be associated with calcifications suggests an older lesion, at least in those cases. They are also often associated with venous hypertension. Thrombi and cushions are most common in placental surface veins and in major villous stem vessels (see Figure 21.10). They often have mural thrombi overlying them. It may be that the cushions form first and then, after much distension and elevated pressure, their endothelial surface degenerates and mural thrombosis develops.

Venoocclusive disease has also been implicated in the development of **hemorrhagic endovasculitis (HEV)**. This entity has aroused much controversy. It was initially identified in the study of many placentas from perinatal deaths and infants with perinatal problems, and it was hypothesized that HEV played an important role in the etiology of these tragedies. HEV is, in effect, a *microangiopathy that etiologically and pathologically resembles the glomerulopathy of the hemolytic uremic syndrome* and is often referred to as a *vasodisruptive* process. It is postulated that, as in frank thrombosis, there is *endothelial injury and vessel necrosis, which leads to fragmentation of RBCs and extravasation of these fragments into the villous stroma.* It is strongly associated with thrombosis as well. The etiology of HEV has been hotly debated and this is, in part, because the histologic picture is often seen in placentas of stillborns and that some of the features can be directly related to loss of fetal circulation to the villous tissue.

Clinical Features and Implications

Venous thrombosis is associated with *compromise of blood flow through the umbilical cord* secondary to cord entanglement, abnormal insertion, and abnormal length or coiling. Thrombosis may also be seen associated with *maternal or fetal thrombophilias* such as the Factor V Leiden mutation, activated protein C resistance, protein S deficiency, protein C deficiency, lupus anticoagulant, and antiphospholipid antibodies (see Chapter 18). *Maternal diabetes* is occasionally associated with thrombosis in the placenta or neonate or both, but there are no other morphologic or clinical features to explain the cause of this fetal vascular coagulation. *Severe chorioamnionitis,* particularly when there is a fetal response, may be associated with thrombosis in fetal vessels. This occurs secondary to damage to the endothelium and vessel wall from the inflammatory changes. Finally, thrombosis has also been associated with *vascular anomalies and various forms of trauma.*

Fetal thrombotic vasculopathy as a whole has been strongly associated with *preeclampsia, intrauterine growth restriction (IUGR), intrauterine fetal demise (IUFD), seizures, and amputation necrosis.* Prenatal and neonatal thrombosis has been described in the central nervous system (CNS), pulmonary circulation, and renal vessels. *Neonatal stroke, cerebral degenerative changes, abnormalities in brain imaging, cerebral palsy, and poor long-term neurologic outcome* have also been described.

> *Suggestions for Examination and Report:*
> *Fetal Thrombotic Vasculopathy*
>
> **Gross Examination:** When gross thrombi are noted or there is a clinical history of cord problem or thrombosis, additional sections of fetal surface vessels should be submitted.
>
> **Comment:** Specific lesions should be listed. Thrombosis may explain poor perinatal outcome, and findings should be correlated with clinical history of coagulopathy, diabetes, or cord problems.

Selected References

PHP4, Chapter 12, pages 375–384.

Baergen RN, Chacko SA, Edersheim T, et al. The placenta in thrombophilias: a clinicopathologic study. Mod Pathol 2001;14:213A.

Baergen RN, Malicki D, Behling CA, et al. Morbidity, mortality and placental pathology in excessively long umbilical cords. Pediatr Dev Pathol 2001; 4:144–153.

Boué DR, Stanley C, Baergen RN. Placental pathology casebook. J Perinatol 1995;15429–25431.

De Sa DJ. Intimal cushions in foetal placental veins. J Pathol 1973;110:347–352.

Fok RY, Pavlova Z, Benirschke K, et al. The correlation of arterial lesions with umbilical artery Doppler velocimetry in placentas of small-for-dates pregnancies. Obstet Gynecol 1990;75:578–583.

Fox H. Thrombosis of foetal arteries in the human placenta. J Obstet Gynaecol Br Commonw 1966;73:961–965.

Heifetz SA. Thrombosis of the umbilical cord: analysis of 52 cases and literature review. Pediatr Pathol 1988;8:37–54.

Kraus FT, Achen VI. Fetal thrombotic vasculopathy in the placenta. Cerebral thrombi, infarct, coagulopathy and cerebral palsy. Hum Pathol 1999;30: 759–769.

Rayne SC, Kraus FT. Placental thrombi and other vascular lesions: classification, morphology, and clinical correlations. Pathol Res Pract 1993;189:2–17.

Redline RW, Pappin A. Fetal thrombotic vasculopathy: the clinical significance of extensive avascular villi. Hum Pathol 1995;26:80.

Sander CH. Hemorrhagic endovasculitis and hemorrhagic villitis of the placenta. Arch Pathol Lab Med 1980;104:371–373.

Sander CM, Gilliland D, Flynn MA, et al. Risk factors for recurrence of hemorrhagic endovasculitis of the placenta. Obstet Gynecol 1997;89:569–576.

Shen-Schwarz S, Macpherson TA, Mueller-Heubach E. The clinical significance of hemorrhagic endovasculitis of the placenta. Am J Obstet Gynecol 1988; 159:48–51.

Section VI

Neoplasms and Gestational Trophoblastic Disease

This section covers primary and metastatic tumors of the placenta and trophoblastic disease. It starts in Chapter 22 with a discussion of the primary tumors seen in the placenta as well as tumors that may metastasize from the mother or the fetus. Gestational trophoblastic disease is discussed in the following chapters. Hydatidiform moles are covered in Chapter 23, choriocarcinoma in Chapter 24, and lesions of extravillous trophoblast in Chapter 25.

Chapter 22

Neoplasms

General Considerations

There are only a few primary neoplasms of the placenta, but there is a wide variety of maternal malignancies that metastasize to the placenta. This reflects the diversity of neoplasms seen in the maternal population. Fetal tumors may also metastasize to the placenta, but these tumors are derived from a smaller group of congenital neoplasms.

Primary Placental Neoplasms

Chorangioma (Angioma)

Pathogenesis

Angiomas are the most common benign tumor of the placenta. Tumors that have been designated **chorioangiomas**, **chorangiomas**, **angiomyxomas**, **fibroangiomyxomas**, and **fibromas** are essentially the same lesion, usually designated simply **chorangioma**. The incidence of these tumors is 1 in 9,000 to 1 in 50,000 placentas. When careful study and sectioning of placentas is undertaken, the prevalence may be as high as 1 in 100. Chorangiomas occur more frequently in Caucasian than in African-American mothers, more often with *multiple gestations*, and more often with *malformed neonates*, particularly infants with hemangiomas. This finding suggests that this tumor may be a congenital malformation or hamartoma, rather than a true neoplasm. Clonal studies, which would differentiate these lesions, have not been done. Interestingly, the incidence of chorangiomas in high-altitude populations such as in Nepal is reported to be from 2.5% to 7.6%, which is much greater than the incidence at lower elevations. In addition, chorangiomas may be associated with *elevated nucleated red blood cells* (*NRBCs*) in the fetal circulation, suggesting that a hypoxic stimulus leads to the excessive villous capillary proliferation. While still speculative, such angiogenesis may well be regulated by vascular growth factors.

Pathologic Features

Grossly, chorangiomas are sharply circumscribed from the surrounding parenchyma and often *bulge from the fetal surface of the placenta* (Figure 22.1). When they are embedded deeper in the villous tissue, they are almost always located closer to the fetal surface. The color and consistency of the cut surface is variable, from a *dark red*, *soft appearance similar to a blood clot to a firm, white lesion similar to an infarct* (Figures 22.2, 22.3). If there is associated fetal hydrops (see below), the entire placenta may be enlarged and edematous. Extremely large tumors may occur (Figure 22.4), and the record is probably held by a 1500-g tumor measuring 30 by 20 by 5 cm. This tumor was associated with placenta previa, hydramnios, preeclampsia, and abruptio placentae. The 32 week gestation fetus weighed 1000 g and died of anemia and hypoxia.

Microscopically, the typical chorangioma is *composed of a proliferation of fetal blood vessels, usually supported by scant connective tissue* (Figures 22.5, 22.6). The vessels comprising the tumor may be capillary or sinusoidal. The *stromal component is frequently abundant*, and the lesion may then resemble a fibroma (Figure 22.7). When Wharton's jelly-like material participates in formation of the tumor, the appearance is that

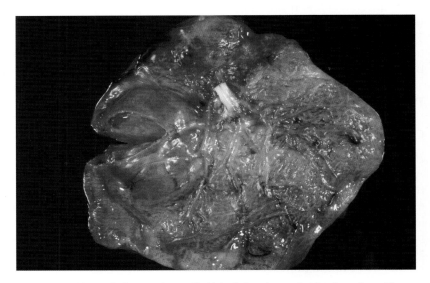

Figure 22.1. Typical chorangioma (left) bulging from the fetal surface. The cut surface is hemorrhagic.

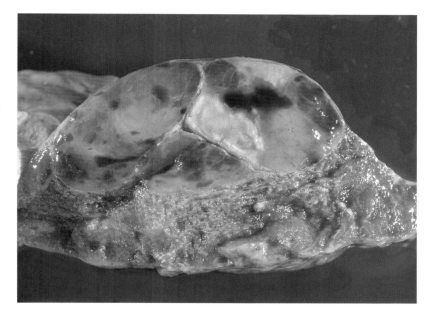

Figure 22.2. Chorangioma. The cut surface is heterogeneous with some areas having the appearance of a blood clot while others appear more fibrous. Normal placental tissue is seen underlying the tumor.

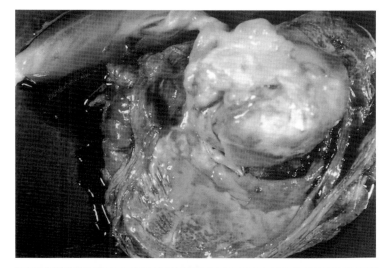

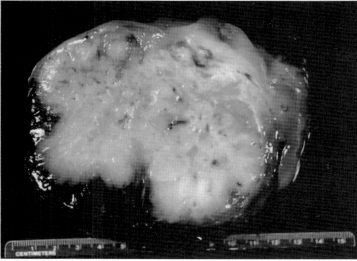

Figure 22.3. A 900-g chorangioma with marked edema of the umbilical cord. There was villous edema and neonatal cardiac failure. Cut section (bottom) appears white and somewhat gelatinous.

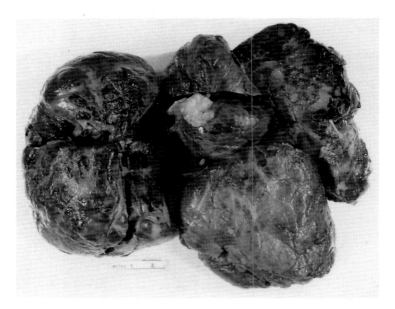

Figure 22.4. Exceptionally large (400-g) chorangioma shelled out from its placenta. The infant was stillborn and had cardiomegaly. The surface in this case had a fibromyxoid appearance.

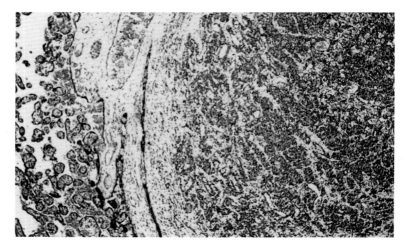

Figure 22.5. Typical microscopic appearance of a chorangioma with marked congestion of the vessels. The convexity of the tumor is covered by syncytiotrophoblast. H&E. ×160.

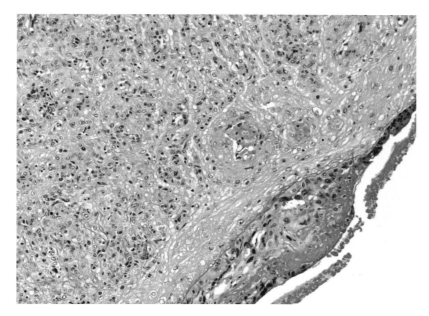

Figure 22.6. This chorangioma has numerous capillaries in an enlarged villus covered by syncytium. The vessels in this case contain little blood. H&E. ×40.

of a *myxomatous neoplasm*. The latter is particularly frequent when a chorangioma arises near the base of the umbilical cord. In such cases, a mucicarmine stain reveals the presence of mucin. *Capillary, cavernous, endotheliomatous, fibrosing*, and *fibromatous* tumors have been differentiated, but such precision is unwarranted as the clinical outcome depends more on the size of the mass than on its composition. Chorangiomas are invariably *covered by trophoblast*, and one may envisage them

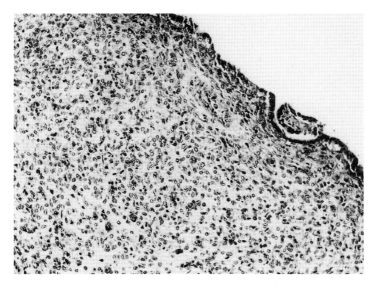

Figure 22.7. Chorangioma with primarily fibromatous appearance. The cellularity of the lesion may suggest a sarcoma. H&E. ×170.

to be the proliferation of vessels within a villus whose surface thus expands. Recent studies have suggested that chorangiomas arise from stem villi rather than terminal villi, as previously thought. These tumors often have *degenerative changes, calcification, infarction, and thrombosis.* They may also be multiple and in some cases have been recurrent. Being characterized by an increase in the villous vessels, chorangiomas have features in common with chorangiomatosis and chorangiosis, both of which are discussed in Chapter 19. Uncommonly, chorangiomas have marked cellularity, cytologic atypia, and prominent mitoses. However, despite this appearance the tumors are invariably benign; metastases and true invasion have never been described.

Clinical Features and Implications

The relation of chorangioma to *hydramnios* and *fetal hydrops,* particularly in large tumors, is well known. Other complications include *stillbirth, fetal growth restriction, anemia, cardiomegaly, heart failure, disseminated intravascular coagulation, transplacental hemorrhage, premature delivery, abruptio, and preeclampsia.* Many complications are secondary to transplacental hemorrhage or sequestration of blood. Thus, large tumors are more likely to be associated with severe complications. *Thrombocytopenia,* which is often observed in these newborns, is secondary to sequestration of platelets within the tumor. Repetitive multiple chorangiomas have been described in several families, sometimes associated with recurrent fetal demise. Whether isolated chorangiomas can occur repetitively is unknown.

Chorangiocarcinoma

Chorangiocarcinoma is a lesion with features similar to both chorangioma and choriocarcinoma. Reported cases have depicted a *solitary lesion typical of a chorangioma whose surface, however, was covered by proliferating trophoblastic cells.* No untoward sequelae have been noted and there is no chemical or cytochemical evidence of choriocarcinoma. Therefore, this tumor is most likely a variant of chorangioma.

Suggestions for Examination and Report: Chorangioma

Gross Examination: Note size, location, and gross appearance of the tumor or tumors. Representative sections of the tumor should be submitted.

Comment: Large chorangiomas may be associated with anemia, thrombocytopenia, hydrops, growth restriction, and stillbirth.

Leiomyoma

There have been several reported cases of tumors morphologically compatible with **leiomyomas**, located within the placental tissue and covered by decidua at the maternal surface. Easy separation of the tumors from the uterus suggests these may not be uterine primaries. However, molecular studies on one reported case confirmed its maternal origin. Furthermore, no intrinsic structures in the placenta contain smooth muscle. For these reasons, it is likely these are *primary uterine leiomyomas that have become parasitic*, losing their vascular connection to the uterus and stealing a new blood supply from the placenta. These tumors have not been associated with adverse outcome.

Teratomas Versus Acardiac Twinning

Masses of tissue composed of *ectodermal, mesodermal, and endodermal elements* have been noted in the fetal membranes, umbilical cord, and chorionic plate of the placenta (see also Chapter 14, Tumors). In cases where either umbilical cord structures or axial skeleton are present, they are usually considered a component of an acardiac twin. There is, however, disagreement over those cases that do not contain either of these elements. Because proof of neoplastic origin has not been presented, we believe that true teratomas of the placenta likely do not exist and that these cases represent variants of acardiac twining.

Hepatocellular Adenoma

Several cases of **hepatocellular adenoma** in the placenta have been reported. Grossly, they have been *tan-white, sharply delimited*, and present in intervillous or subchorionic locations. Microscopically, they *are composed of polyhedral cells with the appearance of hepatocytes*. The cells contain glycogen, and some show reactivity with antibodies to α-fetoprotein, α_1-antitrypsin, and carcinoembryonic antigen, convincing evidence of hepatic differentiation. No portal areas or central veins are seen, but study by electron microscopy has shown structures that resemble bile canaliculi. These lesions may originate from displaced yolk sac structures. The clinical course for both fetus and mother is benign.

Heterotopia

Heterotopic tissues, such as **adrenal gland** and **liver**, occasionally occur in the placenta. Suggested mechanisms for the origin of these tissues have included embolic spread via the fetal vasculature, monodermal teratoma, and abnormal mesodermal differentiation. No sequelae have been reported.

Suggestions for Examination and Report: Miscellaneous Neoplasms and Heterotopia

Gross Examination: Grossly, neoplasms and heterotopias usually present as a mass, which should be liberally sampled for microscopic examination.

Comment: The diagnosis of the various lesions should be given, and a comment may be included indicating the lack of adverse clinical sequelae.

Maternal Neoplasms Metastatic to the Placenta

Clinical Features and Implications
Maternal malignancy occurs in approximately 1 in 1000 pregnancies. Metastasis to the placenta is, however, rare, with only about 70 reported cases in the literature. The most common tumor to metastasize to the placenta is *melanoma*. Carcinomas of the *breast, cervix, gastrointestinal tract, and lung* occur less frequently, and there are rare reports of metastases from the *pancreas, ovary,* and *skin*, as well as metastases from *medulloblastoma* and *rhabdomyosarcoma*. It is interesting to note that melanoma metastasizes so commonly, as it is not frequent in the pregnant population. This phenomenon is probably due to the hematogenous dissemination in melanoma and to the fact that melanoma patients are more likely to have advanced disease. Many placental metastases occur in patients with end-stage disease who presumably had a significant tumor burden, facilitating vascular spread to the placenta.

Transplacental metastasis to the fetus is much rarer than placental metastasis. Here again, *melanoma is most common*, but cases of *lymphoma, leukemia, and pulmonary adenocarcinoma* have been reported. Many cases have resulted in neonatal death, but there are also reports of spontaneous regression. The immunologic ramifications of these cases remain to be studied. *Because of the occurrence of fetal metastasis, although rare, it is recommended that all placentas from patients with a diagnosis of malignancy be examined histologically.*

Pathologic Features
Placental metastases often go unnoticed. In many cases, the lesions are not visible grossly, while in other cases they are overlooked, as they may appear *similar to infarcts*. Microscopically, metastases usually consist of clusters of *malignant cells in the intervillous space* (Figure 22.8). In some cases, *invasion of the villous structures and even the fetal vasculature may occur*. However, the latter feature does not correlate well with the presence of metastasis to the infant. Often these intervillous collections do not show vascularization, leading some authors to call them "pseudometastases." In the case of maternal **leukemia**, metastasis cannot be documented merely by the presence of leukemic cells in the intervillous space, but must be made by the presence of leukemic cells in the villous tissue and/or fetal vessels.

Suggestions for Examination and Report: Maternal Metastasis to the Placenta

Gross Examination: Metastatic lesions are usually not grossly visible, but, if large, may appear similar to an infarct. In the context of a maternal malignancy, any parenchymal lesion should be sampled. If no gross lesions are present, additional random sections should be submitted.

Comment: If metastases are present, characterization of the type of metastasis and comparison with the maternal primary is

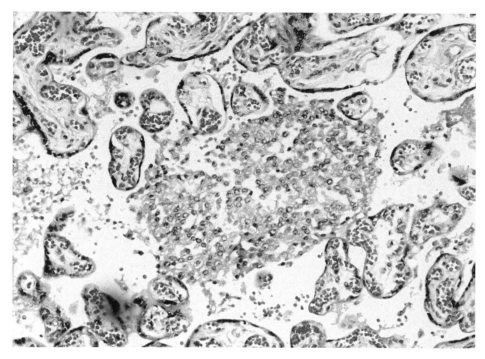

Figure 22.8. Metastatic melanoma to the placenta. Note the large, atypical cells present in the intervillous space. The mother had widespread metastases at the time of delivery and died 1 month later. H&E. ×200.

optimal. Immunohistochemistry may be necessary to fully evaluate the malignant cells. In addition, involvement of the villous stroma or fetal vessels should also be noted. The fact that fetal metastasis is a possible, although rare, complication may also be stated.

Fetal Neoplasms Metastatic to the Placenta

Malignant Fetal Tumors

Congenital malignancies include **neuroblastoma**, **lymphoma**, **leukemia**, **sarcomas**, **brain tumors**, **hepatoblastoma**, and **teratomas**. Metastases from these neoplasms to the placenta are rare but do occur. Congenital **neuroblastoma** has repeatedly been shown to cause fetal heart failure, hydrops, and death, but the pathogenesis of hydrops remains to be identified. Grossly, the *placenta is markedly enlarged.* On histologic examination, the villi are *enlarged, edematous, and have increased numbers of Hofbauer cells with persistent villous cytotrophoblast. Cords of neuroblastoma cells may be found in fetal capillaries,* sometimes accompanied by erythroblasts (Figure 22.9). Neuroblastoma cells may also infiltrate the villous tissue. Fetal hydrops and placentomegaly may also be seen in association with fetal **hepatoblastoma**. Similar to neuroblastoma, the placental metastases consist of *malignant, immature-*

appearing cells filling the villous capillaries. Due to the lack of differentiation, immunohistochemistry may be necessary to identify the true nature of these cells. **Sacrococcygeal teratomas** may produce *placentomegaly, fetal edema, hydramnios, and elevated human chorionic gonadotropin (hCG) levels.* On histologic examination, one sees only large numbers of *nucleated red blood cells in the villous capillaries.* There is one reported case of a teratoma with placental metastasis within villous vessels. Last, fetal **leukemia** occurs rarely and placental involvement is even rarer. When it does occur, it is also associated with placentomegaly. On microscopic examination, villous capillaries are packed with leukemic cells, which may extend into the villous stroma (Figure 22.10). Diagnosis can be quite difficult on placental tissue alone.

Benign "Metastatic" Lesions

Fetal giant pigmented nevi have been described in the placenta, usually as *multiple foci of pigmented nevus cells in the villi.* Occasionally, there is extensive placental involvement but the lesions are considered benign. The cells may derive from early neural crest cell migration.

> ### Suggestions for Examination and Report: Fetal Neoplasms Metastatic to the Placenta
>
> **Gross Examination**: When a fetal malignancy is known, additional sections of placenta should be submitted for identification of metastases.
>
> **Comment**: Diagnosis of the neoplasm is essential and may require immunohistochemistry. As with maternal malignancy, the location and extent of involvement should also be mentioned.

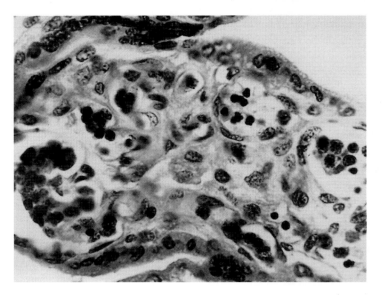

Figure 22.9. Villus from a case of congenital neuroblastoma. The enlarged villus has numerous neuroblastoma cells within the villous capillaries, some of which show rosetting. H&E. ×400.

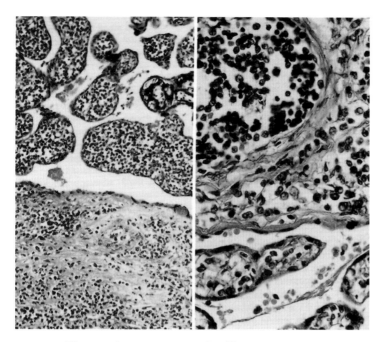

Figure 22.10.   Placenta from a macerated stillborn with presumed leukemia. The villous capillaries are packed with leukemic cells, and some stromal infiltration is seen. H&E. Left ×60; right ×160.

Selected References

PHP4, Chapter 16, pages 471–472 (Fetal Tumors); Chapter 24, pages 778–789 (Benign Tumors).

Baergen RN, Johnson D, Moore T, et al. Maternal melanoma metastatic to the placenta. Arch Pathol Lab Med 1997;121:508–511.

Benirschke K. Recent trends in chorangiomas, especially those of multiple and recurrent chorangiomas. Pediatr Dev Pathol 1999;2:264–269.

Doss BJ, Vicari J, Jacques SM, et al. Placental involvement in congenital hepatoblastoma. Pediatr Dev Pathol 1998;1:538–542.

Ernst LM, Hui P, Parkash V. Intraplacental smooth muscle tumor: a case report. Int J Gynecol Pathol 2001;29:284–288.

Guschman M, Vogel M, Urban M. Adrenal tissue in the placenta. A heterotopia caused by migration and embolism? Placenta 2000;21:427–431.

Khalifa MA, Gersell DJ, Hansen CH, et al. Hepatic (hepatocellular) adenoma of the placenta: a study of four cases. Int J Gynecol Pathol 1998;17:241–244.

Lentz SE, Coulson CC, Gocke CD, et al. Placental pathology in maternal and neonatal myeloproliferative disorders. Obstet Gynecol 1998;91:863–864.

Leung JC, Mann S, Salafia CM, et al. Sacrococcygeal teratoma with vascular placental dissemination. Obstet Gynecol 1999;93:856.

Lynn AA, Parry SI, Morgan M, et al. Disseminated congenital neuroblastoma involving the placenta. Arch Pathol Lab Med 1997;121:741–744.

Majlessi HF, Wagner KM, Brooks JJ. Atypical cellular chorangioma of the placenta. Int J Gynecol Pathol 1983;1:403–408.

Qureshi F, Jacques SM. Adrenocortical heterotopia in the placenta. Pediatr Pathol Lab Med 1995;15:51–56.

Chapter 23

Hydatidiform Moles

General Considerations

Understanding early trophoblastic development is essential to the discussion and categorization of trophoblastic lesions. Therefore, a brief review is presented here (see also Chapter 8, Extravillous Trophoblast). After fertilization, the blastocyst differentiates into embryonic and extraembryonic cells, the latter becoming **trophoblast**, the forerunner of the placenta. The trophoblastic cells further differentiate into villous and extravillous trophoblast. **Villous trophoblast** consists of *villous cytotrophoblast and syncytiotrophoblast.* **Extravillous trophoblast** is composed of the trophoblast of the *chorionic plate, chorion laeve, cell islands, septa, implantation site*, and *basal plate*. Currently, the term "intermediate" trophoblast is commonly used to represent all types of extravillous trophoblast. Unfortunately, however, it has also been used to refer to a type of *villous* trophoblast that is transitional between cytotrophoblast and syncytiotrophoblast. This is incorrect because extravillous trophoblast, or "intermediate trophoblast," by definition **cannot** be villous trophoblast. Therefore, the use of the term "intermediate tro-

Table 23.1. WHO classification of gestational trophoblastic disease

Hydatidiform mole
  Complete mole
  Partial mole
  Invasive mole
  Metastatic mole

Trophoblastic neoplasms
  Choriocarcinoma
  Placental site trophoblastic tumor
  Epithelioid trophoblastic tumor

Nonneoplastic, nonmolar trophoblastic lesions
  Placental site nodule and plaque
  Exaggerated placental site

Source: From Tavassoli FA, Devilee P. World Health Organization classification of tumours: pathology and genetics. Tumours of the breast and female genital organs. Lyon, France: IARC Press, 2003.

phoblast" should be abandoned. Simply stated, *villous and extravillous trophoblast are derived from different pathways of trophoblastic differentiation, and lesions arising from these cells have different morphologic features, clinical attributes, and biologic behavior.*

Trophoblastic lesions comprise a complex and challenging group of lesions that are unique in pathology for the following reasons:

- They are composed, partly or exclusively, of genetic maternal derived from another individual.
- They have counterparts that arise from gonadal germ cells rather than a conceptus.
- The nonneoplastic cells have features usually only associated with malignancy:
  - Destructive **stromal invasion** (in the implantation site),
  - Distant **deportation** of cells into the maternal circulation during pregnancy, and
  - **Cytologic features of malignancy.**

Trophoblastic lesions are classified as into several groups (Table 23.1). Hydatidiform moles are nonneoplastic lesions derived from villous trophoblast. They are divided into complete, partial, and invasive types. Choriocarcinoma, a malignant tumor of gestational trophoblastic origin, also derives from villous trophoblast. The remaining lesions, placental site trophoblastic tumor, exaggerated placental site, and placental site nodule, derive from extravillous trophoblast.

Hydatidiform Moles

Pathogenesis

Hydatidiform moles are not neoplasms. They are, however, *associated with an increased risk for the development of neoplasms*, specifically **choriocarcinoma**, a highly malignant tumor of trophoblastic origin (see Chapter 24). Traditionally, moles have been subdivided into complete and partial hydatidiform moles. **Complete hydatidiform moles** have a genetic complement that is *androgenetic, that is, all the genetic material is paternally derived.* In most instances, they result from *an ovum that has lost its nucleus, an "empty egg," and then is fertilized by a single sperm. Subsequent duplication of the haploid spermatozoal complement* leads to a diploid genotype (Figure 23.1 A). Thus, complete moles are usually

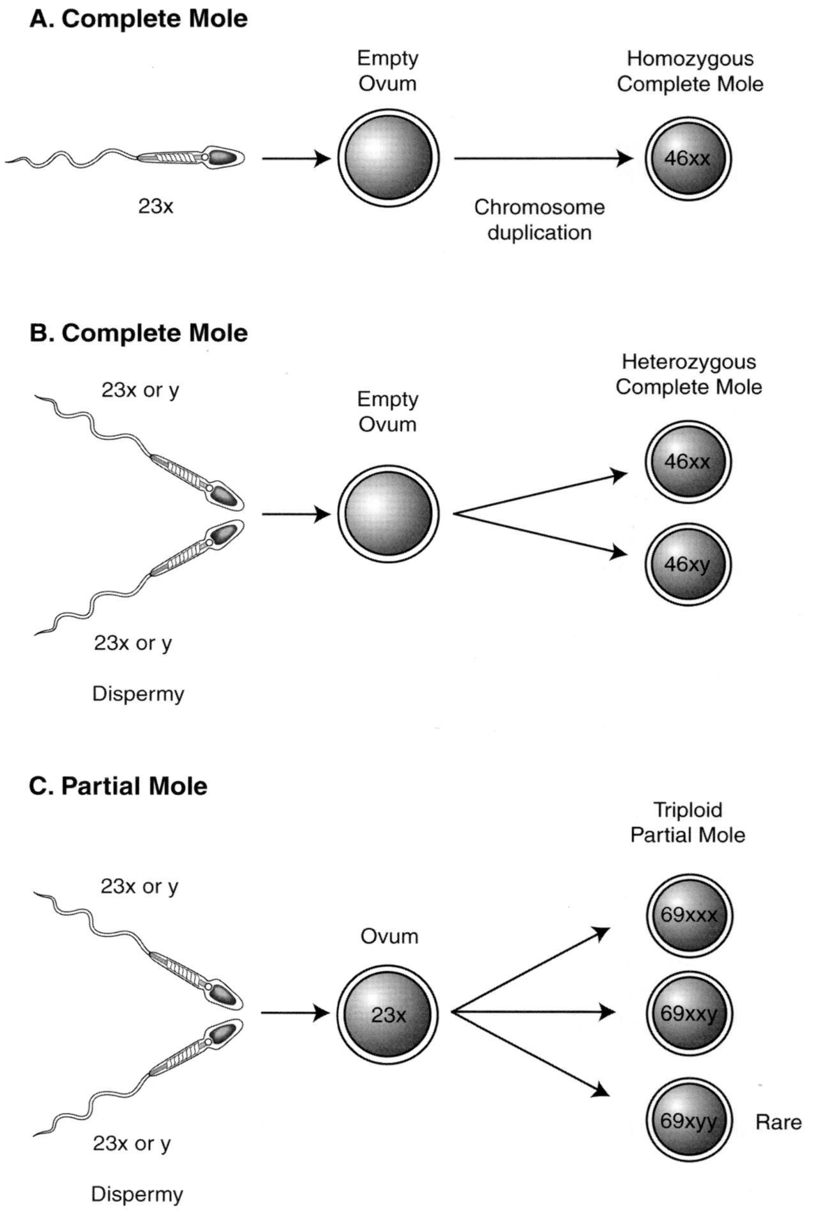

A. Complete Mole

B. Complete Mole

C. Partial Mole

Figure 23.1. Origin of complete and partial hydatidiform moles. (A) Complete moles most commonly arise from fertilization of an empty ovum by a single sperm that then undergoes duplication of its chromosomes. (B) Less commonly, complete moles arise from dispermy in which two sperm fertilize an empty ovum. (C) Partial moles arise from two sperm fertilizing a single ovum.

46XX. A small number of complete moles are 46XY. These, along with a minority of 46XX moles, arise from *dispermy, that is, fertilization of an empty egg by two sperm with fusion of the two male pronuclei* (Figure 23.1 B). Moles with a 46YY karyotype are not found, and it is assumed that this is a lethal condition with limited survival. Dispermy represents about 15% of all complete moles. Triploid and tetraploid complete moles occur rarely; these are also derived solely from paternal DNA. In comparison, **partial hydatidiform moles** are *usually triploid.* They develop from *fertilization of an ovum by two sperm, leading to a paternal to maternal chromosome ratio of 2:1* (Figure 23.1 C). Thus, partial moles are generally 69XXX, 69XXY, or rarely 69XYY. Tetraploid partial moles have also been described and have a paternal to maternal chromosome ratio of 3:1.

Imprinting plays a pivotal role in the development of hydatidiform moles. Studies in mice have shown *that paternally derived genes are important for placental development, whereas maternal genes have more influence over fetal development.* Therefore, excess paternal genetic material leads to excessive growth of trophoblastic over fetal tissues, which is the sine quo non for the diagnosis of molar pregnancies. The fetus, if identifiable, is usually small and stunted. Complete moles, having *only* paternal DNA, have more extreme trophoblastic proliferation than partial moles, which maintain some maternal DNA, albeit in the minority. On the other hand, *nonmolar triploid abortuses have a 2:1 maternal to paternal chromosome ratio* and derive from nondisjunction of maternal chromosomes. Because there is a maternal excess of genetic material, they do not show the trophoblastic proliferation seen in moles. Furthermore, in contrast to partial moles, the placenta is often quite small and stunted whereas the fetus is relatively normal in size, even though congenital anomalies are the rule. Maternal triploidy represents only about 10% to 15% of triploid conceptuses overall.

Because identification of an excess paternal contribution is *essential* in the diagnosis of molar pregnancies, various techniques have been developed to confirm paternal origin. These include **polymerase chain reaction, DNA fingerprinting, restriction fragment length polymorphism (RFLP) assessment**, and use of **short tandem repeat-derived DNA polymorphisms**. In addition, **flow cytometry** readily allows the diagnosis of triploidy.

Incidence and Epidemiologic Factors

The incidence of molar pregnancies in the United States is approximately 1 in 1000 to 1 in 2000 pregnancies. There are clear ethnic and geographic differences, with complete moles being particularly common in Hawaii, the Philippines, India, and Japan. The frequency is higher toward the beginning and the end of childbearing age, with the highest incidence in women over 45, but moles have been described in women as young as 12 and as old as 60 years of age. Many other epidemiologic factors have been associated with an increased risk of molar pregnancy. These include race, ethnicity, ABO blood groups, diet, and previous treatment with certain drugs. However, no specific etiologic factor has been confirmed. There *is* an increased incidence of moles with a history of a previous molar pregnancy, which may be explained by a *genetic propensity for loss of chromosomal material from ova*. This is supported by reports of women with multiple recurrent moles from different fathers.

Complete Hydatidiform Moles

Pathologic Features

Macroscopically, complete moles have abundant tissue with *grossly identifiable translucent vesicles* that represent enlarged, hydropic villi. The vesicles are classically described as "grapelike" and may measure 2 cm in diameter or more (Figures 23.2, 23.3). Most or all of the villi show hydropic swelling, and often the uterine cavity is filled with molar tissue (Figure 23.3). Procedural manipulation may, at times, result in collapse of some or all of the vesicles.

On microscopic examination, the villi are *diffusely hydropic* due to massive fluid accumulation, primarily in the terminal villi. *Cisterns are present that consist of central acellular spaces within the hydropic villi.* They form when the connective tissue of the villi dissociates (Figure 23.4). *Trophoblastic hyperplasia is universally present and is a requirement for diagnosis.* Proliferation varies from villus to villus, but is usually *circumferential around the entire villous perimeter and involves both cytotrophoblast and syncytiotrophoblast* (Figure 23.5). *Trophoblastic atypia* is present, manifesting as nuclear pleomorphism and cytoplasmic vacuolization in syncytiotrophoblast. Mitotic figures may be present. Focally, degenerative change of the trophoblast may be present; the villous surface becoming enmeshed in fibrinoid. Many Hofbauer cells may be identified in the villous stroma. *Intervillous thrombi* are also common due to

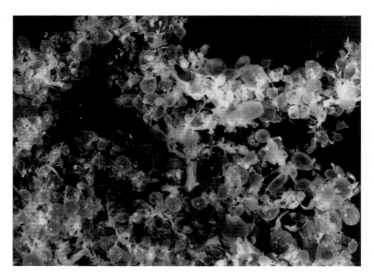

Figure 23.2. Complete hydatidiform mole photographed under water. Note bulbous swelling of terminal villi.

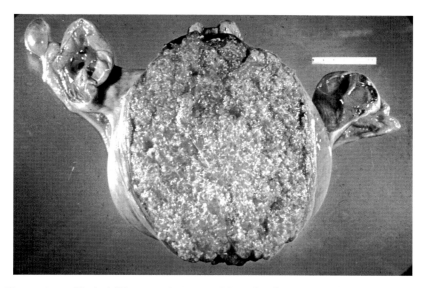

Figure 23.3. Hydatidiform mole in situ. Note the distension of the uterus and the bilateral theca lutein cysts of the ovaries. The vesicular nature of the molar villi is apparent grossly.

the aberrant intervillous circulation. The implantation site frequently shows an exuberant proliferation of implantation trophoblast. This exaggerated physiologic response, called an **exaggerated placental site** (see Chapter 25), is seen commonly enough in complete moles for its presence to be helpful in the differential diagnosis.

There have been many attempts at grading molar pregnancies in an effort to determine which moles are most likely to develop choriocar-

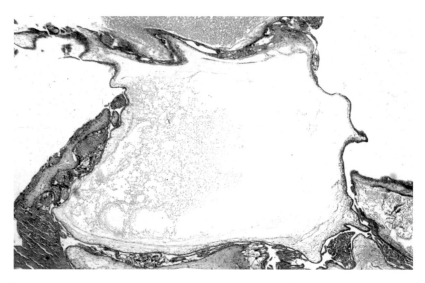

Figure 23.4. Complete mole demonstrating marked villous edema with cistern formation. Note the acellular central region surrounded by edematous, loose stroma, which is usually devoid of blood vessels. H&E. ×120.

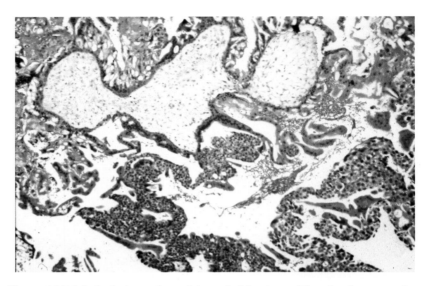

Figure 23.5 Marked circumferential trophoblastic proliferation in a complete mole. H&E. ×100.

cinoma. Classifications based on trophoblastic atypia, proliferation, and so on have been proposed. However, grading has not been found to be of use in predicting behavior. The most important criterion in predicting prognosis is differentiation between partial and complete moles.

Embryonic and Fetal Tissue in Complete Hydatidiform Moles: Traditional teaching has been that complete moles are never associated with an embryo. Even though in the majority of cases embryos are absent, fetal blood vessels and fetal nucleated red blood cells may be encountered in many complete moles and, in rare cases, an embryo may be present. This is logical because the stroma of the villi in complete moles, as with other conceptuses, is derived from **embryonic** mesenchyme. Thus, an embryo must have been present, at least initially. There are several reasons that embryos are rarely seen in complete moles. First, it is quite likely that early embryonic death is common in complete moles. As most moles are homozygous for all their genes, and most individuals have several recessive lethal genes, it makes sense that some of these lethal genes would lead to early death. Second, small, stunted embryos may not be identified in the massive villous tissue and so they may be missed. Last, it is clear from studies of early abortion that the incidence of complete moles is much lower than would be expected. This is probably due to the subtlety of diagnostic features seen in early moles (see below). Therefore, early on when an embryo might still be visible, the diagnosis of a mole is less likely to be made. A documented case is shown in Figure 23.6 in which a complete mole was identified with a tiny embryo and in which the patient later developed disseminated choriocarcinoma. The conclusion is that although embryonic or fetal tissue is rare in complete moles, it is does occur. Therefore, the presence of these elements **does not rule out a complete mole**.

Clinical Features and Implications

Patients with complete moles usually present between the 11th and 25th week of pregnancy with a markedly elevated serum β-hCG. The levels are much higher than expected for the gestational age, in some reaching more than 1,000,000 mI/mL. There may be associated *vaginal bleeding or with an enlarged and distended uterus* ("size greater than dates"). Sonographically, there is *usually* no embryo or demonstrable heart activity and the presence of multiple echogenic signals described as a *"speckled" or "snowstorm."* Sonographic examination used in conjunction with serum β-human chorionic gonadotropin (β-hCG) levels gives a diagnostic accuracy reaching 90%.

Complete moles have been associated with various clinical conditions in the mother, some of which are attributable to the elevated hCG levels. **Multiple theca lutein cysts** or **hyperreactio luteinalis** in the ovary are present in 25% to 60% of patients with complete moles. These "functional" ovarian cysts may grow up to 35 cm in diameter, causing significant ovarian enlargement (see Figure 23.3). The cysts are usually multiple, with thin walls and filled with clear or hemorrhagic fluid. Microscopically, *multiple follicle cysts are lined by luteinized theca cells.*

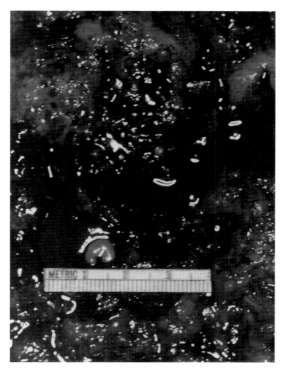

Figure 23.6. Hydatidiform moles with degenerating embryo. This was the third consecutive complete mole and was followed by fatal choriocarcinoma. The tiny embryo is visible above the ruler.

Granulosa cells may also show luteinization. The *ovarian stroma is usually edematous and contains scattered luteinized cells as well* (Figure 23.7). The cysts regress spontaneously after termination of the pregnancy. Moles are also associated with *preeclampsia, eclampsia, pregnancy-induced hypertension, hyperemesis gravidarum, hyperthyroidism, and pulmonary edema,* conditions that spontaneously resolve after evacuation. At least some of these conditions are attributable to the elevated β-hCG levels.

Development of **persistent gestational trophoblastic disease** occurs in approximately 20% of women with a diagnosis of complete mole. Most develop persistent or invasive moles (see below), and 1% to 2% develop **choriocarcinoma**. Early and complete evacuation of the mole is the first line of therapy. Patients with a complete mole are usually followed with serial serum β-hCG levels and concurrent contraception for 6 months to a year or until they fall within the normal range. The reason for contraception is that rises in the titers caused by pregnancy may be confused with the development of persistent disease. If the β-hCG titers do not normalize, or if they rise, persistent trophoblastic disease is usually diagnosed without the benefit of a tissue diagnosis, and chemotherapy is given without pathologic confirmation.

Early Complete Hydatidiform Moles

With the advent of sonography and the early diagnosis and evacuation of moles, specimens at younger gestational ages are being sent for

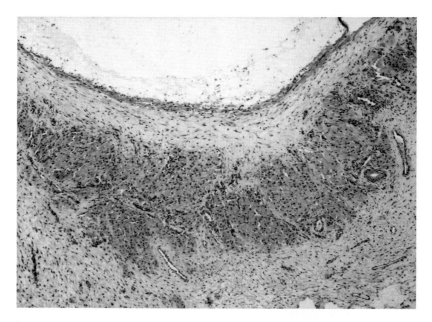

Figure 23.7. Hyperreactio luteinalis of the ovary in a patient with a complete mole. The ovaries are markedly enlarged by numerous luteinized follicle cysts and many luteinized cells in the stroma. A portion of a follicle cyst wall is seen here. H&E. ×40.

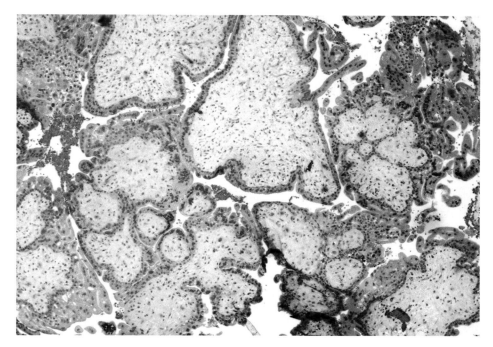

Figure 23.8. Early complete mole with clublike villi and moderate trophoblastic proliferation. The stroma has a myxoid appearance. H&E. ×100.

pathologic evaluation with increasing frequency. **Early complete hydatidiform moles** represent a greater challenge in diagnosis, as *the pathologic features are more subtle and less well developed.* They are thus more difficult to differentiate from partial moles and hydropic abortuses. It is likely that many of these have gone unrecognized in the past. Younger moles tend to have *smaller, less edematous villi, which are more bulbous, club shaped, or "cauliflower" shaped* than older moles (Figure 23.8). The *villous stroma often shows a light blue discoloration or myxoid-like change. Cisternae are poorly formed, and trophoblastic proliferation is not as pronounced* as in the more "mature" mole. Capillary remnants and fetal blood vessels are also more easily found.

Biparental Complete Hydatidiform Moles

Recently, families have been described in which recurrent moles are common. Further study revealed that unlike the usual complete moles, which are completely androgenic, these were **biparental**. This phenomenon results from an abnormal, autosomal recessive gene affecting imprinting. Although the underlying mutation has not been fully described, linkage studies have shown that the gene, which lies on the long arm of chromosome 19, allows greater expression of paternal genes leading to, morphologically, a complete mole. Further study is ongoing.

Ectopic Molar Pregnancy

Partial and complete moles may arise in the fallopian tube, ovary, or other ectopic sites. Moles arising in the fallopian tube are likely to result in *tubal rupture* if not treated promptly. The practice of administering methotrexate to patients with early ectopic pregnancies has interesting implications in the development and behavior of ectopic moles that have yet to be studied. *Overall, moles arising in ectopic locations have similar recurrence rates and risk of development of persistent gestational trophoblastic disease as their intrauterine counterparts.*

Partial Hydatidiform Mole

Pathologic Features

Partial hydatidiform moles are *most commonly triploid with two sets of paternal genes and one set of maternal genes.* The gross and microscopic features are *similar to the complete mole but the features are less striking.* The partial mole is less voluminous and is composed of *normal-appearing villous tissue intermixed with larger, distended villi or vesicles.* An associated embryo or fetal tissue is identified more commonly than in complete moles. Microscopically, partial moles have *an admixture of relatively normal immature villi and distended hydropic villi.* The villous outlines are scalloped and the villi are irregularly edematous. *Although cisterns are present, they tend to be scarce.* Trophoblastic pseudoinclusions, which are due to tangential sectioning of the irregular villous outlines, are easily identified (Figure 23.9). *Focal villous fibrosis may be present.* As

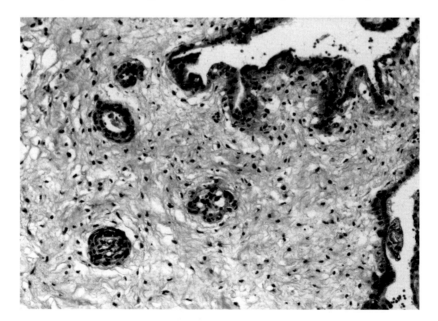

Figure 23.9. Partial hydatidiform mole showing trophoblastic "pseudoinclusions" and irregular invaginations of the villi with moderate edema. H&E. ×200.

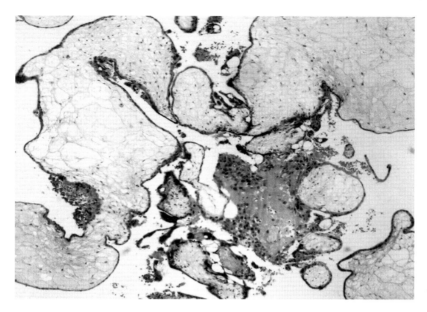

Figure 23.10. Partial mole demonstrating only modest, circumferential trophoblastic proliferation. Two populations of villi are seen here, typical of partial moles. H&E. ×40.

with complete moles, trophoblastic proliferation is required for diagnosis, but *the degree of trophoblastic proliferation and atypia is less* in partial moles (Figure 23.10). *Villous capillaries can usually be found.* Many features, such as trophoblastic pseudoinclusions, are occasionally seen in the chromosomally abnormal abortus.

Four major features have been suggested for partial moles, and if the following diagnostic criteria are not met, consideration should be given to ancillary studies:

- An **admixture of two populations of villi** (normal and hydropic)
- **Enlarged villi with "cavitation"**
- **Irregular villi with scalloped borders and trophoblastic pseudoinclusions**
- **Focal, mild trophoblastic hyperplasia**

Clinical Features and Implications
Patients with partial moles usually present between the 18th and 20th week of gestation with *vaginal bleeding suggestive of a missed abortion,* "size *less* than dates," and *moderate elevations in serum β-hCG.* They also may show findings on sonographic examination similar to that seen for complete moles. Partial moles are associated with **persistent gestational trophoblastic disease** in less than 5% of cases, usually in the form of persistent molar tissue. These patients are generally treated with chemotherapy. There is only one well-documented case of a patient with a partial mole who developed a subsequent malignancy, that is, choriocarcinoma. After a partial mole, patients are followed

with serial β-hCG levels for variable periods, usually at least until it reaches normal levels.

Differential Diagnosis

There is much overlap in the histologic appearance of partial and complete moles, and even experienced pathologists may have difficulty in differentiating between them. Problems usually occur between complete and partial moles, between partial moles and hydropic abortuses, and in diagnosing early moles. These differential diagnoses are discussed below and summarized in Table 23.2.

Table 23.2. Differential diagnosis of complete and partial hydatidiform moles

Characteristic	Hydropic abortus	Complete mole	Early complete mole	Partial mole
Ploidy[a]	Diploid	Diploid	Diploid	Triploid
Paternal: maternal chromosome ratio[a]	1:1	2:0	2:0	2:1
Embryo/fetus	May be present	Rarely present	Rarely present	Often present
Clinical presentation	Missed abortion	Size > dates	±Missed abortion	Size < dates
Serum β-hCG	Normal or low	Markedly elevated	Moderately to markedly elevated	Moderately elevated
Histology				
Villous enlargement	Moderate	Marked	Mild to moderate	Moderate with admixture of normal villi
Villous population	Range of villi from small to hydropic	Relatively uniform population of large hydropic villi	Relatively uniform population of mildly enlarged villi	Two populations of villi, one normal and one moderately hydropic
Villous shape	Round	Round	Clubbed or bulbous	Scalloped with trophoblastic pseudoinclusions
Cisterns	Usually absent	Common	Rare	Rare
Trophoblastic proliferation	None	Marked Circumferential	Moderate Circumferential	Mild to moderate and focal
Trophoblastic atypia	None	Common	Common	Minimal
Fetal blood vessels/ nucleated red blood cells	Usually absent	Rare	May be present	Common
Persistent GTD	No	Up to 20%, may develop choriocarcinoma	Up to 20%, may develop choriocarcinoma	Less than 5%, usually not requiring chemotherapy

[a] Most common presentation, but variations may occur. See text for more information.

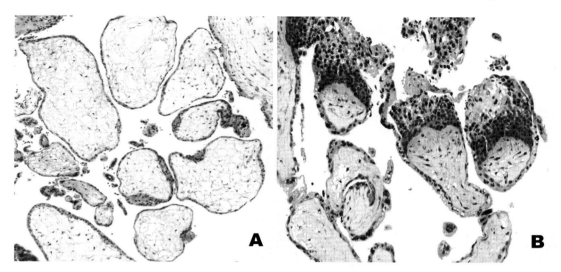

Figure 23.11. (A) Hydropic abortus with marked swelling of the villi. In contrast to a molar pregnancy, the trophoblastic cover is thin and attenuated. H&E ×40. (B) "Polar" proliferation of trophoblast, rather than circumferential proliferation may be present and is a feature which distinguishes hydropic abortuses from partial moles. H&E. ×100.

Hydropic Abortus Versus Partial Mole

Hydropic abortuses tend to have *less tissue than partial moles and do not show grossly identifiable vesicles.* The latter are not present in all partial moles, but are usually present admixed with more normal-appearing tissue. Microscopically, hydropic abortuses and partial moles both show moderate *hydropic change in a portion of the chorionic villi.* The swollen villi of the abortus will be covered by thinned and *attenuated trophoblast* (Figure 23.11 A), and this occurs when the villi swell after embryonic death and the trophoblast is literally stretched over the circumference of the villus. Proliferation of trophoblast may be seen in early abortuses but is clearly *polar,* growing from one aspect of the villus (Figure 23.11 B). These are usually anchoring villi and represent an area of growth in the early placenta (see Chapter 8). In partial moles, there is *proliferation of trophoblast, which although focal is circumferential* around the villous perimeter (Figure 23.10). The abortus will show a spectrum of villi, from small normal villi all the way to large hydropic villi, while *the partial mole shows two distinct populations of villi.*

Partial Mole Versus Complete Mole

Complete moles tend to have more *voluminous tissue* than partial moles, with *easily identifiable vesicles* on gross examination (see Figure 23.2). Microscopically, the complete mole shows significantly *more trophoblastic proliferation that involves all the villous tissue* rather than the *focal proliferation* seen in partial moles. Complete moles have more *nuclear pleomorphism and anaplasia as well.* The proliferation in partial

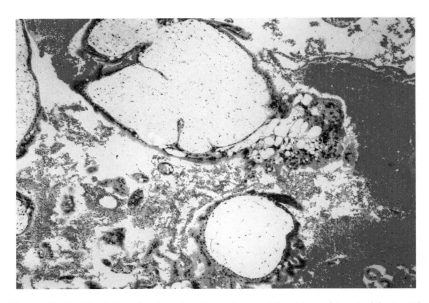

Figure 23.12. Partial mole showing irregular proliferation of trophoblast with lacy extensions. H&E. ×40.

moles is *clubbed or lacy* (Figure 23.12) rather than the more solid prolifations seen in complete moles. Partial moles also have *two distinct populations of villi*; one population of normal villi, and the other, villi with *edema, irregular villous contours, invaginations, and trophoblastic pseudoinclusions* (see Figure 23.9). The latter are not generally seen in complete moles. Finally, although embryonic or fetal tissue, blood vessels, and nucleated red blood cells may be seen in both complete and partial moles, these are much more common in partial moles.

Early Mole Versus Hydropic Abortus

In early moles (particularly those less than 10 weeks), the histologic features are more subtle and therefore may be confused with hydropic abortuses. The latter has a complete range of villi, from large hydropic villi to small, normal villi. The hydropic villi may have *cisterns*, but these are covered by *thin, attenuated trophoblast*. On the other hand, early moles have a uniform population of villi with *bulbous, cauliflower-like or clubbed villi, myxoid-like stroma, and poorly formed cisterns*. Blood vessels are more common and the villous stroma is more cellular than in older moles, and the villi have an appearance typical of mesenchymal villi (see Chapter 7). The most important feature in differentiating an abortus from an early mole is that the latter shows *trophoblastic proliferation*, albeit less than an older mole.

Partial Mole Versus Twin Pregnancy with Complete Mole

Rarely, in twin pregnancy, one of the twins is a mole and the other normal. The distinction from a partial mole may be quite difficult, particularly if the tissue is disrupted. Both will have two populations of villi, some hydropic and some normal (Figure 23.13), and both may have fetal tissue. *The most important feature in differentiation is the presence of marked trophoblastic proliferation and atypia* in the complete mole. Of course, twin pregnancies occur in which a partial mole is combined with a normal pregnancy. Accurate diagnosis may be impossible unless the placentas may be grossly differentiated from each other.

Ancillary Testing

As the histologic features are not completely reliable, in certain cases accurate categorization may be improved by performing ploidy analysis. Ploidy may be helpful in the following situations:

- Partial versus complete mole:
  - Diploid → complete mole
  - Triploid → most likely a partial mole
- Partial mole versus hydropic abortus:
  - Diploid → hydropic abortus
  - Triploid → most likely a partial mole

Caution is advised, as these rules are not strict. Particularly, *rare* complete moles are triploid or tetraploid. In addition, nonmolar triploidy

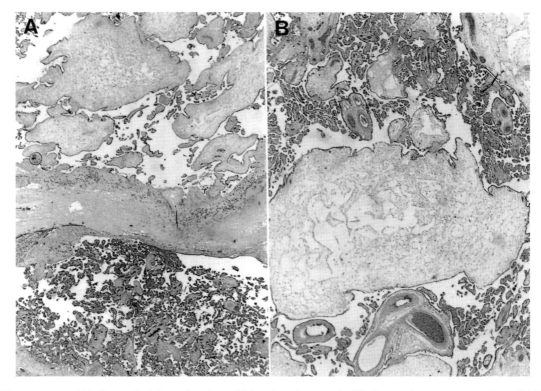

Figure 23.13. (A) Sharp division of molar villi (top) and normal villi (bottom) in twin gestation. H&E. ×16. (B) Focal admixture of molar and normal villi. H&E. ×16.

may occur with a maternal excess of DNA, or **maternal triploidy**. These do not show the trophoblastic proliferation typical of moles and so are not usually confused histologically with moles. If flow cytometry or other methods are not available or the diagnosis is still unclear, a report reflecting uncertainty may be prudent and the patient may then be followed with β-hCG monitoring.

Recently, *a maternally transcribed but paternally imprinted gene* has been described that is a cyclin-dependent kinase (CDK) inhibitor p57[KIP2] protein, referred to as **p57KIP2 or p57**. This protein is strongly expressed in maternal tissues such as decidua and is expressed in cytotrophoblast and villous stromal cells if a maternal component is present, such as in partial moles and hydropic abortuses. However, it is **not** expressed in androgenetic complete moles, or in the rare biparental complete moles. Therefore, since this antibody is commercially available, immunohistochemistry for p57 may be helpful in the differential diagnosis of difficult cases.

Suggestions for Examination and Report: Hydatidiform Moles

Gross Examination: The presence of enlarged villi or vesicles should be noted and is most consistent with a molar pregnancy. If the clinical history suggests molar pregnancy (elevated hCG or typical sonography), and vesicles are not visible grossly, additional sections should be submitted. Identification of fetal or embryonic tissue should also be documented.

Comment: If the diagnosis is equivocal, additional sections should be submitted. If the issue is not then clarified, additional testing such as flow cytometry or p57 immunostaining should be employed. If the diagnosis is still in question or if ancillary testing is not available, and the differential is between complete and partial mole, the diagnosis of a "**hydatidiform mole**" can be made with a comment that differentiation between partial and complete is not possible. A suggestion should also be made for serial β-hCG testing, at least until the levels normalize. If the differential is between a hydropic abortus and a partial mole and cannot be resolved, a descriptive diagnosis should be rendered such as "**chorionic villi with hydropic change and trophoblastic proliferation, see comment.**" The comment should then address the differential, again with the suggestion for serial β-hCG measurements.

Invasive Hydatidiform Mole

Pathogenesis
Invasive mole is a rare entity composed of *trophoblastic cells and molar villi, which invade the uterus and have the potential for invasion of adjacent structures.* Invasive moles usually develop subsequent to a molar preg-

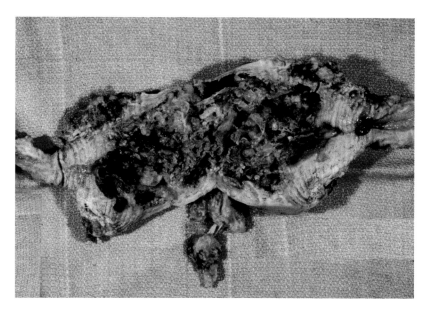

Figure 23.14. Hysterectomy specimen with a small subendometrial hemorrhagic lesion containing molar tissue. (From Lage JM, Driscoll SG, Yavner DL, et al., Hydatidiform moles: application of flow cytometry in diagnosis. Am J Clin Pathol 1988;89:596–600, with permission.)

nancy and are most often diagnosed by ultrasonography or other imaging technique. As they are characterized by molar villi invading through the myometrium, they may be viewed as *the molar equivalent of a placenta increta* (see Chapter 12). However, their behavior has more similarities to choriocarcinoma.

Pathologic Features

Microscopically, *molar villi are admixed with proliferating cytotrophoblast and syncytiotrophoblast.* The villi invade the myometrium without intervening decidual tissue (Figures 23.14, 23.15). *Deep myometrial invasion is typical and uterine perforation may occur.* Invasive moles are often associated with abundant hemorrhage and necrosis, similar to that seen in choriocarcinoma. Differentiation between an invasive mole and choriocarcinoma is straightforward as, by definition, molar villi are present in invasive moles and not in choriocarcinoma.

Clinical Features and Implications

Invasive moles usually occur after a previously diagnosed molar pregnancy, and most commonly a rise in the serum β-hCG heralds the onset. Their behavior is similar to choriocarcinoma and usually requires similar therapy with chemotherapeutic agents. They may develop metastases, usually to the lungs, and late metastases have been reported. Prognosis is based on the nature of the mole and the efficacy of its initial removal. Rare cases of spontaneous regression have been described.

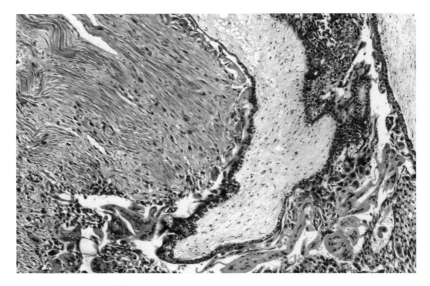

Figure 23.15. Invasive mole showing a molar villus invading the myometrium. Note the trophoblastic proliferation at the right. H&E. ×200.

Suggestions for Examination and Report:
Invasive Hydatidiform Mole

Gross Examination: When an invasive mole is suspected, generous sampling of the endomyometrium is advised as well as any grossly identifiable molar villi.

Comment: If an invasive mole is diagnosed, a comment on the extent of involvement is suggested.

Selected References

PHP4, Chapter 22, pages 718–753.

Ambrani LM, Vaidya RA, Rao CS, et al. Familial occurrence of trophoblastic disease: report of recurrent molar pregnancies in sisters in three families. Clin Genet 1980;18:27–29.

Baergen RN, Kelly T, McGinnis MJ, et al. Complete hydatidiform mole with a coexisting embryo. Hum Pathol 1996;27:731–734.

Fukunaga M. Immunohistochemical characterization of p57^{KIP2} expression in early hydatidiform moles. Hum Pathol 2002;33:1188–1192.

Gardner HAR, Lage JM. Choriocarcinoma following a partial hydatidiform mole. A case report. Hum Pathol 1992;23:468–471.

Genest DR. Partial hydatidiform mole: clinicopathologic features, differential diagnosis, ploidy and molecular studies, and gold standards for diagnosis. Int J Gynecol Pathol 2001;20:315–322.

Genest DR, Laborde O, Berkowitz RS, et al. A clinicopathologic study of 153 cases of complete hydatidiform mole (1980–1990): histologic grade lacks prognostic significance. Obstet Gynecol 1991;78:402–409.

Jacobs PA, Szulman AE, Funkhouser J, et al. Human triploidy: relationship between parental origin of the additional haploid complement and development of partial hydatidiform mole. Ann Hum Genet 1982;46:223–231.

Kajii T, Ohama K. Androgenetic origin of hydatidiform mole. Nature (Lond) 1977;268:633–634.

Kajii T, Kurashige H, Ohama K, et al. XY and XX complete moles: clinical and morphological correlations. Am J Obstet Gynecol 1984;150:57–64.

Keep D, Zaragoza MV, Hassold T, et al. Very early complete hydatidiform mole. Hum Pathol 1996;27:708–713.

Lage JM, Driscoll SG, Yavner DL, et al. Hydatidiform moles: application of flow cytometry in diagnosis. Am J Clin Pathol 1988;89:596–600.

Lawler SD, Fisher RA, Dent JA. prospective genetic study of complete and partial hydatidiform moles. Am J Obstet Gynecol 1991;164:1270–1277.

Li HW, Tsao SW, Cheung ANY. Current understandings of the molecular genetics of gestational trophoblastic diseases. Placenta 2002;23:20–31.

Muto MG, Lage JM, Berkowitz RS, et al. Gestational trophoblastic disease of the fallopian tube. J Reprod Med 1991;36:57–60.

Ohama, K, Kajii T, Okamoto E, et al. Dispermic origin of XY hydatidiform moles. Nature (Lond) 1981;292:551–552.

Szulman AE, Surti U. The syndromes of hydatidiform mole. I. Cytogenetic and morphologic correlations. Am J Obstet Gynecol 1978;131:665–671.

Szulman AE, Surti U. The syndromes of hydatidiform mole. II. Morphologic evolution of the complete and partial mole. Am J Obstet Gynecol 1978;132:20–27.

Vassilakos P, Riotton G, Kajii T. Hydatidiform mole: two entities. A morphologic and cytogenetic study with some clinical considerations. Am J Obstet Gynecol 1977;127:167–170.

Zaragoza MV, Keep D, Genest DR, et al. Early complete hydatidiform moles contain inner cell mass derivatives. Am J Med Genet 1997;70:273–277.

Chapter 24

Choriocarcinoma

General Considerations

Choriocarcinoma is a rare tumor with an incidence of 1 in 25,000 to 40,000 pregnancies. It may develop after an abortion, a term or preterm pregnancy, an ectopic pregnancy, or a hydatidiform mole. In their oft-depicted diagram (Figure 24.1), Hertig and Mansell estimated that the lesion was preceded by a *complete hydatidiform mole in 50%, an abortion in 25%, a normal pregnancy in 22.5%, and an ectopic pregnancy in 2.5%*. Choriocarcinoma is more common in young women and in those 40 years of age or older. There is as wide a geographic variation in its incidence as there is for hydatidiform moles.

Clinical Features and Implications
The most common presenting symptom is *abnormal vaginal bleeding*, usually developing several months following a pregnancy. Long latency periods up to 14 years or more have been reported. Some patients present with *elevated serum β-human chorionic gonadotropin (β-hCG), a radiographically detectable lesion, or metastatic disease* with symptoms reflecting the site of the metastasis.

Before the advent of chemotherapy, the prognosis of choriocarcinoma was dismal with a 5-year survival rate of 32%, which dropped to 19% if metastatic disease were present. Survival has improved dramatically since the introduction of efficacious chemotherapeutic agents, and the *overall survival for all gestational trophoblastic disease (GTD) is greater than 90%*. Some women successfully treated for choriocarcinoma have gone on to have normal pregnancies. Prognosis is primarily based on the stage (Table 24.1). A staging system for gestational trophoblastic disease devised by the International Federation of Gynecology and Obstetrics has been recently revised to include the modi-

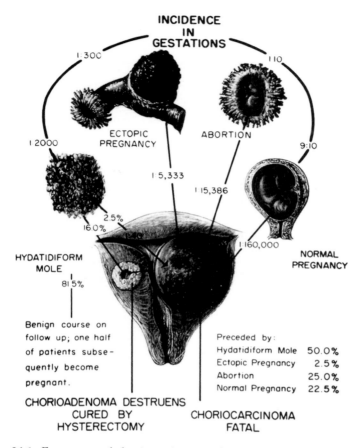

INCIDENCE
IN
GESTATIONS

1:300

1:10

ECTOPIC
PREGNANCY

ABORTION

1:2000

9:10

1:5,333

1:15,386

2.5%
16.0%

HYDATIDIFORM
MOLE

1:160,000

NORMAL
PREGNANCY

81.5%

Benign course on
follow up; one half
of patients subse-
quently become
pregnant.

Preceded by:
Hydatidiform Mole   50.0%
Ectopic Pregnancy   2.5%
Abortion   25.0%
Normal Pregnancy   22.5%

CHORIOADENOMA DESTRUENS
CURED BY
HYSTERECTOMY

CHORIOCARCINOMA
FATAL

Figure 24.1. Frequency of choriocarcinoma relative to its various precursors. (From Hertig AT, Mansell H. Tumors of the female sex organs. I. Hydatidiform mole and choriocarcinoma. In: Atlas of Tumor Pathology, Sect. IX, Fasc. 33. Washington, DC: Armed Forces of Pathology, 1956, with permission.)

fied World Health Organization risk factor scoring system (Table 24.2). *Older age, longer interval from preceding pregnancy, antecedent term pregnancy, high serum β-hCG levels, location and number of metastases, and history of failed treatment are all poor prognostic indicators.* This scoring system along with staging forms the basis for treatment. In general, patients with a score of seven or more are considered high risk and are treated with more aggressive multiagent chemotherapy.

Table 24.1. Staging of gestational trophoblastic disease[a]

Stage	Definition
I	Disease confined to the uterus
II	Disease outside the uterus but limited to the genital structures (i.e., pelvis, vagina)
III	Metastatic disease to the lungs
IV	Metastatic disease to sites other than the lungs

[a] Data taken from Kohorn, 2001.

Table 24.2. International ederation of gynecology and obstetrics (FIGO) 2000 scoring system for gestational trophoblastic disease[a]

FIGO score	0	1	2	3
Age at diagnosis	≤39 years	>39 years		
Type of antecedent pregnancy	Hydatidiform mole	Abortion	Term pregnancy	
Interval from antecedent pregnancy	<4 months	4–6 months	7 to 12 months	>12 months
Serum β-hCG mIU/mL	<1000	1000–10,000	10,000–100,000	>100,000
Tumor size	≤4 cm	>4 cm		
Sites of metastases	None	Spleen or kidney	Gastrointestinal trace	Brain or liver
Number of metastases	0	1 to 3	4 to 8	>8
Response to chemotherapy	Full response	Full response	Failure with single- drug chemotherapy	Failure with multiagent chemotherapy

Risk is assessed by adding factors according to the above system. Scores of 7 or greater constitute a high-risk group that is treated more aggressively.
[a] Data taken from Kohorn, 2001.

Pathologic Features

Grossly, choriocarcinoma may vary from an inconspicuous tumor only a few millimeters in diameter to large, bulky tumors. They present as a *friable, hemorrhagic, and often necrotic mass* with an infiltrating border (Figure 24.2). The tumors may be so large as to completely fill the uterine cavity (Figure 24.3). On microscopic examination, choriocarcinoma consists of *solid sheets of cytotrophoblast and multinucleated syncytium without stroma* (Figure 24.4). As the tumor has no intrinsic vascular stroma, it takes its blood supply from invasion of host vessels. This great propensity for *vascular invasion* leads to the prominent *hemorrhage and necrosis* characteristic of choriocarcinoma (Figure 24.5). So much blood may be present in some tumors that one may have to search long for the tumor cells, which are often at the periphery of the lesion. Classically, *broad sheets or smaller nests of cytotrophoblast form the central portions of the tumor, the periphery being syncytium*, recapitulating the normal relationship of trophoblast in the early embryo (Figure 24.6). Commonly, there is a completely haphazard mixture of trophoblastic cells that irregularly infiltrate the surrounding tissue. The **syncytiotrophoblast** contain *multiple irregular, hyperchromatic nuclei with dense, eosinophilic cytoplasm*. Nuclear pleomorphism is common. Because of its dilated cytoplasmic cisternae, the *syncytium is frequently vacuolated* (Figure 24.7). The **cytotrophoblastic cells** are *large, with moderate clear to lightly eosinophilic cytoplasm, large round nuclei, clumped chromatin, and one or more nucleoli*. A few **transitional trophoblastic cells** may be present in choriocarcinoma, even though they are not the hallmark of the lesion. Those cells are truly intermediate between cytotrophoblast and syncytium but are **not** the "intermediate trophoblast" of the implantation site (extravillous trophoblast). Differentiation of choriocarcinoma from lesions of extravillous trophoblast is discussed in Chapter 25 and summarized in Tables 25.1 to 25.3.

Occasionally confusion with early abortion specimens may occur as the latter will contain sheets of proliferating trophoblastic cells with mitotic activity. Choriocarcinoma has no villous stroma or blood vessels, and these can easily be found in the early abortus. One does not usually make the diagnosis of a choriocarcinoma in the presence of chorionic villi. The exception is choriocarcinoma in a term or near-term placenta (see below).

Metastasis: **Metastases** occur largely from *hematogenous dissemination through the venous system to the lungs* and in some cases into the systemic circulation. Therefore, metastatic lung lesions are present in 94% of patients with metastases. The *vagina* is also often involved. Other, less common metastatic sites include *brain, liver, kidney, spleen, intestines,*

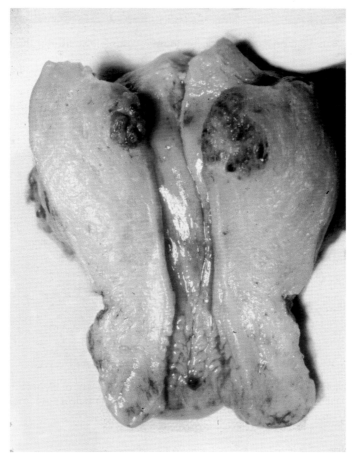

Figure 24.2. Opened uterus showing an irregular, hemorrhagic tumor involving endomyometrium. (From Baergen RN, Rutgers JL. Trophoblastic lesions of the placental site. Gen Diagn Pathol 1997;143:143–158, with permission.)

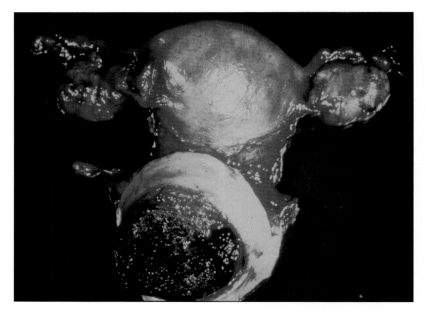

Figure 24.3. Hemorrhagic choriocarcinoma completely filling the uterine cavity.

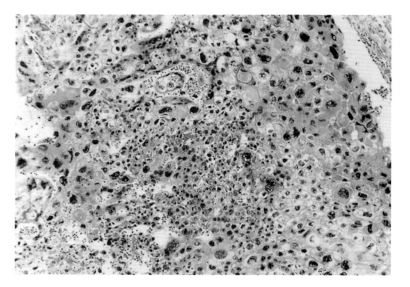

Figure 24.4. Choriocarcinoma of the uterus. Solid sheets of neoplastic cytotrophoblast and syncytiotrophoblast with marked nuclear pleomorphism. H&E. ×160.

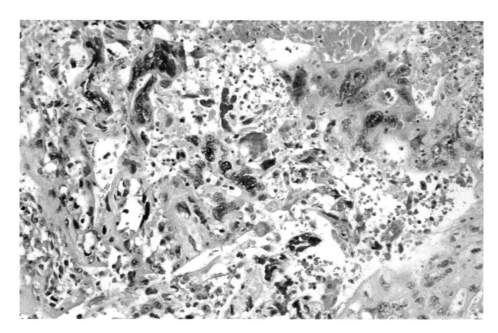

Figure 24.5. Choriocarcinoma demonstrating the characteristic hemorrhage and necrosis. H&E. ×200.

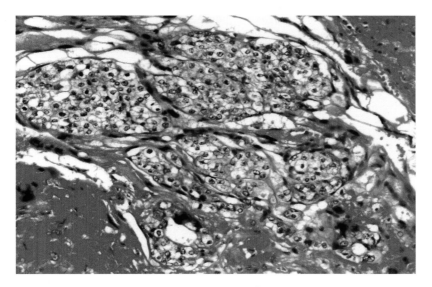

Figure 24.6. Choriocarcinoma, recapitulating the normal arrangement seen in chorionic villi with syncytial cells surrounding groups of cytotrophoblast. H&E. ×150.

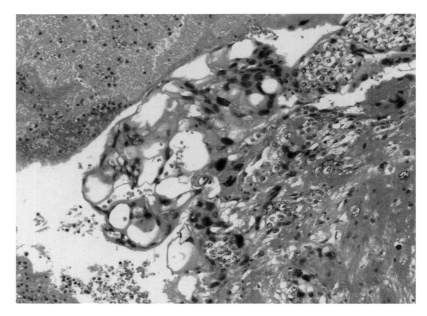

Figure 24.7. Vacuolated syncytiotrophoblast with marked atypia, characteristic for choriocarcinoma. H&E. ×200.

broad ligament, ovary, pelvis, and cervix. Rarely metastases have occurred in the *oral gingival, subungual region, gastrocnemius muscle, coronary artery, aorta, and choroid of the eye.* Histologically, metastatic lesions tend to be *better circumscribed* but are otherwise histologically similar to the primary (Figures 24.8, 24.9). Occasionally a metastasis is identified without an identifiable primary. Spontaneous resolution of the primary

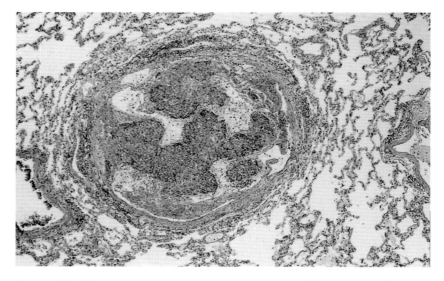

Figure 24.8. Choriocarcinoma metastatic to the lungs. This vessel is filled with solid nodules of choriocarcinoma. Some inflammatory reaction is also present in the vascular wall. H&E. ×40.

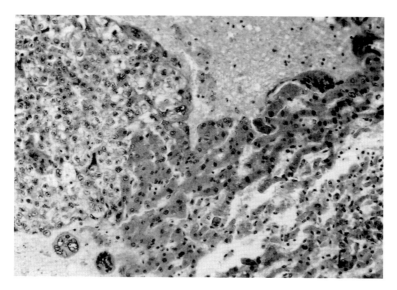

Figure 24.9. Metastatic choriocarcinoma in the liver. Cords of disrupted liver cells are seen at right; a large tumor mass is present at the left consisting primarily of cytotrophoblast. H&E. ×160.

lesion may be the explanation. Spontaneous remission of a metastasis has also been reported infrequently.

Choriocarcinoma-In-Situ—Placental Choriocarcinoma

Pathogenesis

When choriocarcinoma develops during a term or near-term pregnancy, an intraplacental lesion may be identified. This lesion has been referred to as **choriocarcinoma-in-situ**. The lesion clearly arises in the placenta (Figure 24.10), but these intraplacental lesions are usually

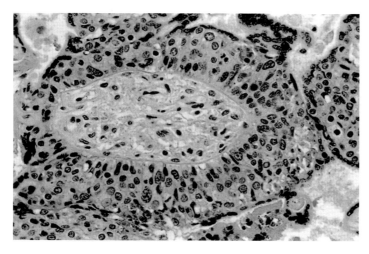

Figure 24.10. A single villus in a term placenta shows proliferation of trophoblast with several mitoses. This may represent the precursor lesion of placental choriocarcinoma. H&E. ×400.

invasive within the placenta and often metastatic. Therefore, a pre-ferred designation is **placental choriocarcinoma**. These lesions are the probable origin of many of the choriocarcinomas that develop after a term pregnancy. As routine placental examination is not performed on every placenta, it is quite likely that many of these lesions are missed.

Pathologic Features

Placental choriocarcinomas are usually *inconspicuous grossly and are often mistaken for an infarct.* Microscopically, they show *proliferation of both cytotrophoblast and syncytiotrophoblast in the intervillous space* (Figures 24.11, 24.12). Usually there is focal involvement of the adjacent chorionic villi. Invasion of the villous stroma or fetal vessels may also be present.

Clinical Features and Implications

The reported cases of placental choriocarcinoma have had a varied outcome. In some cases, mother and infant showed no ill effect, while in other cases metastatic lesions, particularly to the lungs, required treatment. Placental choriocarcinoma can *metastasize to both the mother and the fetus,* and may be fatal to both. *Massive transplacental fetal hem-orrhage* has also been reported. Occasionally, tumor in the placenta is not identified despite metastasis in the neonate. In some of these cases, this was certainly due to lack of placental examination. Due to the subtle nature of the gross appearance of these lesions, it is likely that many cases go undiagnosed.

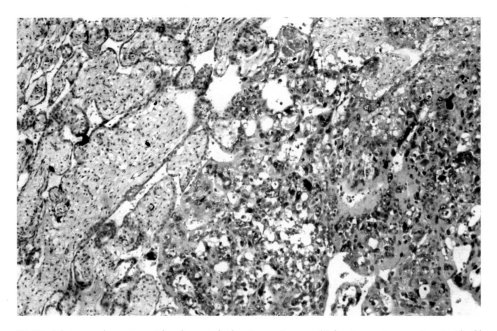

Figure 24.11. Mature placenta with placental choriocarcinoma ("choriocarcinoma-in-situ"). Sheets of atypical trophoblast proliferate between the chorionic villi within the intervillous space. H&E. ×200.

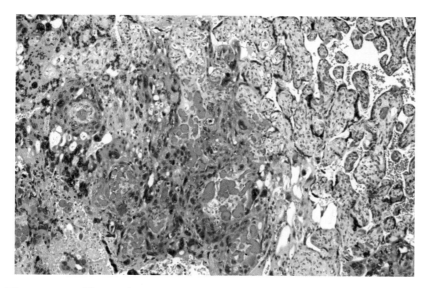

Figure 24.12. Placental choriocarcinoma demonstrating the cytologic atypia pleomorphism. H&E. ×200.

Suggestions for Examination and Report: Choriocarcinoma

Gross Examination: Uterine choriocarcinomas are hemorrhagic and necrotic and may require many sections for identification of viable tumor cells. Often, the primary lesion is not resected or even noted and it is the metastatic lesions that find its way to the pathology laboratory. Generous sampling is advised. Placental choriocarcinomas are not usually visible grossly or have an inconspicuous appearance.

Comment: If placental choriocarcinoma is present, a comment may be made about the possibility of maternal or fetal metastases. In the rare case of a resection of a primary uterine choriocarcinoma or a metastasis, information about the extent of disease spread is necessary in order that proper staging be performed (see Table 24.1).

Selected References

PHP4, Chapter 23, pages 754–761, 767–777.

Baergen RN. Gestational choriocarcinoma. Gen Diagn Pathol 1997;143:127–142.

Driscoll SG. Choriocarcinoma: an "incidental finding" within a term placenta. Obstet Gynecol 1963;21:96–101.

Gardiner HAR, Lage JM. Choriocarcinoma following a partial hydatidiform mole: a case report. Hum Pathol 1992;23:468–471.

Jacques SM, Qureshi F, Doss BJ, et al. Intraplacental choriocarcinoma associated with viable pregnancy: pathologic features and implications for the mother and infant. Pediatr Dev Pathol 1998;1:380–387.

Kendall A, Gillmore R, Newlands E. Chemotherapy for trophoblastic disease: current standards. Curr Opin Obstet Gynecol 2002;14:33–38.

Kohorn EI. The new FIGO 2000 staging and risk factor scoring system for gestational trophoblastic disease: description and critical assessment. Int J Gynecol Cancer 2001;11:73–77.

Lage JM, Roberts DJ. Choriocarcinoma in a term placenta: pathologic diagnosis of tumor in an asymptomatic patient with metastatic disease. Int J Gynecol Pathol 1993;12:80–85.

Seckl MJ, Newlands ES. Treatment of gestational trophoblastic disease. Gen Diagn Pathol 1997;143:159–171.

Silverberg SG, Kurman RJ. Tumors of the uterine corpus and gestational trophoblastic disease. Atlas of tumor pathology, third series, fascicle 3. Washington, DC: Armed Forces Intitute of Pathology, 1992.

Scully RE, Bonfiglio TA, Kurman RJ, et al. Histologic typing of female genital tract tumours, 2nd edition. New York: Springer-Verlag, 1994.

Chapter 25

Lesions of Extravillous Trophoblast

General Considerations

Lesions of extravillous trophoblast (EVT) have been known for over 100 years. The first lesion that was described, "syncytial endometritis," is a nonneoplastic lesion that is merely an exuberant proliferation of the EVT in the implantation site. It was later renamed **exaggerated placental site**. Another lesion of EVT was described shortly thereafter, the "syncytioma." Other designations such as chorioma, atypical chorionepithelioma, chorionepitheliosis, and trophoblastic pseudotumor have also been used. It was first thought that it was also a benign, nonneoplastic proliferation of EVT, hence the designation of pseudotumor. Reports of lesions with aggressive behavior and metastasis, however, have led to its reclassification as a potentially malignant neoplasm. It is since been renamed **placental site trophoblastic tumor**. Much more recently, two additional lesions of EVT have been described; a benign nonneoplastic lesion called the **placental site nodule** and a variant of placental site trophoblastic tumor, the **epithelioid trophoblastic tumor**.

Placental Site Nodule

Clinical Features and Implications

The **placental site nodule** (PSN) is a benign, nonneoplastic lesion thought to represent EVT retained in the uterus after pregnancy. PSNs occur primarily in reproductive-age patients, but may be seen in post-menopausal patients. PSNs may follow a normal pregnancy, abortion, or mole and may be diagnosed several weeks to many years after the preceding pregnancy. Many patients have a history of previous gynecologic surgery such as cesarean section, therapeutic abortion, or curettage. In one study, a significant number of patients had a history of bilateral tubal ligation. One-half of the patients present with *abnormal bleeding*, and in the remainder, the lesions are *incidental findings in curettage or hysterectomy specimens*. Serum β-hCG levels are not elevated. *Follow-up on patients with PSNs has been benign*, and no progression to any gynecologic malignancy or trophoblastic disease has been reported.

Pathologic Features

PSNs are usually *too small to be visible by gross inspection*. When they are visible, they consist of single or multiple, small, focally *hemorrhagic pale-tan nodules in the endometrium or the superficial myometrium measuring from 1 to 4 mm in diameter*. They are commonly located in the lower uterine segment or the cervix. Microscopically, PSNs consist of *well-circumscribed, rounded nodules or plaques with prominent hyalinization and fibrinoid deposition* (Figure 25.1). They may have *central hyalinization with a more cellular peripheral zone of EVT* (Figure 25.2). The cells are arranged singly or in clusters, and contain *eosinophilic or amphophilic cytoplasm*

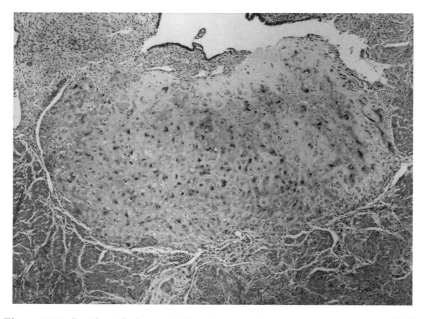

Figure 25.1. Incidental placental site plaque in a hysterectomy specimen. H&E. ×40.

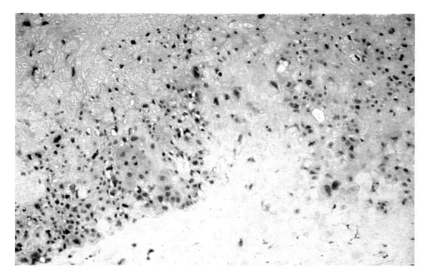

Figure 25.2. Placental site nodule showing prominent hyalinization and peripheral EVT. H&E. ×200.

that is often vacuolated. The cell borders are often indistinct, merging with the extracellular material. The *nuclei may be degenerative or smudgy* in appearance (Figure 25.3). Occasionally they are pale and vesicular, lobulated, or, infrequently, bizarre. *Mitotic activity is minimal or absent,* and nodules stained immunohistochemically for Ki-67 show positivity in less than 5% of cells (the Ki-67 labeling index). The nodule also may contain scattered chronic inflammatory cells and fibroblasts. In more

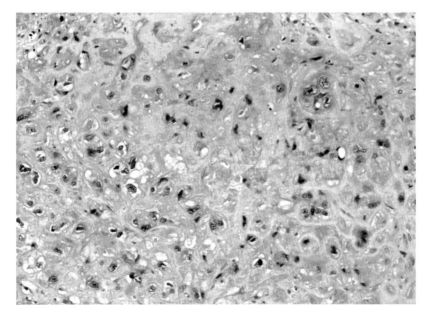

Figure 25.3. Placental site nodule with degenerated and vacuolated nuclei. H&E. ×200.

than one-half of the cases, small extensions or *"pseudopods" consisting of EVT admixed with eosinophilic, fibrinoid material extend into the surrounding tissue*. The fibrinoid material in particular is similar to keratinization and may mimic invasive squamous carcinoma. The frequent location of PSNs in the cervix may thus be problematic. The adjacent endometrium is usually proliferative or secretory. PSNs are not associated with chorionic villi.

Exaggerated Placental Site

Clinical Features and Implications

Exaggerated placental site (EPS) is a *nonneoplastic, albeit exuberant, proliferation of EVT in the implantation site, associated with pregnancy*. It occurs in approximately 1.6% of first trimester abortion specimens and represents an *"excessive" physiologic response* of EVT. The original name of syncytial endometritis for lesion reflects the presence of many placental site giant cells in the implantation site.

Pathologic Features

EPS is *not identifiable on gross examination*. On microscopic examination, the architecture of the endometrial and myometrial tissue in the placental site is maintained. The trophoblastic cells *proliferate in and around the endometrial glands and smooth muscle fibers without destructive invasion* (Figure 25.4). The extravillous trophoblastic cells have moderately

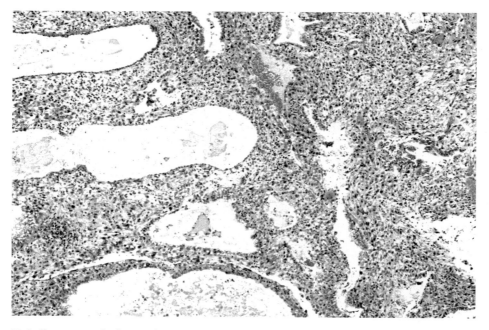

Figure 25.4. Exaggerated placental site. Note preservation of glandular architecture and the exuberant trophoblastic proliferation. Multinucleated trophoblast are also present. H&E. ×20.

abundant *eosinophilic or amphophilic cytoplasm and nuclei that are some-times irregular or hyperchromatic.* Occasional multinucleated cells are also present. *Mitotic activity is minimal or absent.* Intermixed with the trophoblastic cells are variable numbers of smooth muscle cells, decid-ual cells, and inflammatory cells and the *fibrinoid material* that is so char-acteristic of EVT. These lesions occur concomitant with pregnancy and therefore *chorionic villi are almost always present.* Their presence is an important clue in diagnosis. The significance of this lesion lies prima-rily in its common association with complete hydatidiform moles and in its differentiation from other trophoblastic lesions. *Differentiation of EPS from a normal implantation site is rather arbitrary as there are no spe-cific criteria.* This is in part because "normal" placental sites are rarely sampled or observed by pathologists. Diagnosis may be made when the proliferation of EVT is significantly more prominent than usual.

Placental Site Trophoblastic Tumor

Clinical Features

Placental site trophoblastic tumor (PSTT) is a rare gestational tumor with only 200 or so cases reported in the English literature. As with other trophoblastic lesions, PSTTs occur predominantly in reproduc-tive-age women and have been reported in patients as young as 18 and as old as 62 years of age. PSTTs may occur after abortions, term preg-nancies, or moles. In contrast to choriocarcinoma in which 50% develop after a hydatidiform mole, only 5% to 8% of PSTTs develop after a molar pregnancy. The interval from the previous known pregnancy has been reported to be as little as several months to as long as 18 years.

Patients most commonly present with *abnormal uterine bleeding and/or amenorrhea.* In comparison to choriocarcinoma, in which virtually all patients have marked elevations in serum β-hCG levels, in PSST, β-hCG *levels are only moderately elevated and only in 80% of patients.* The pres-ence of *uterine enlargement, abnormal bleeding, and a positive pregnancy test* often leads to the presumptive diagnosis of pregnancy, missed abortion, or ectopic pregnancy. In rare cases, patients may present with abdominal pain, virilization, spider angiomata of the skin, infertility, galactorrhea, or renal failure.

Pathologic Features

Lesions arise primarily in the *myometrium and endomyometrium* but occasionally may involve, or extend to, the cervix. They vary in size from a *few millimeters to large, bulky masses measuring up to 10 cm in diam-eter.* Most commonly, they have ill-defined borders (Figure 25.5). Occa-sionally they may be grossly well circumscribed. On cut section, the tumor is generally *soft, tan-white to yellow. Focal hemorrhage and necrosis are sometimes identified;* however, the hemorrhage and necrosis is much less conspicuous than in choriocarcinoma. PSTTs are deeply invasive into the uterine wall in 60% of patients, and extension to the serosa may result in *uterine perforation* at presentation or curettage. Some tumors have extended through the uterine wall to involve the fallopian tube or broad ligament.

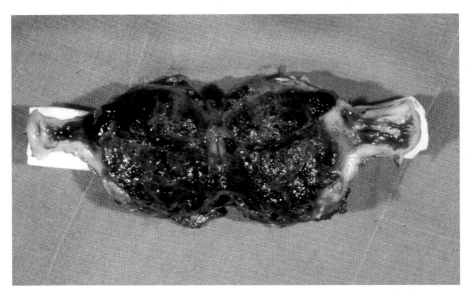

Figure 25.5. Placental site trophoblastic tumor (PSTT). An ill-defined, hemorrhagic and necrotic tumor fills the endometrial cavity. (From Baergen RN. Gestational choriocarcinoma. Gen Diagn Pathol 1997:143:127–141, with permission.)

Microscopic examination typically reveals an *infiltrative mass* within the endomyometrium composed of *infiltrating sheets and cords of predominantly mononuclear EVT, which separate and split apart individual smooth muscle fibers.* (Figure 25.6). *The histologic appearance is quite variable*, both from tumor to tumor and within the same tumor. The tumor

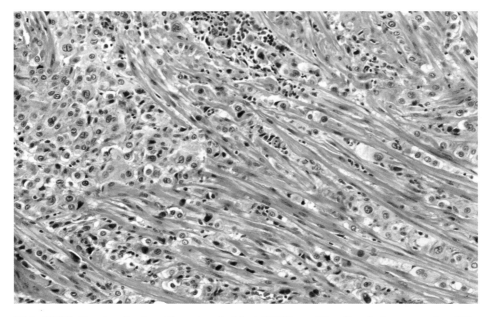

Figure 25.6. PSTT. Sheets of extravillous trophoblast (EVT) proliferating between and splitting apart smooth muscle fibers. H&E. ×40.

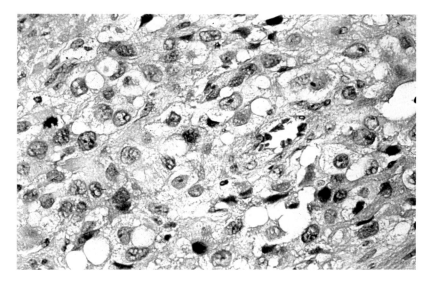

Figure 25.7. Variant of PSTT with clear cytoplasm. H&E. ×200.

cells are predominantly *polygonal with moderately abundant dense amphophilic, eosinophilic, or clear cytoplasm* (Figure 25.7). Tumor cells may also be *spindled*, and in some tumors, the majority of cells are spindled. A minority of the EVT may be binucleated or trinucleated, and contain nuclei similar to those within the mononuclear cells. Often scattered throughout the tumor are multinucleated cells with irregular, hyperchromatic, or smudgy nuclei similar to syncytiotrophoblast; however, these are generally scarce. The cells may be relatively monomorphic (Figure 25.8) or show marked nuclear pleomorphism and atypia

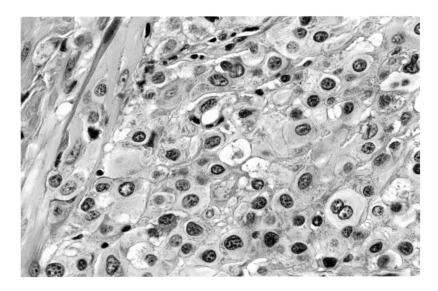

Figure 25.8. Relatively monomorphic population of EVT with minimal atypia in PSTT. H&E. ×160.

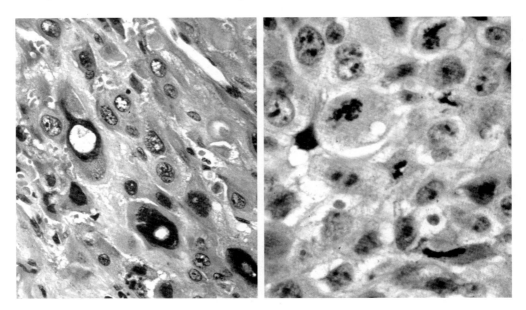

Figure 25.9. PSTT. Marked nuclear pleomorphism (left) is present in this tumor which also shows easily identifiable mitotic figures (right). H&E. ×400.

(Figure 25.9). Nuclear folding and intranuclear pseudoinclusions may also be seen. *Nucleoli, however, are usually small and indistinct*, but focally may be quite large and prominent. The mitotic rate ranges from less than 1 to more than 30 mitoses per 10 hpf. Atypical mitotic figures are seen in as many as 90% of cases.

Coagulative tumor cell necrosis, hemorrhage, and focal inflammation are seen in over two-thirds of these tumors. One of the *most characteristic features is the presence of extracellular fibrinoid material* similar to that present in the normal implantation site. This feature is also present in more than 90% of cases (Figure 25.10). In approximately two-thirds of cases, there is a peculiar form of *vascular invasion* that recapitulates the normal implantation site in that there is replacement of the vascular wall by trophoblast and the presence of intraluminal trophoblast (Figure 25.11). The uninvolved endometrium is usually decidualized or secretory, but occasionally it is proliferative or inactive.

Clinical Implications
Most PSTTs behave in a benign manner. The remaining 10% to 15% of patients shows aggressive disease with metastasis and even death. Metastases have been reported in the *lungs, liver, vagina, gastrointestinal tract, pelvis, bladder, brain, ovary, omentum, diaphragm, spleen, pancreas, pelvic lymph nodes, and bone marrow.* Lung metastases are the most common. Metastasis to the brain is usually fatal due to intracranial hemorrhage. Late metastasis or recurrence has been reported 5 years after initial diagnosis.

Unfortunately, at present there is no way of accurately predicting which tumors will behave in a malignant manner. Recent attempts to

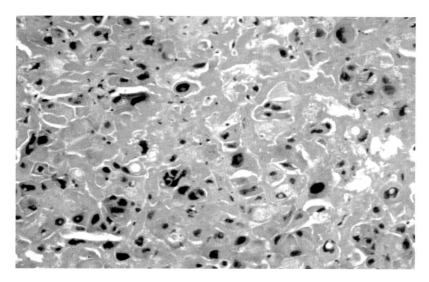

Figure 25.10. PSTT. Prominent fibrinoid deposition is present. H&E. ×200.

find clinical and histologic features that could serve as prognostic factors have generally been disappointing. This having been said, some features are more common in patients that develop distant metastases. The most important prognostic factor is International Federation of Gynecology and Obstetrics (FIGO) trophoblastic staging. Histologic factors that have been associated with poor prognosis are *deep myometrial invasion, cervical involvement, increased mitotic activity, and clear cytoplasm*. Clinical factors associated with a poorer prognosis are *more advanced age at diagnosis, increased interval from preceding pregnancy, pre-*

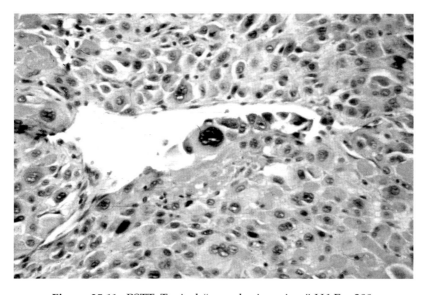

Figure 25.11. PSTT. Typical "vascular invasion." H&E. ×200.

ceding term pregnancy, and high maximum serum levels of β-hCG. Caution must be used when predicting the behavior of individual tumors, as some tumors with low mitotic rates have metastasized and some with pelvic extension or metastasis have ultimately had an indolent or even benign course without treatment.

In most patients with disease confined to the uterus, the treatment of choice is *hysterectomy*. Conservative local excision has been advocated for some patients with limited disease. Unfortunately, patients with metastatic PSTT have not experienced the success seen in patients with choriocarcinoma who have been treated with chemotherapy. Some patients with advanced disease have been cured, but outcome is variable. Patients may be followed for treatment response or to monitor the disease with serial serum β-hCG determinations because the levels fall to normal in remission and rise with disease recurrence or metastasis. This is not useful in all patients, as 20% of patients do not have an elevation in serum β-hCG.

Differential Diagnosis

Placental site trophoblastic tumor (PSTT) must be distinguished from other lesions of EVT, from choriocarcinoma and from nontrophoblastic lesions, particularly poorly differentiated carcinomas. Clinical features that may be used in differentiating extravillous trophoblastic lesions are summarized in Tables 25.1, pathologic features in Table 25.2, and immunohistochemical findings in Table 25.3.

Table 25.1. Clinical features of trophoblastic lesions

	PSN	EPS	PSTT/ETT	CCA
H/O Previous mole	—	—	5%–8%	50%
Serum β-hCG	Normal	Appropriate for pregnancy	Moderately elevated in 80%	Markedly elevated
Symptoms	50% have abnormal uterine bleeding	Related to pregnancy	Bleeding, uterine enlargement, or mass	Bleeding, uterine enlargement
Location	Often in lower uterine segment or cervix	Endometrium	Endomyometrium	Endomyometrium
Treatment	None	None	Hysterectomy; chemotherapy if malignant	Chemotherapy
Metastasis	None	None	Occurs in 10%–15% of cases	Potential for metastasis
Prognosis	No sequelae	No sequelae	Guarded if malignant	More than 90% responsive to chemotherapy

PSN, placental site nodule; EPS, exaggerated placental site; PSTT, placental site trophoblastic tumor; ETT, epithelioid trophoblastic tumors; CA, choriocarcinoma.

Table 25.2. Histopathologic features of trophoblastic lesions

	PSN	EPS	PSTT	ETT	CCA
Forms a mass	–	–	+	+	±
Chorionic villi present	–	+	Very rare	Very rare	–[a]
Fibrinoid	+	+	+	–	–
Hemorrhage	–	±	+	+	++
Necrosis	–	±	+	++	++
Vascular invasion	–	+	+	+	+
Degenerative changes	–	–	–	–	+
Extravillous trophoblast	+	+	+	+	–
Syncytiotrophoblast	–	+	–[b]	–	++
Nuclear pleomorphism	–	–	++	–	++
Mitotic activity	Minimal or absent	Minimal or absent	+	+	+

PSN, placental site nodules; EPS, exaggerated placental site; PSTT, placental site trophoblastic tumor; ETT, epithelioid trophoblastic tumor; CCA, choriocarcinoma.
[a] Villi are present only in placental or "in situ" choriocarcinoma (see Chapter 24).
[b] Multinucleated cells similar to syncytiotrophoblast may be present.

Differentiation Between Lesions of EVT

Because PSN, EPS, and PSTT derive from EVT, differentiation between lesions may sometimes be difficult. PSTTs are infiltrative tumors with mitotic activity, hemorrhage, necrosis, and vascular invasion and are quite cellular. PSNs, on the other hand, are well-circumscribed nodules with hyalinization and a degenerative appearance that can usually be recognized as benign lesions, despite the presence of irregular extensions into the adjacent tissue or pseudopods. Neither EPSs nor PSNs produce a mass lesion or grow in an infiltrative pattern. Neither PSTT nor PSN contain chorionic villi, a feature that usually distinguishes both from an EPS.

Immunohistochemical studies of PSN, EPS, and PSTT confirm origin from EVT, with positivity for epithelial markers such as cytokeratin

Table 25.3. Immunohistochemistry of trophoblastic lesions

	PSN	EPS	PSTT	ETT	CCA
Cytokeratin	+	+	+	+	+
EMA	+	+	+	+	+
hCG	Weak focal	+	Weak focal	Weak focal	+++
hPL	Focal	Diffuse	Diffuse	Focal	Focal
PLAP	Diffuse	Focal	Focal	Diffuse	
Mel-CAM	Focal	Diffuse	Diffuse	Focal	
Major basic protein	±	+	+	+	–
α-Inhibin	+	+	+	+	–
Ki-67	<5%		5–15%	5–15%	

PSN, placental site nodules; EPS, exaggerated placental site; PSTT, placental site trophoblastic tumor; ETT, epithelioid trophoblastic tumor; CCA, choriocarcinoma.

and early membrane antigen (EMA), positivity for trophoblastic markers such as human placental lactogen (hPL), human chorionic gonadotropin (hCG), placental alkaline phosphatase (PLAP), Mel-CAM (CD146), and α-inhibin. PSNs show diffuse positivity for PLAP and only focal positivity for hPL and Mel-CAM, while PSTTs show the opposite pattern with diffuse positivity for hPL and Mel-CAM and only focal positivity for PLAP and hCG. Thus, staining of PSNS is similar to the staining pattern of *EVT in the chorion laeve and it has been suggested that PSNs derive from those cells.* The difference in immunohistochemical profiles is summarized in Table 25.3. Ki-67 is also useful as PSN has a labeling index of less than 5% while PSTT may have a labeling index of up to 14%.

Clinical information may be essential in the differentiation of these lesions. PSTT usually presents clinically as a mass, so information gained from physical examination or various types of imaging studies may be very helpful in adjudicating difficult cases. Patients with PSN do not have elevations in serum β-hCG, while those with EPS will have elevations consistent with an intrauterine pregnancy. As 80% of patients with PSTT have elevations, this may help distinguish these lesions. *When it is difficult to distinguish PSTT from a PSN, serum β-hCG levels should be requested.*

Differentiation of Placental Site Trophoblastic Tumor from Choriocarcinoma

The main difference between *choriocarcinoma and PSTT is that the former consists almost exclusively of villous trophoblast while the latter consists almost exclusively of extravillous trophoblast.* Although rare "monophasic" variants of choriocarcinoma have been described, choriocarcinoma typically consists of cytotrophoblast and syncytiotrophoblast with a typical biphasic pattern, as opposed to the monophasic proliferation of the EVT seen in PSTT.

Immunohistochemistry is helpful in differentiating EVT from villous trophoblast as PSTTs will be positive for markers of EVT, while mononuclear cytotrophoblast is generally negative for those markers and hCG. Syncytiotrophoblast is not difficult to distinguish from EVT due to its multinucleation, the presence of atypical hyperchromatic nuclei, and strong immunoreactivity for hCG. However, occasional multinucleated syncytial cells may be seen in PSTT that stain positive for hCG. In addition, rare trophoblastic tumors have been described that have features of both PSTT and choriocarcinoma. These may represent tumors of stem cell trophoblast that have divergent differentiation.

Differentiation of Placental Site Trophoblastic Tumor from Other Tumors

Often, the infiltrative and malignant nature of PSTT is obvious, but its origin remains obscure. It may be misinterpreted as a type of poorly differentiated carcinoma or even a sarcoma. *The fibrinoid produced by EVT often suggests keratin, and as a result PSTT may be confused with squamous cell carcinoma.* This is particularly problematic when the tumor is present in the cervix. Although both tumors are cytokeratin positive, markers for EVT will be negative in squamous carcinomas. Occasionally, *PSTT may be confused with a sarcoma, in particular epithelioid leiomyosarcoma or with a mesothelioma showing deciduoid morphology.* Immunohistochemistry will also easily differentiate between these tumors.

Epithelioid Trophoblastic Tumor

Clinical Features and Implications
The **epithelioid trophoblastic tumor** (ETT) is a recently described tumor believed to *arise from EVT of the chorion laeve.* It has immunohistochemical similarities to PSN and thus may represent its neoplastic equivalent. Clinical features are indistinguishable from PSTT. Patients generally are in the reproductive-age group and present with vaginal bleeding. Most patients have an elevated β-hCG. The interval from preceding pregnancy is up to 18 years. *Approximately 25% of the reported cases have been malignant,* similar to that reported for PSTT. *Treatment and follow-up have also been similar to PSTT.*

Pathologic Features
On gross examination, ETTs are *tan to yellow, fleshy, infiltrative nodules in the endomyometrium* measuring up to 5 cm in diameter. Like PSNs, they are *commonly seen in the lower uterine segment.* They tend to show more necrosis than typical PSTTs. On histologic section, ETTs have a distinctive appearance with nests of *small, relatively uniform trophoblastic cells clustered around small vessels with surrounding geographic necrosis* (Figure 25.12). The tumor cells are smaller and more monomorphic compared to those in a typical PSTT. The cells usually have *clear or vacuolated cytoplasm, and the nuclei contain finely dispersed chromatin with identifiable nucleoli.* The mitotic rate is variable. Many ETTs focally show a pattern reminiscent of typical PSTT. Differential diagnosis is shown in Tables 25.1 to 25.3.

Extrauterine Lesions of Extravillous Trophoblast

As with hydatidiform moles and choriocarcinoma, *lesions of EVT may occur in ectopic locations such as the fallopian tube, ovary, mesosalpinx, and broad ligament.* Reported cases have included both PSNs and PSTTs. They are similar in appearance and behavior to their uterine counterparts and are *presumed to arise from previous ectopic pregnancies.* They are frequently associated with chronic salpingitis and endometriosis.

Another lesion called "**trophoblastic implants**," "residual trophoblastic tissue," or "persistent ectopic pregnancy" has also been described. Trophoblastic implants occur in up to 29% of patients with ectopic pregnancies treated conservatively with laparoscopic salpingostomy. They may be found in the adnexa, pelvic peritoneum, or even the omentum and are *thought to represent residual extrauterine implantation sites that have not undergone full involution or excision.* Grossly, they appear as *hemorrhagic nodules* and may be confused with

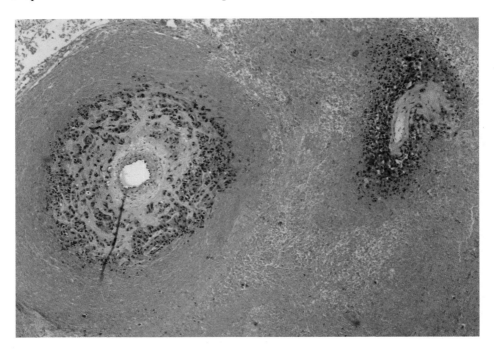

Figure 25.12. Epithelioid trophoblastic tumor consisting of a relatively monomorphic population of extravillous trophoblast surrounded by geographic necrosis. H&E. ×100.

endometriosis by the surgeon. Microscopically, they consist of *degenerative nodules composed of EVT admixed with chorionic villi*. They do not show the hyalinization of PSNs, nor the infiltrative features, cytologic atypia, and proliferative activity of PSTTs. Serum β-hCG levels are often elevated. Patients may require additional surgery for excision of the lesions, but clinical follow-up has been benign.

> *Suggestions for Examination and Report:*
> *Extravillous Trophoblastic Lesions*
>
> **Gross Examination:** PSN and EPS are not grossly identifiable. PSTTs and ETTs are generally evident as infiltrative masses in the endomyometrium. Sufficient sections should be taken to adequately sample the tumor, given its variable histologic pattern, and to provide sufficient information for staging.
>
> **Comment:** Immunohistochemistry is particularly useful in the diagnosis of these lesions. If diagnosis of a PSTT or ETT cannot definitely be made, serum β-hCG levels may be requested. If positive, it is helpful in making the diagnosis as well as for follow-up. If negative, a neoplastic process cannot be ruled out. With PSN and EPS, a comment may be made about the benign nature of the lesion.

Selected References

PHP4, Chapter 23, pages 761–767.

Baergen RN, Rutgers JL, Young RH. Extrauterine lesions of intermediate trophoblast. Int J Gynecol Pathol 2003;22:362–367.

Baergen RN, Rutgers JL. Trophoblastic lesions of the placental site. Gen Diagn Pathol 1997;143:143–158.

Finkler NJ, Berkowitz RS, Driscoll SG, et al. Clinical experience with placental site trophoblastic tumors at the New England Trophoblastic Disease Center. Obstet Gynecol 1988;71:854–857.

Huetter PC, Gersell DJ. Placental site nodule: an analysis of 40 cases. Mod Pathol 1993;4:74A; abstract 422.

Kurman RJ, Main, CS, Chen H-C. Intermediate trophoblast: a distinctive form of trophoblast with specific morphological, biochemical and functional features. Placenta 1984;5:349–370.

Roberts JP, Lurain JR. Treatment of low-risk metastatic gestational trophoblastic tumors with single-agent chemotherapy. Am J Obstet Gynecol 1996;174:1917–1924.

Rutgers JL, Baergen RN, Young RH, et al. Placental site trophoblastic tumor: clinicopathologic study of 64 cases. Mod Pathol 1995;8:96A.

Scully RE, Young RH. Trophoblastic pseudotumor: a reappraisal. Am J Surg Pathol 1981;5:75–76.

Shih I-M, Kurman RJ. Epithelioid trophoblastic tumor. A neoplasm distinct from choriocarcinoma and placental site trophoblastic tumor simulating carcinoma. Am J Surg Pathol 1998;22:1393–1403.

Shitabata PK, Rutgers JL. The placental site nodule: an immunohistochemical study. Hum Pathol 1993;25:1295–1301.

Young RH, Kurman RJ, Scully RE. Placental site nodules and plaques. A clinicopathologic analysis of 20 cases. Am J Surg Pathol 1990;14:1001–1009.

Section VII

Legal Aspects and Future Directions

This final section differs from the previous sections in that it discusses the application of placental pathology rather than pathology itself. Chapter 26 discusses legal aspects to placental examination. It is not intended as advice on how to perform expert review in legal cases, but rather as a guide for the practicing pathologist. It is hoped that it will give the reader a sense of the importance of placental pathology in understanding perinatal outcome and provide guidance on maximizing the benefit to the patient as well as the potential expert who might examine the case in the future. The subject of Chapter 27 is future directions and is written by Kurt Benirschke. This chapter covers new and fascinating discoveries and advances in the field of placental pathology.

Chapter 26

Legal Considerations

General Considerations

Numerous litigations against hospitals, obstetricians, and other physicians take place in which the placental findings become an important participant in advising the disputing parties on perinatal circumstances. These are initiated most often on behalf of children with cerebral palsy, children with malformations, stillborns, or children with other less than optimal or unexpected outcomes. Weinstein (1988), who wrote a concise review on the topic, asserted that such litigation is principally the result of the following:

- Society's belief that all wrongs must have a reason and that the wrongs must be put right
- The pervasive lottery mentality
- The inability of individuals to accept responsibility for themselves or their actions
- An increasing incidence of true medical negligence

Thus, many lawsuits are filed merely because there is an unexpected or poor outcome and not by the perception that medical negligence has occurred. This is unfortunately fueled by the increasing incidence of true medical negligence. In addition, many pregnant patients continue the use of alcohol, tobacco, cocaine, crack, and other agents that endanger their fetuses. Unfortunately, these facts are rarely taken into serious consideration when malpractice claims are litigated, or they are casually dismissed as likely not being contributory. The oversimplified allegations of intrapartum hypoxia and its assumed relationship to neonatal pH, Apgar score, and ultimate outcome are often incorrectly assessed, and assumption of negligence or guilt on the part of a physician is frequently not justified.

It has been estimated that 2.7 of 1000 children aged 5 to 7 years suffer a form of cerebral palsy. There is no doubt that there has been an increase in the overall incidence of cerebral palsy because of the increasingly smaller babies for whom care is provided. Moreover, with increased usage of assisted reproductive technology, there are more multiple births, which are often preterm. They are also delivered by much older women, and these are all factors of importance in cerebral palsy. Nearly 36% of cases occur in children with birth weights of less than 2500 g, and it is estimated that 70% have an antenatal onset. However, our understanding of how cerebral palsy develops is still imperfect. The study of the causes of cerebral palsy is a difficult aspect of medicine, as no single etiology can possibly be assigned. Conclusions made from the 56,000 pregnancies in the Collaborative Perinatal Study were that chronic, rather than acute hypoxia has a greater influence in causing abnormal brain development. Cerebral palsy obviously has obviously great social importance; the disease represents often a major tragedy to the families involved, let alone to the child.

The Placenta in Litigation

The placenta is a reflection of intrauterine life, providing a wealth of information on prenatal events. It may be helpful in understanding adverse outcome in several ways. First, the *placenta itself may be abnormal and thus the cause of the adverse outcome*. This is the case in primary lesions of the placenta such as maternal floor infarction as well as maternal diseases such as preeclampsia. At times, the placenta itself is functionally normal, but *reflects an adverse intrauterine environment*. Such is the case with severe fetomaternal hemorrhage in which the placenta is markedly pale and hydropic due to the severe fetal anemia. Finally, the placenta may *show no abnormality* and thus is not helpful in determining causation. In the latter case, the answer must be sought elsewhere.

It is now apparent to many health care providers that, when caring for problematic neonates or when difficulties in labor and delivery are encountered, the placenta should be examined professionally. The recognition that placental examination is helpful in adjudicating perinatal "asphyxia" litigations has also been recognized by the legal profession. Although experts in perinatal pathology may be asked to review these cases, the general pathologist usually receives the placenta and examines it first. All too often, when placental consultation is requested, the placental material available is insufficient for an expert opinion. Recommendations have been made (Chapter 3) on how to collect and examine placentas. It is regrettable that, occasionally, erroneous testimony is given in good faith because the consultant did not have the benefit of a complete gross examination and was not made aware of the perinatal circumstances. Of course, a pathologist should not be put into the position of making judgments on fetal monitor strips and the like but must have a general idea of the entirety of these complex cases before the placental examination can be meaningfully interpreted.

It is most important that placentas be *adequately sampled for histology.* When selecting the villous tissue, it is important that more than the obviously infarcted or pathologic areas be sampled; most infarcts look alike microscopically. For an appreciation of the placental status, *the more normal-appearing villous tissue is usually most informative.* It is often beneficial to have *photograph of the placenta* available, particularly when confronted with the record of a poorly described or inadequately studied placenta. If photography is impractical, a drawing of salient findings, for example, to indicate the insertion of the umbilical cord or the presence of twin vascular anastomoses is often more helpful than a poor description of the gross features. Another important aspect to gross examination is the evaluation of the *extent or involvement of any macroscopic lesions.* The percentage of villous tissue involved as well as the location (peripheral versus central) of the lesions should always be noted.

Twinning Problems

Multiple births have not only a much higher incidence of prematurity and demise, but suffer an increased frequency of cerebral palsy compared with singletons. It should be understood that the umbilical cords of twins must be labeled at delivery, so that it becomes possible to assign specific placental lesions to individual infants. Central nervous system damage of prenatal onset appears to be more common in **monozygotic, monochorionic** twins than in dizygotic twins, and this is primarily *due to the vascular anastomoses* between the placentas. If one wants to understand the origin of the lesions, *it is imperative that the membrane relation and vascular anastomoses of all twins be firmly established during placental study.* The anastomoses are best recorded by making a drawing of these connections; they cannot otherwise be easily reconstructed. This point is particularly important when one twin has died prenatally. Coagulative, destructive events in the survivor are then especially common due to **acute twin-to-twin transfusion** (see Chapter 10) commencing soon after the death of the co-twin. The notion that "thromboplastic" substances are released from the circulation of the dead twin and cause strokes and other adverse events in the survivor has been shown to be incorrect.

Twins also suffer from **chronic twin-to-twin transfusion syndrome**, an important aspect of monozygotic twinning (Chapter 10). Firm diagnosis requires the demonstration of dominant arteriovenous shunts in the placenta. Chronic twin-to-twin transfusion usually leads to polyhydramnios in the recipient twin and oligohydramnios in the donor. It is associated with premature delivery and often results in fetal demise, usually of the donor twin. When this occurs, the chronic transfusion is reversed and the plethoric recipient twin becomes the anemic donor twin as it acutely exsanguinates into the stillborn twin. This is often referred to as **"acute-on-chronic" twin-to-twin transfusion**. Brain damage or death is often the fate of the surviving twin.

The highest mortality in twins attends **monoamnionic-monochorionic** twins due to *frequent entanglement of their cords*. This complication often kills one or both fetuses; in others, venous return problems are evident by the presence of fetal vascular thrombosis. Monoamnionic twins also have vascular anastomoses and thus may suffer from rapid shifts of blood from one twin to the other, which may lead to acute anemia and hypotension in utero.

Acute Chorioamnionitis

Ascending infections, as evidenced by the presence of **acute chorioamnionitis** and **acute funisitis**, *are much overrepresented in children who develop cerebral palsy*. These pathologic findings have also been correlated with prenatal cystic lesions in the brain. Studies have suggested that the mechanism may be the result of vasoconstriction, engendered by the release of prostaglandins, tumor necrosis factor, or other vasoactive agents and cytokines that come either from the inflammatory exudate or from bacterial products in the amniotic cavity. Moreover, various inflammatory mediators have been shown to cause direct neuronal injury, astrogliosis, and inhibition of oligodendrocyte maturation. Because ascending infection often leads to premature delivery, the infants are also susceptible to the risk factors associated with prematurity. Chorioamnionitis is an occasional cause of thrombosis in fetal surface vessels (Chapter 16). The correlation with cerebral palsy is stronger is cases in which there is a fetal inflammatory response, that is, when there is inflammation in the chorionic vessels, inflammation in the umbilical vessels, and particularly when there is thrombosis of these vessels. Adequate sampling of the membranes, fetal surface, and fetal surface vessels is essential to determining the extent of the infection and its possible impact on fetal morbidity and mortality.

Chronic Villitis

Chronic villitis may be of infectious or of unknown etiology. In suspected viral infections, it is difficult to identify the specific infection by histopathologic study alone. Immunohistochemistry, polymerase chain reaction (PCR), DNA hybridization, or other methods may then be used to identify specific organisms. Unfortunately, some viruses, such as human immunodeficiency virus, leave no characteristic alterations in the placenta. **Cytomegalovirus** infection is perhaps the most common prenatal virus infection of relevance to cerebral palsy-type lesions. Significant damage to the fetal brain and other organs occurs frequently from this infection, and the placenta often shows characteristic chronic villitis with plasma cells (see Chapter 16). Nevertheless, these changes are frequently widely scattered in the placenta, sometimes affecting only a few villi, and thus may be difficult to find. Infection with **herpesvirus** before birth may lead to destructive encephalopathy, porencephaly, and neonatal death. However, when these infants come to autopsy, neither culture nor electron microscopy may identify the now-vanished agent.

Villitis of unknown etiology (VUE) is an alteration of villi in which there is an infiltrate of lymphocytes, macrophages, and rare plasma cells, and it is associated with villous destruction (see Chapter 16). It is often indistinguishable from infectious villitis. VUE reduces the area of placental exchange and, if severe, may be associated with *fetal death and with growth restriction*. The etiology of VUE is unknown at this time, but its dire significance is not in doubt, and it has a tendency to recur in future pregnancies. It may be difficult at times to differentiate VUE from infectious villitis and adequate sectioning of the villous tissue is essential.

Meconium or the "Green" Placenta

Prenatal meconium discharge is common and occurs in about 17% of all births. Its presence at birth is a frequent reason for allegations that birth was delayed or inappropriately handled, the suggestion being that it is evidence of fetal distress. In fact, **meconium** staining of the placental surface, in most cases, is **not** associated with fetal distress or cerebral palsy. *In a mature placenta, meconium discharge occurs primarily because the fetus is mature enough to discharge meconium and not because of intrauterine stress.* Meconium is extremely rare in immature placentas, and when present **may** be an indication of intrauterine hypoxia. However, when a damaged or stillborn infant is under consideration and its birth is not accompanied by meconium discharge, the question of why the baby did not release meconium is never asked. Interestingly, most stillbirths have no meconium staining, even though, ultimately, anoxia was the cause of their death. The legal profession often overemphasizes the importance of meconium discharge, without appreciating the complexity of this process and of cerebral palsy.

Rather than meconium discharge occurring because of fetal distress, it is likely that the *meconium damages the fetus by acting as a vasoconstrictive agent on the umbilical and superficial placental vessels.* In so doing, it may reduce the venous return of oxygenated blood from the placenta. These avenues are now being explored experimentally. Therefore, when the umbilical cord is meconium stained, *additional sections of the discolored cord should be submitted to identify meconium-induced myonecrosis of the umbilical vessels* (see Chapter 14). Furthermore, there is some speculation that the real damage of the "meconium aspiration syndrome" in neonates is a chemical injury to the alveolar epithelium, similar to its effect on amnion and cord vessels leading to a chemical pneumonitis. It is noteworthy that not all meconium-stained placentas are accompanied by fetal meconium aspiration. It must also be emphasized that meconium may have been discharged many hours before delivery, and most of it may already have been transported away from the fetal surface when the placenta becomes available for study. It is also probable that repeated meconium discharge could occur in utero, which would be most difficult to discern from placental examination alone.

When a placenta from a premature infant has a green surface, one must consider the possibility that this discoloration is due to **hemosiderin** and related precursor pigments. Hemosiderin deposits frequently accompany the *peripheral hemorrhages of circumvallate placentas, retromembranous hematomas, marginal hemorrhage, and fetal hemolysis* (see Chapter 14). An iron stain of the placenta quickly reveals the nature of the pigment when doubt exists.

Vascular Abnormalities

Abnormalities of the umbilical cord and placental surface vessels are important findings in placental examinations. It is particularly important to look for thromboses in the fetal surface vessels of every placenta. Many surface **vascular thrombi** are evident macroscopically by the yellow-white streak that is present in a chorionic vessel. Thrombi are more difficult to spot in the umbilical cord. Thrombi may be associated with *cord entanglements, velamentous cords, excessively long cords, or markedly twisted cords* (see Chapter 15). They are also associated with *maternal lupus anticoagulant, maternal diabetes, and thrombophilias*. Vascular thrombosis may be a feature of certain infections such as *acute chorioamnionitis, cytomegalovirus infection, and toxoplasmosis*. There are many other placentas with extensive thrombosis in which the etiology of the thrombi remains obscure. Thrombosis may be associated with CNS damage and the thrombi may embolize to the fetus, causing tissue infarcts and strokes. However, unless such an infant comes to autopsy, embolic sequelae are usually not evident. Complete vascular obliteration leads to "atrophy" of the villous district subserved by the vessel. It is the frequent cause of **avascular hyalinized villi** (Chapter 21), which may thus reduce the quantity of available "exchange membrane"; for this reason, chronic thrombosis correlates with *growth restriction and hypoxia*. For the purpose of legal adjudication, it is important to recognize this point and to acknowledge that thrombosis is usually a long-standing event and that it can usually not be anticipated before birth.

Recently, **hemorrhagic endovasculitis** (Chapter 21) has been associated with adverse neurologic outcome. Some changes associated with "bland" hemorrhagic endovasculitis may be indistinguishable from degenerative changes seen after intrauterine demise. However, the "active" form has been not been described in stillborns and has a stronger association with adverse outcome.

Umbilical Cord

The cord displays many lesions that have a significant impact on fetal well-being (Chapter 15). It may also be discolored from hemolysis, especially when thrombi are present or when prenatal bleeding has occurred. True cord **hematomas**, often caused by other lesions in the cord such as **hemangiomas, aneurysms**, etc., may lead to hypoxia and subsequent neurologic injury primarily caused by *compression of the umbilical vessels* and embarrassment of blood flow through the cord. These are uncommonly seen. Compression from **true knots** or **prolapsed cords** may cause significant obstruction and may be accompanied by *marked distension of blood vessels on one side but not the other*, betraying the prenatal compromise of the circulation. The cord may also show **excessive twisting** or **excessive length**. That such excessive spiraling *can lead to fetal death* is not in doubt. More problematic is the chronic effect that may ensue from cord obstruction such as reduced venous return and subsequent fetal *surface vessel (venous) thrombi*. *Associations with neurologic injury are seen with excessively short cords, excessively long cords, excessively twisted cords, minimally twisted cords, cord entanglements, cord prolapse, and true knots*. **Velamentous insertion** of the umbilical cord and marginal insertions with membranous vessels may also cause significant anemia and hypoxia if the membranes vessels rupture or *thrombose*. Dire fetal sequelae may occur, including death and/or neurologic injury. The abnormalities of the umbilical cord that are associated with adverse outcome are often macroscopic lesions and so adequate documentation of these findings in the gross description is essential. Photographs are especially helpful.

Placental Pallor

The color of the villous tissue reflects the fetal hemoglobin content. Placentas of diabetic mothers are dark and congested because of fetal plethora, and those of immature infants are lighter. **Pale placentas** occur primarily from infants with hydrops or severe anemia. The latter may be due to *fetomaternal hemorrhage, fetal bleeding from ruptured velamentous vessels*, or, rarely, from a *ruptured umbilical cord*. If fetomaternal hemorrhage is suspected, an immediate Kleihauer-Betke stain on maternal blood is strongly suggested (Chapter 20) to assess the amount of fetal blood loss. Significant hypotension and hypoxia may transpire, and this is an important cause of brain injury, but unfortunately the diagnosis cannot be made until after delivery. If the amount of fetal blood present in the maternal circulation exceeds 50% of the fetal blood volume, the hemorrhage is likely chronic in nature as an acute hemorrhage of this magnitude would lead to fetal death. The adjustment of the fetal hematocrit may take some time after fetal blood loss, but we have only the most superficial knowledge of how quickly the hematocrits adjust after fetal bleeding. Occasionally infants become hydropic due to high-output cardiac failure from large **placental chorioangiomas**, and these are readily apparent when the placenta is examined and sectioned.

Maternal Floor Infarction

Maternal floor infarction is strongly correlated with fetal growth restriction and demise (Chapter 19), and recently an association with adverse neurologic outcome has been demonstrated. Appropriate histologic study verifies the existence of excessive fibrinoid deposits. It is clear from histologic examination that the surface exchange area in these placentas is severely limited, and so it is easy to understand how this condition could lead to growth restriction or other sequelae. The disorder is of unknown etiology and has a tendency to recur in subsequent pregnancies. Descriptions of the percentage of tissue involvement is key to evaluating this lesion.

Abruptio Placentae

Most cases of placental separation are clinically silent and can be observed only when the maternal surface is carefully scrutinized. A fresh **retroplacental hematoma** will show *indentation of the villous tissue*. In an older lesion, the clot will be drier, stringy, and compacted. When placental separation is focal and has occurred long before delivery, the clot may have largely disappeared, or is replaced by a brown, filmy material. After placental separation, a retroplacental clot forms. It will become adherent to the placental surface within a few hours and then will begin to compress the placental surface. The underlying villous tissue becomes ischemic immediately on separation of the placenta; however, the effects are not visible under the microscope until almost a day later with collapse of the intervillous space and villous agglutination. Therefore, in abruptios less than 24 hours old, identification of the retroplacental clot is much easier on gross examination. With increasing time, infarction develops with smudging of the trophoblast nuclei and loss of nuclear basophilia, and eventually the villous tissue becomes pale and ghostlike (Chapter 18). Sudden separation of more than 50% of the placenta usually results in fetal death. If an abruptio develops over time, the fetus can adjust somewhat and so larger, but more slowly developing, abruptios may not result in stillbirth. Neurologic injury may still occur.

Infarcts

Small infarcts at the edge of the placenta at term are common and are of little significance. **Multiple infarcts** scattered throughout the placenta, however, signify maternal disease of some sort. This finding assumes particular importance in prematurely delivered infants in whom infarcts are rare. Most commonly, the cause of such infarcts is *preeclampsia*, but the lesions due to *lupus anticoagulant* and *thrombophilia* may have a similar appearance (Chapter 18). When infarcts are found in the absence of signs of pregnancy toxemia, their cause requires further study. To understand the fetal impact of infarcts, it is necessary that a *percentage estimate of the amount of infarcted villous tissue* be recorded. If sufficient placental tissue is infarcted, fetal hypoxia develops with the potential for brain injury and even death.

Chorangiosis

Chorangiosis is an abnormal condition correlated with *prolonged fetal oxygen deprivation*. It has been associated with *many perinatal problems* and is never found in normal cases. Although minor forms of chorangiosis are reasonably common, its value for our understanding of the fetal–placental–maternal relations has so far been underestimated. That it is associated with hypoxia is supported by the finding of chorangiosis in women gestating at very high altitude and the fact that it is often present peripheral to avascular villi when thrombi have occluded the fetal vascular bed. Other correlations exist with *fetal death, diabetes, umbilical cord problems, and other perinatal problems*. It is important to realize that because chorangiosis involves proliferation and formation of new capillaries, it must take weeks to develop.

Nucleated Red Blood Cells

After approximately 28 weeks, the fetal circulation of the placenta contains very few **nucleated red blood cells** (NRBCs). When they are found in sections of the placenta, the pathologist must seek an explanation for their presence. It may be obvious that there is evidence of *hemolytic disease or that transplacental bleeding or chronic infection* existed, but often the cause of an excessive number of NRBCs is not immediately evident. Presumably, the human fetus reacts to oxygen deficiency, as he or she does to anemia, by first releasing and then increasing production of NRBCs from the hepatic or bone marrow stores. There is no consensus as to exactly how acutely this reaction occurs, and to what degree. Probably there is an initial release of already formed, slightly immature NRBCs within a relatively short period. If hypoxia is sustained, the production of red cells is increased and the immature forms are produced and released in increasing numbers. In the case of fetal hemorrhage, some degree of an initial NRBC response may be detectable already *within an hour*. It is thought that the rise of NRBC count is much slower when due to hypoxia. When the initial NRBC count is very high, it indicates a more severe and prolonged hypoxia.

Villous Changes

Another relevant feature is **villous dysmaturity**, the discrepancy of apparent villous maturation with chronologic age. In delayed maturation, there is *an increase in villous size, an increase in stromal cells, decreased* *syncytial knots, and frequently increased vascularity*. Irregularly matured villi are frequent in the placentas of a variety of chromosomal abnormalities (see Chapter 11) and maternal diabetes. Alternatively, accelerated villous maturity, as evidenced by **increased syncytial knotting** or **terminal villus deficiency**, signifies deficient uteroplacental blood flow of some duration and thus reduced oxygen to the fetus. The implication to the fetus must be made in light of other pathologic findings and clinical history. Focal **villous edema** has been associated with *premature delivery, neonatal hypoxia, and neonatal death*. However, further studies are needed to clarify the importance of villous edema as a correlate of fetal well-being and its pathogenesis.

Timing of Fetal Death

In cases of fetal death, the timing of intrauterine death is important to determine. Genest (1992) has depicted the changes seen after fetal death and, based on cases in which the time of fetal death was known, has provided a timeline on their occurrence. The evaluation is based on the fact that autolysis of fetal organs occurs at differing rates. By evaluating the loss of nuclear basophilia in various organs, one can estimate the time of fetal death and intrauterine retention.

Conclusion

During legal proceedings, the pathologist is frequently asked to place a time frame for the lesion under discussion. He or she may be required to specify how quickly villi can become infarcted, what is the exact temporal evolution of thrombi, how long has acute chorioamnionitis been present, and so on. These and other probing questions are often difficult to adjudicate and the answers may present problems for a conscientious witness. It requires experience, and it may be best to state the lack of our knowledge than to express unwarranted opinions that are contradicted in the courtroom or by other experts. This uncertainty is also an indication for the pathologist to seek new information from appropriate cases in which clinical data corroborate a particular finding.

Selected References

PHP4, Chapter 26, pages 903–916.
Altshuler GA. Conceptual approach to placental pathology and pregnancy outcome. Semin Diagn Pathol 1993;10:204–221.
Altshuler G. Some placental considerations related to neurodevelopmental and other disorders. J Child Neurol 1993;8:78–94.
Bejar R, Vigliocco G, Gramajo H, et al. Antenatal origin of neurologic damage in newborn infants. Part II. Multiple gestations. Am J Obstet Gynecol 1990; 162:1230–1236.
Benirschke K. The placenta in the litigation process. Am J Obstet Gynecol 1990; 162:1445–1450.
Benirschke K. Intrauterine death of a twin: mechanisms, implications for surviving twin, and placental pathology. Semin Diagn Pathol 1993;10:222–231.

Benirschke K. The use of the placenta in the understanding of perinatal injury. In: Fisher DSM (ed) Risk management techniques and neonatal practice. Armonk, NY: Futura, 1996:325–345.

Depp R. Perinatal asphyxia. Assessing its causal role and timing. Semin Pediatr Neurol 1995;2:3–36.

Fleischer LD. Wrongful births: when is there liability for prenatal injury? Am J Dis Child 1987;141:1260–1265.

Genest DR. Estimating the time of death in stillborn fetuses: II. Histologic evaluation of the placenta; a study of 71 stillborns. Obstet Gynecol 1992; 80:585–592.

Grafe MR. The correlation of prenatal brain damage with placental pathology. J Neuropathol Exp Neurol 1994;53:407–415.

Kaplan CG. Forensic aspects of the placenta. In: Dimmick JE, Singer DB (eds) Forensic aspects in pediatric pathology. Perspectives of pediatric pathology, vol 19. Basel: Karger, 1995:20–42.

Kraus FT. Cerebral palsy and thrombi in placental vessels of the fetus: insights from litigation. Hum Pathol 1997;28:246–248.

Kuban KCK, Leviton A. Cerebral palsy. N Engl J Med 1994;330:188–195.

Marin-Padilla M. Developmental neuropathology and impact of perinatal brain damage. II: White matter lesions of the neocortex. J Neuropathol Exp Neurol 1997;56:219–235.

Naeye RL, Localio AR. Determining the time before birth when ischemia and hypoxemia initiated cerebral palsy. Obstet Gynecol 1995;86:713–719.

Naeye RL, Peters EC, Bartholomew M, et al. Origins of cerebral palsy. Am J Dis Child 1989;143:1154–1161.

Nelson KB, Dambrosia JM, Ting TY, et al. Uncertain value of electronic fetal monitoring in predicting cerebral palsy. N Engl J Med 1996;334:613–618.

Redline RW, Wilson-Costello D, Borawski E, et al. Placental lesions associated with neurologic impairment and cerebral palsy in very low-birth-weight infants. Arch Pathol Lab Med 1098;122:1091–1098.

Weinstein L. Malpractice: the syndrome of the 80s. Obstet Gynecol 1988; 72:130–135.

Chapter 27

New Directions

Kurt Benirschke

What Is New in Placental Studies?

The answer to that, of course depends very much on the preferences of the beholder but, from my perspective, perhaps the most interesting aspects have been the placental changes that are now being observed in multiple gestations and resulting from the different practices of assisted reproductive technology (ART), especially, the intracytoplasmic sperm injection (ICSI). The increased frequency with which excessive numbers of multiples are produced has been widely commented upon and, in recent publications, it has been recommended that single ovum transfer only be practiced in ART, rather than the common multiple blastocyst transfer. The attending prematurity rate and the often serious sequelae of marked prematurity are the principal reasons for this recommendation. Additionally, because of uterine space limitations when multiple blastocysts compete for implantation sites, some placentas become "squeezed" by the other placenta and thus acquire less room for expansion. This may then lead to fetal growth restriction and the more frequent abnormal (velamentous) cord insertion seen in multiples. We studied 127 sets of triplet placentas recently that had more single umbilical arteries (SUAs), more circumvallation, more chorangiomas, and, interestingly, more placentas with increased syncytial knots.

Even more interesting, however, is the increased frequency of monochorionic placentas developing with these practices. Thus, when three blastocysts were transferred, four embryos may develop. Apparently, one of the embryos has split to result in monozygotic twins. We also found that when three embryos were implanted, sometimes we ended up with two of the triplets being monochorionic–probably due to the death of one embryo with splitting of another former quadruplet. The reason for this apparent induced "splitting" have been difficult to explain, but Steinman (2003) has suggested a model that needs future investigation. He proposed that adhesion molecules that normally keep the blastomeres together are weakened in their effectiveness. He believes that this is dependent on the calcium concentration in the culture media used and that contain the blastocysts before their transfer; he incriminates the anticoagulant EDTA (ethylenediaminetetraacetic acid) used for the prevention of coagulation as a possible culprit. Because we still do not have any reliable cause for the process of monozygotic twinning in general, this suggestion needs serious consideration by the community of physicians employing ART.

Another development recently discovered in several placental studies is the discovery of dizygotic twins (DZ) with monochorionic placentation (DiMo) and also possessing vascular anastomoses (Souter et al., 2003). The finding of DiMo placentas has, in the past, been held to be diagnostic of MZ twinning. That notion now needs revision. Moreover, the cases of blood chimerism, starting with Mrs. McKay many years ago, need reexamination, and new care needs to be exercised by the placental pathologist. This patient (Mrs. McK.) was found to be a blood chimera while pregnant, and when asked about having possibly had a twin, she recalled that her male co-twin had died while very young (Dunsford et al., 1953). His blood group could then still be ascertained and, presumably, she would also still have had a chimeric XY lymphocyte cell line. Similar cases have since come to light, but truly competent placental studies demonstrating the anastomoses are rare.

In the recent past much progress has also been made in the therapy of the twin-to-twin-transfusion syndrome (TTTS). It has emerged that serial amniocentesis for the relief of hydramnios is not truly efficacious in the treatment of the "disease," and more centers now have gone over to the more effective laser coagulation of the causative A-V shunts in the placenta. They are not always easy to identify through the small optics during fetoscopy, and selecting the right ones is a challenge. It is therefore strongly recommended that future fetoscopic surgeons familiarize themselves with the vascular anatomy of the placental surface before attempting this challenging procedure. It has also emerged that artery-to-artery anastomoses are largely protective; they generally prevent the TTTS. What is less well appreciated, however, is that the neonatal diagnosis of TTTS may be difficult, as blood shifts rapidly during delivery between the twins' circulations. Thus, false hematologic values emerge that may not betray the prenatal, in utero, circumstances. This has particular legal ramifications, and we have repeatedly suggested that it is imperative to adjudicate the cases through an examination of the twins' heart sizes (Benirschke and Masliah, 2001). In the true TTTS, there is a major discrepancy of the heart sizes beginning already prior to hydramnios or other symptoms of TTTS, especially when they are adjusted for gestational age. This cardiac size discrepancy, rather than hematologic values, is a more reliable measure for the existence of the TTTS. Also, it has now become well established that the prenatal CNS damage that may occur, especially when one twin dies in utero, is the result of a transient severe hypotension because transplacental "hemorrhage" into the dead twin occurs from which the living twin may recover, albeit with CNS damage. This CNS damage is not the result of a coagulation syndrome as was formerly suspected. It has even been witnessed sonographically as a reversal of flow in such cases. Indeed, prenatal sonography has become an essential tool also in the assessment of the "dividing membranes" of twins, with the twin peak sign in DiDi twins and the ascertainment of possible disruption of the amnionic membranes. Attempts at defining heart sizes of twins should be the next goal.

While speaking of chimerism, the other notable development is the recognition of several maternal autoimmune diseases as being the result of maternal blood chimerism that was initiated during the woman's prior pregnancy. It is envisaged that fetal lymphocytes (even stem cells) transfer to the mother, and that this occurs most likely, in small numbers, regularly during all gestations. When significant HLA diversity is present, perhaps these transferred white blood cells direct their attention against the maternal antigens later in life and "reject" them. Indeed, an important case reported by Srivatsa et al. (2001) indicates that, in a case of postpartum thyroiditis, even the maternal thyroid epithelium may be replaced by fetal cells. The magnitude of this process is under active investigation, but a correlation with the type and possible complications of prior gestations has rarely been possible. Thus, in view of the occasionally massive fetal hemorrhage (into maternal blood with Kleihauer-positive maternal blood), the result that we occasionally witness in the perinatal period, it might be asked whether the resultant induced chimerism is perhaps more often responsible for maternal autoimmune diseases in the future of those particular mothers (Johnson et al., 2001). Therefore, attention might be paid more specifically to the future diseases that might affect the mothers with major fetal blood transfer.

There has been a remarkable reduction of perinatal mortality since the development of surfactant therapy for prematurely born infants. The old "hyaline membrane disease" has virtually disappeared in our perinatal autopsies consequently. Neonatal autopsies are now largely limited to significant structural abnormalities, to chromosomal errors, and to severely premature infants, those weighing less than 1000 g. The placental pathologist notices that the latter infants are almost always associated with chorioamnionitis, or the placentas show at least a significant deciduitis. Remarkable progress has been made clinically in identifying the presence of this ascending infection (e.g., sonographic assessment of the cervix, interferon measurements, and identification of the many interleukins present), but little advance has been made in the precise identification of the responsible organisms, let alone in the therapy for these frequently recurrent infections. It has been our contention that the process is initiated by the existence of chronic endocervicitis that is then followed by deciduitis of the "forelying" membranes. Subsequently, local phospholipid production leads to cervical dilatation, to foreshortening of the cervix, and to premature labor. Cerclage, occasionally practiced in this clientele, has not been effective nor has the initiation of antibiotic therapy at the time of cervical "incompetence," This disease process has not diminished in frequency and is now the most important cause of significant prematurity. It needs additional attention by the reproductive specialists. Because of the frequent recurrence of this cause of significant prematurity, these patients may benefit from antibiotic therapy **in between** pregnancies, and this probably should include the husbands, because nongonorrheal urethritis may accompany these gestations. At least it is worthy of a major clinical trial. We also need to make much greater efforts in identifying the organisms that cause the inflammation.

Much progress is being made in the identification of genes that regulate placental development–in the mouse, that is (Cross et al., 2003). Despite all the publications on putative causes of pregnancy-induced hypertension (PIH) (preeclampsia), we are not truly closer to understanding its etiology. It is often speculated that PIH relates to the immunologic disparity of placental and maternal genotypes, but this has not been borne out with sufficient clarity, despite the occasional mutations occurring in the HLA-G complex. Hope exists that, once genetic regulation of murine placentation is better understood, we can decipher human placental development also. But we are not there yet. Microarrays are beginning to be employed without yet defining genes for specific diseases. This regulation is of more than casual interest as it also involves the determinants of paternal placental "imprinting" and may be of concern to those of us with an interest in cloning and interspecific embryo transfers and, of course, in hopes to understanding the complex mechanisms that must underlie the evolution of the many different types of placentas. Aspects of comparative placentation and their evolution have long been hotly debated without clear resolution, and they are currently mostly descriptive (http://medicine.ucsd.edu/cpa). Greater attention might profitably be paid to the often deeply invasive trophoblast in South American rodents, and the possible immunologic consequences. The genetic disparity of these litters from the dams should be more fully investigated because they have claimed little attention to date.

We have made remarkably little progress concerning the etiology of chromosomal errors and their correlation with placental phenotype. For one thing, the high frequency of spontaneous abortions due to aneuploidies in the human population is not mirrored in other species that have been studied. In fact, it seems to be low in Primate Research Centers where breeding is supervised and conceptions are known (Small and Smith, 1983), and this is also true from my observations with wild animals at the San Diego Zoo; abortions occur extremely rarely and chromosomal errors as their cause are practically unknown or they can be enumerated easily. The reasons for these discrepancies are of potential importance to our own reproductive performance and need better explanations than they now receive. But it is also true that we lack an understanding why major trisomies cause often specific congenital anomalies in the embryo, but they appear to cause few if any characteristic placental changes. To be sure, the "partial mole" (PHM) due to triploidy can be cited as an exception; but other major chromosomal errors are not known to be reflected in specific placental phenotypes. Perhaps we need to make a greater effort in their recognition and must more carefully compare cytogenetic findings with placental characteristics. Other than sporadic villous changes or the presence of a single umbilical artery, not much is known; not even a correlation with placental weights exists. In addition, the same applies to "confined placental mosaicism"; no good histology supports the abnormal placental regions. When unusual moles have been characterized cytogenetically, a number of mosaic or chimeric genotypes have been identified. A beginning is made by the methods of differentiating PHM from CHM through the employment of chromosomal in situ hybridization (Lai et al., 2004). And while it is easy to state that complete hydatidiform moles have an exclusively paternal genome, the reasons for this feature (other than speculations about imprinting) are unknown. It has become clear now that all complete moles must have had an embryo, at least at one time in early development. Not only have some been demonstrated but this is also to be deduced because of the connective tissue these moles contain. But what are the precise reasons (? structural anomalies or imprinting) for the death of these embryos? And why are moles so much more common in the Oriental populations, and why have they never been seen in any other species? These are questions to which a placental pathologist should address some of his thoughts and research efforts.

Another important "black box" at present is the etiology of "maternal floor infarction" (MFI), a condition that can occasionally now be recognized sonographically. In this condition, excessive amounts of fibrinoid are deposited, and frequently it is associated with excessive proliferation of extravillous trophoblast. First, the precise nature of the fibrinoid has not been sufficiently explored, and then, the reasons for the frequent recurrences are similarly unknown. It is here where more definitive knowledge of trophoblast regulation that we hope to obtain from the mouse model might be applied. Perhaps the same can be said of "villitis of unknown etiology." As with MFI, the condition is occasionally recurrent and leads to growth restriction and may lead to fetal death. Search for an infectious etiology has been negative and the only detailed study that has attempted to identify the population of inflammatory cells within the villi is incomplete (Redline and Patterson, 1993). It suggested that, in male births, there was no Y-signal in the affected villous inflammatory cell population. But that was done on histologic sections, not on fresh material. Thus, the exact nature of the infiltrating cell population remains unknown. Clearly, immunologists need to participate in identifying these cells more precisely than we have been able to do so far. A much more intensive study of this problem is now in order.

Years ago, placenta accreta was rare and placenta percreta was virtually unheard of. Now, both play an important role in gynecologic pathology. We see many cases of placenta percreta annually, and most are identified sonographically long before labor commences. Usually, the uterus is removed; the placenta is found to lie anteriorly and has dehisced through a former cesarean section scar. It has not usually "invaded"; it just sticks out of the uterus because the thin scar tissue has become even thinner as the uterus expands in all directions. Most of this of course is the result of the greater frequency with which cesarean section delivery is done, and the frequently practiced avoidance of a trial of labor after one cesarean section. Are there other causes? Certainly, there is no evidence that the trophoblast is truly invasive and destructive to the implantation site; abdominal pregnancies alone support that notion. But perhaps the uteri are less adequately repaired after cesarean section. At least that is what we believe; that the rapidity of closure, the single stitch approach, and the nature of the suture material may be responsible for the higher frequency of percretas. One fact is certain, however; the progress made in sonography techniques, the recognition of placental "lakes," apparent hemangiomas, or abnormal-appearing implantation sites by ultrasound has much enhanced early recognition of this potentially serious complication of pregnancy.

Other advances in sonography might be highlighted as they also affect placental pathology studies and give insight into prenatal life. The coiling and entanglement of the umbilical cord (especially in MoMo twins) are recognized; blood flow can be adjudicated (and reversal can be documented–end-diastolic flow), we will learn to identify more precisely the sites of twin anastomoses, and perhaps with color power angiography we will even better assess the development and abnormalities of the villous tree (Konje et al., 2003). The prospects are excellent, and the placental pathologist should stay abreast of these developments to enable him/her to make more meaningful studies and diagnoses.

References

Benirschke K, Masliah E. The placenta in multiple pregnancy: outstanding issues. Reprod Fertil Dev 2001;13:615–622.

Cross JC, Baczyk D, Dobric N, et al. Genes, development and evolution of the placenta. Placenta 2003;24:123–130.

Dunsford I, Bowley CC, Hutchison AM, et al. A human blood group chimera. Br Med J 1953;2:81.

Johnson KL, Nelson JL, Furst DE, et al. Fetal cell microchimerism in tissue from multiple sites in women with systemic sclerosis. Arthritis Rheum 2001; 44:1848–1854.

Konje JC, Huppertz B, Bell SC, et al. 3-dimensional colour power angiography for staging human placental development. Lancet 2003;362:1199–1201.

Lai CYL, Chan KYK, Khoo U-S, et al. Analysis of gestational trophoblastic disease by genotyping and chromosome *in situ* hybridization. Mod Pathol 2004;17:40–48.

Redline RW, Patterson P. Villitis of unknown etiology is associated with major infiltration of fetal tissue by maternal inflammatory cells. Am J Pathol 1993;143:473–479.

Small MF, Smith DG. Chromosomal analysis of perinatal death in *Macaca mulatta* and *Macaca radiata*. Am J Primatol 1983;5:381–384.

Souter VL, Kapur RP, Nyholt DR, et al. A report of dizygous monochorionic twins. N Engl J Med 2003;349:154–158.

Srivatsa B, Srivatsa S, Johnson KL, et al. Microchimerism of presumed fetal origin in thyroid specimens from women: a case-control study. Lancet 2001; 358:2034–2038.

Steinman G. Mechanism of twinning VI. Genetics and the etiology of monozygotic twinning in in vitro fertilization. J Reprod Med 2003;48:583–589.

Appendix

Abbreviations

ACLA	anticardiolipin antibodies
AEDF	absent end-diastolic flow
AFI	amniotic fluid index
AFLP	acute fatty liver of pregnancy
AGA	appropriate for gestational age
APLA	antiphospholipid antibodies
AROM	artificial rupture of membranes
ART	assisted reproductive technology
BPD	biparietal diameter
BPP	biophysical profile
BTBV	beat-to-beat variability
CPD	cephalopelvic disproportion
CPM	confined placental mosaicism
CS	cesarean section
CVS	chorionic villus sampling
EDC	estimated date of "confinement"
EDD	estimated date of delivery
EFW	estimated fetal weight
EGA	estimated gestational age
FGR	fetal growth restriction
FHR	fetal heart rate
FLM	fetal lung maturity
FM	fetal movement
FMH	fetomaternal hemorrhage
FW	fetal weight
GBBS	group B beta *Streptococcus*
GBS	group B *Streptococcus*
GDM	gestational diabetes mellitus
GDMA1	non-insulin-dependent diabetes mellitus
GDMA2	insulin-dependent diabetes mellitus
GTD	gestational trophoblastic disease

GxPxxxx	gravity, parity; numbers after parity indicate—term, preterm, abortion, living
HELLP	hemolysis, elevated liver enzymes, low platelets
hPL	human placental lactogen
ICSI	intracytoplasmic sperm injection,
IDM	infant of diabetic mother
IUFD	intrauterine fetal demise
IUGR	intrauterine growth restriction (formerly "retardation")
IUP	intrauterine pregnancy
IVDA	intravenous drug abuse
IVF	in vitro fertilization
LAC	lupus anticoagulant
LFCS	low flap cesarean section
LGA	large for gestational age
LOF	low outlet forceps
LTCS	low transverse cesarean section
MFI	maternal floor infarction
MSAFP	maternal serum alpha fetoprotein
MSF	meconium-stained (amniotic) fluid
NIHF	nonimmune hydrops fetalis
NRNST	nonreactive nonstress test
NST	nonstress test; antenatal test of fetal well-being
NSVD	normal spontaneous vaginal delivery
OA	occiput anterior (presenting part)
OCT	oxytocin challenge test
OP	occiput posterior (presenting part)
PEC	preeclampsia
PET	preeclampsia, toxemia
PIH	pregnancy-induced hypertension
PLAP	placental alkaline phosphatase
PNC	prenatal care
PPROM	preterm premature rupture of membranes; may be prolonged (>24 hours) as well
PROM	preterm (prior to term) or premature (prior to labor) rupture of membranes
PTL	preterm labor
PUBS	percutaneous umbilical blood sampling
PUPPP	pruritic urticarial papules and plaques of pregnancy
REDF	reversed end-diastolic flow
SGA	small for gestational age
SROM	spontaneous rupture of membranes
SVD	spontaneous vaginal delivery
TTTS	twin-to-twin transfusion syndrome
UC	uterine contractions
UC	umbilical cord
UPD	uniparental disomy
US	ultrasound
VAVD	vacuum-assisted vaginal delivery
VBAC	vaginal birth after cesarean delivery
Vtx	vertex presentation of the fetus during delivery.
VUE	villitis of unknown etiology

Clinical Terms

Amnioinfusion Fluid, usually saline, injected intraamniotically in situations with thick meconium in an attempt to dilute the meconium.

Apgar scores Evaluation of infant after delivery and used as a predictor of fetal well-being. Commonly done at 1 and 5 min. Zero, one, or two points given for color, tone, cry, respiratory effort, and reflex irritability.

Biophysical profile Test of fetal well-being. Includes nonstress test (NST, see below) and assessment of amniotic fluid volume. Highest is 10; 7 and above is considered reassuring.

Beat-to-beat variability In fetal heart monitoring. Normally strip should show a certain amount of variability in rate from beat to beat. Lack of this variability is an indication of "nonreassuring fetal status."

Cord prolapse When the cord is the presenting part and precedes the fetus during delivery. Results in cord occlusion if the head is allowed to compress the cord against the cervix.

Deceleration Fetal heart monitoring abnormality. May be early, variable, or late. Variable usually considered due to cord compression. Late decelerations commonly thought to be "uteroplacental insufficiency" and are ominous findings.

Doppler velocimetry Studies of blood flow, usually through the umbilical artery, to measure systolic and diastolic flow (see end-diastolic flow).

End-diastolic flow End-diastolic blood flow through the umbilical artery may be absent or reversed with significant placental malperfusion. Absent or reversed EDF has been associated with IUGR and poor outcome.

Incompetent cervix Defined as painless cervical dilation in the second trimester or early third trimester, with prolapse and ballooning of the membranes into the vagina, followed by ruptured membranes and delivery. Often recurs and is maybe due to an anatomical defect.

L/S ratio Lecithin/sphingomyelin ratio, used to evaluate fetal lung maturity, measured on samples of amniotic fluid.

Nonstress test Evaluation of fetal well-being by assessment of fetal heart rate acceleration detected by Doppler coordinated with fetal movements as perceived by the mother. It is a test of fetal well-being.

Placenta previa Placental implantation over the cervical os, may be partial.

Percutaneous umbilical cord sampling Sampling of fetal blood by introduction of a needle through the abdomen into the umbilical cord.

Quadruple screen Prenatal screen for anomalies performed on maternal serum; includes beta-hCG, estriol, alpha fetoprotein, and dimeric alpha inhibin; reported as multiples of the median.

Stress test Also called contraction stress test, is a test of uteroplacental function. Contractions are enhanced by IV oxytocin and fetal heart rate is monitored. A positive or abnormal test is when fetal heart rate decelerations are noted.

Tocolysis Use of various drugs to inhibit preterm labor.

Triple screen   Prenatal screen for anomalies performed on maternal serum. Includes beta-hCG, estriol, and alphafetoprotein. Reported as multiples of the median.

Twin peak sign   Peak seen on the fetal surface of twin placentas that represents the fibrin ridge seen between fused diamnionic-dichorionic twin placentas.

Vasa previa   Velamentous vessels over cervical os.

Index